T0211879

Lecture Notes of the Institute for Computer Sciences, Social Informatics and Telecommunications Engineering   320

More information about this series at http://www.springer.com/series/8197

Gregory M. P. O'Hare ·
Michael J. O'Grady · John O'Donoghue ·
Patrick Henn (Eds.)

Wireless Mobile Communication and Healthcare

8th EAI International Conference, MobiHealth 2019
Dublin, Ireland, November 14–15, 2019
Proceedings

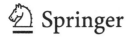 Springer

Editors
Gregory M. P. O'Hare 🆔
School of Computer Science and Informatics
University College Dublin
Dublin 4, Ireland

Michael J. O'Grady
School of Computer Science and Informatics
University College Dublin
Dublin, Dublin, Ireland

John O'Donoghue
Malawi eHealth Research Center
Cork, Ireland

Patrick Henn
University College Cork
Cork, Ireland

ISSN 1867-8211   ISSN 1867-822X (electronic)
Lecture Notes of the Institute for Computer Sciences, Social Informatics
and Telecommunications Engineering
ISBN 978-3-030-49288-5   ISBN 978-3-030-49289-2 (eBook)
https://doi.org/10.1007/978-3-030-49289-2

This Springer imprint is published by the registered company Springer Nature Switzerland AG
The registered company address is: Gewerbestrasse 11, 6330 Cham, Switzerland

Preface

MobiHealth 2019 was the 8th in a series of scientific conferences seeking to bring together transdisciplinary expertise from the technological, physiological, medical, and AI domains among others. The conference took place on the campus of University College Dublin (UCD), Ireland, during November 14–15, 2019. Many timely and pertinent mHealth topics covered included: activity recognition, wearable devices, Apps, and sensor platforms, among others. The conference compromised 6 sessions incorporating 26 papers and attracted over 40 attendees from all over the world.

The MobiHealth conference series has been in existence for almost a decade; its commencement closely aligned with the launch of the smartphone and it has continued to remain aligned with many vital developments during this time, in particular sensors and wearable computing. This current time juncture may be especially auspicious for future mobile healthcare paradigms; 5G networks are being launched and offer significant potential to successfully usher in a new era of innovative mobile health services. Such a profound development will undoubtedly give rise to new technical, ethical, legal, and social challenges. Looking forward, future meetings of MobiHealth must seek to keep abreast of these developments, as well as promote innovate pathways for the realization of impactful research and solutions in the mobile health space.

All accepted papers underwent a triple-blind review process, involving members of the Technical Program Committee (TPC) and other external experts. This highly selective review process increased the scientific level of all papers accepted for presentation and subsequent publication. This current volume includes all papers presented during the conference in Dublin.

The editors wish to express their gratitude to the European Alliance for Innovation for their sponsorship and to UCD for hosting the event. The efforts of the TPC in reviewing manuscripts in a timely and professional manner was indispensable to the quality of the conference, and these proceedings. The dedicated efforts of the Local Organizing Committee members for the efficient operation of the conference is acknowledged. We wish to thank all the participants for their efforts in preparing and revising their manuscripts and then making their way to Dublin to present and discuss their work. The editors are acutely aware of the effort expended by the authors, reviewers and Organizing Committee, and consider the publication of these proceedings the culmination of a creative but collaborative journey. It is our fervent hope that these proceedings will serve as an invaluable resource for community and society on the state of the art in mHealth technologies. Finally, we wish to thank the local UCD team on the ground – Eleanor, Nestor, and Karl – for their dedication and efforts to ensure the smooth operation of the conference on the day.

December 2019

Michael O'Grady
Gregory O'Hare
Patrick Henn
John O'Donoghue

Organization

Steering Committee

Chair

Imrich Chlamtac   University of Trento, Italy

Founding Chair

James C. Lin   University of Illinois at Chicago, USA

Members

Dimitrios Koutsouris	National Technical University of Athens, Greece
Janet Lin	University of Illinois at Chicago, USA
Arye Nehorai	Washington University in St. Louis, USA
Konstantina S. Nikita	National Technical University of Athens, Greece
George Papadopoulos	University of Cyprus, Cyprus
Oscar Mayora	CREATE-NET, Italy

Organizing Committee

General Chairs

Gregory O'Hare	University College Dublin, Ireland
Patrick Henn	University College Cork, Ireland
Simon Smith	University College Cork, Ireland
Michael O'Grady	University College Dublin, Ireland

Program Chair

John O'Donoghue   University College Cork, Ireland

Workshops Chair

David Power   University College Cork, Ireland

Sponsorship and Exhibits Chairs

David Power	University College Cork, Ireland
John O'Donoghue	University College Cork, Ireland

Publications Chair

John O'Donoghue   University College Cork, Ireland

Local Arrangement Chair

Patrick Henn   University College Cork, Ireland

Web Chairs

Kevin McGuire   University College Cork, Ireland
John O'Donoghue   University College Cork, Ireland

Conference Manager

Dominika Belisova   EAI

Technical Program Committee

Alessandro Tognetti	Università di Pisa, Italy
Angelo Basteris	Griffith University, Australia
Anja Exler	Karlsruhe Institute of Technology (KIT), Germany
Athanasios Kakarountas	University of Thessaly, Greece
Benard Bene	Imperial College London, UK
Bo Andersson	Lund University, Sweden
Carlo Emilio Standoli	Politecnico di Milano, Italy
Chipo Kanjo	Chancellor College of the University of Malawi, Malawi
Chris Watson	Queen's University Belfast, UK
Daniel Carter	University of Limerick, Ireland
Gregory O'Hare	University College Dublin, Ireland
Griphin Baxer	Mzuzu University, Malawi
Henry Potts	University College London, UK
Holger Kunz	University College London, UK
Jane Walsh	NUI Galway, Ireland
John O'Donoghue	University College Cork, Ireland
John Nelson	University of Limerick, Ireland
Kevin Balanda	University College Cork, Ireland
Liam Glynn	University of Limerick, Ireland
Mary Sibande	Livingstonia University, Malawi
Michael O'Grady	University College Dublin, Ireland
Nikolaos Papachristou	University of Surry, UK
Patrick Henn	University College Cork, Ireland
Peter Harrington Palms	GP Surgery, Ireland
Philip Fadahunsi	Imperial College London, UK
Salma Kammoun	Abdulaziz University Jeddah, Saudi Arabia
Simon Smith	University College Cork, Ireland
Siobhan O'Connor	University of Edinburgh, UK
Zuhal Hussein	Universiti Teknologi MARA, Malaysia

Contents

Mobility and Real-Time Assessment

Remote Testing of Usability in Medical Apps.................... 3
Janina Sauer, Alexander Muenzberg, Laura Siewert, Andreas Hein,
and Norbert Roesch

Mobile Application for Celiac Disease Patients' Wellness and Support 18
Sara Altamirano, Gudrun Thorsteinsdottir, and Verónica Burriel

Real-Time Continuous Monitoring of Cerebral Edema Based on a Flexible
Conformal Coil Sensor 36
Jingbo Chen, Gen Li, Mingsheng Chen, Jun Yang, and Mingxin Qin

Remote Patient Monitoring

Evaluating End-User Perception Towards a Cardiac Self-care
Monitoring Process... 43
Gabriella Casalino, Giovanna Castellano, Vincenzo Pasquadibisceglie,
and Gianluca Zaza

Walking Pace Induction Application Based on the BPM and RhythmValue
of Music 60
Atsushi Otsubo, Hirohiko Suwa, Yutaka Arakawa, and Keiichi Yasumoto

User-Oriented Interface for Monitoring Affective Diseases in Patients
with Bipolar Disorder Using Mobile Devices 75
Salvador Prefasi-Gomar, Teresa Magal-Royo, Elisa Gallach-Solano,
Pilar Sierra San Miguel, Humberto Echevarria Mateu,
and Nieves Martínez-Alzamora

The PERFORM Mask: A Psychophysiological sEnsoRs Mask
FOr Real-Life Cognitive Monitoring 86
Danilo Menicucci, Marco Laurino, Elena Marinari, Valentina Cesari,
and Angelo Gemignani

Patient Monitoring and Assessment of ICT Solutions

The Design of a Holistic mHealth Community Library Model
and Its Impact on Empowering Rural America 97
Guy C. Hembroff, Daniel Boyle, and Timothy Van Wagner

Stop Anxiety: Tackling Anxiety in the Academic Campus Through an
mHealth Multidisciplinary User-Centred Approach   112
   David Ferreira, Daniela Melo, Andreia Santo, Pedro Silva,
   Sandra C. Soares, and Samuel Silva

Using Data Distribution Service for IEEE 11073-10207 Medical
Device Communication   127
   Merle Baake, Josef Ingenerf, and Björn Andersen

Enabling Multimodal Emotionally-Aware Ecosystems Through
a W3C-Aligned Generic Interaction Modality   140
   David Ferreira, Nuno Almeida, Susana Brás, Sandra C. Soares,
   António Teixeira, and Samuel Silva

A SmartBed for Non-obtrusive Physiological Monitoring During Sleep:
The LAID Project   153
   Marco Laurino, Nicola Carbonaro, Danilo Menicucci, Gaspare Alfì,
   Angelo Gemignani, and Alessandro Tognetti

A Prototype System of Acute Stroke Type Discrimination and Monitoring
Based on a Annulus Antenna Array: A Pilot Study   163
   Mingsheng Chen, Jia Xu, Jingbo Chen, Haisheng Zhang,
   and Mingxin Qin

Patient Monitoring and Robotics

Smart System for Supporting the Elderly in Home Environment   171
   Eleni Boumpa and Athanasios Kakarountas

A Wearable Exoskeleton for Hand Kinesthetic Feedback
in Virtual Reality   186
   Emanuele Lindo Secco and Andualem Maereg Tadesse

Development of an Intuitive EMG Interface for Multi-dexterous
Robotic Hand   201
   Emanuele Lindo Secco, Daniel McHugh, David Reid,
   and Atulya Kumar Nagar

Kinesthetic Feedback for Robot-Assisted Minimally Invasive Surgery
(Da Vinci) with Two Fingers Exoskeleton   212
   Emanuele Lindo Secco and Andualem Maereg Tadesse

Wearable Technologies and Smart Measurement

Evaluating the Requirements of Digital Stress Management Systems:
A Modified Delphi Study   229
   Kim Janine Blankenhagel, Miriam Linker, and Rüdiger Zarnekow

Preliminary Assessment of a Smart Mattress for Position
and Breathing Sensing.   249
    Lucia Arcarisi, Carlotta Marinai, Massimo Teppati Losè,
    Marco Laurino, Nicola Carbonaro, and Alessandro Tognetti

Preliminary Investigation on Band Tightness Estimation
of Wrist-Worn Devices Using Inertial Sensors   256
    Masayuki Hayashi, Hiroki Yoshikawa, Akira Uchiyama,
    and Teruo Higashino

Artificial Intelligence at the Edge in the Blockchain of Things   267
    Tuan Nguyen Gia, Anum Nawaz, Jorge Peña Querata,
    Hannu Tenhunen, and Tomi Westerlund

Continuous Wellness Tracking with Firstbeat – Usability, User Experience,
and Subjective Wellness Impact   281
    Timo Partala, Laura Saar, Minna Männikkö, Maarit Karhula,
    and Tuulevi Aschan

Developing a Novel Citizen-Scientist Smartphone App for Collecting
Behavioral and Affective Data from Children Populations   294
    Christos Maramis, Ioannis Ioakimidis, Vassilis Kilintzis,
    Leandros Stefanopoulos, Eirini Lekka, Vasileios Papapanagiotou,
    Christos Diou, Anastasios Delopoulos, Penio Kassari,
    Evangelia Charmandari, and Nikolaos Maglaveras

Data Management within mHealth Environments

Intelligent Combination of Food Composition Databases and Food Product
Databases for Use in Health Applications.   305
    Alexander Muenzberg, Janina Sauer, Andreas Hein, and Norbert Roesch

Labeling of Activity Recognition Datasets: Detection
of Misbehaving Users   320
    Alessio Vecchio, Giada Anastasi, Davide Coccomini,
    Stefano Guazzelli, Sara Lotano, and Giuliano Zara

Mobile App for Optimizing Home Care Nursing.   332
    Virginia Sandulescu, Sorin Puscoci, Monica Petre, Sorin Soviany,
    Mirabela Chirvasa, and Alexandru Girlea

Author Index   341

Mobility and Real-Time Assessment

Remote Testing of Usability in Medical Apps

Janina Sauer[1,2(✉)], Alexander Muenzberg[1,2], Laura Siewert[1], Andreas Hein[2], and Norbert Roesch[1]

[1] University of Applied Sciences Kaiserslautern, Kaiserslautern, Germany
{janina.sauer,alexander.muenzberg,norbert.roesch}@hs-kl.de
[2] Carl von Ossietzky University of Oldenburg, Oldenburg, Germany
{janina.sauer,alexander.muenzberg,andreas.hein}@uni-oldenburg.de

Abstract. Usability tests play an important role in any kind of software, as they limit errors and misunderstandings. Especially in the growing market of medical applications it is indispensable, but time-consuming and expensive. In order to improve the quality of medical applications and remove obstacles for developers, a method has been developed that simplifies testing the usability of mobile medical applications and provides additional data on compliance and effectiveness. Because this test method is remote-controlled and asynchronous, finding examiners is simplified. It also allows more subjects to be found and more data to be collected. This increases user experience and achieves more natural results as study participants act in their natural environment. In order to decide whether the app developed is suitable for this remote testing method, a questionnaire was developed to assist in the decision-making process. The described method will be tested in a study.

Keywords: Medical app · Usability · Remote testing · App testing · Mobile health

1 Introduction

The market for mobile healthcare has grown steadily in recent years and continues to grow. In 2017, 325,000 health, fitness and medical apps are available in all major app stores. Last year, 78,000 new health apps were launched in the major app stores. Estimated 3.7 billion downloads of health apps in 2017 [1].

Within the European Union (EU), medical apps have to be considered as medical device and are entitled under the European Medical Device Regulation (93/42/EEC) if the intended use is linked with medical purposes. But even in other cases, comprehensive tests are mandatory to improves product quality, reduce user errors, increase customer loyalty and satisfaction. It's also reduces support costs and increases the recommendation rate [2].

Regarding the United States (US) market and according to the US Food and Drug Administration, most errors are only discovered at the end of development, so special attention should be paid to formative testing during development. Regardless of when the tests are performed, the type of test is crucial.

G. M. P. O'Hare et al. (Eds.): MobiHealth 2019, LNICST 320, pp. 3–17, 2020.
https://doi.org/10.1007/978-3-030-49289-2_1

Therefore, usability planning should be considered from the beginning. There are different guidelines for this, also special ones for apps in the health sector. After comparing several existing guidelines, the following aspects occur frequently:

- "Representation of Elements" (I, II, III, IV, VI, IX)
  Information should be presented effectively and clearly formulated. In some cases, images and icons are more appropriate than words, as long as they are unambiguous.
- "Learning facilitation and support" (I, II, III, IV, V, VII)
  The app should be intuitive to use and contain a logic in the process.
- "Consistency and predictability" (I, II, III, V, X)
  All parts of the app should look and feel the same. The action of different buttons should be predictable.
- "Giving feedback" (I, II, V, VII)
  The user should always be informed of what is happening and should always be given the opportunity to correct possible errors.
- "Clarity and Functionality" (I, II, III, IV, VI)
  The app should be as simple as possible and make all important functionalities clearly visible to the user.
- "Metaphors" (I, II, III)
  Virtual objects and actions should be represented as metaphors from the real world.
- "Self-description" (I, III, X)
  The user should always know where he or she is. The navigation of the app should be uniform and comprehensible.
- "Effective Use of Language" (I, III, IX)
  Developers should use short phrases with simple words.
- "Fastest way" (I, V, IX)
  The user should always be clearly offered the fastest way to the desired destination and clearly represented.
- "Direct manipulation" (II, III, X)
  Direct manipulation of onscreen content engages people and facilities understanding. Icons from the real world are helpful.
- "Give the user control" (II, III, V)
  Users have control without receiving unwanted outcome.
- "Use platform specific functions" (III, IX, X)
  The developers must be aware of the platform or platforms for which they are developing.

The following guidelines and principles were taken into consideration:

   I.   HIMSS Guidelines [3]
   II.   iOS Design Principles [4]
  III. Android Principles [5]
  IV. MARS [6]
   V.   Sheiderman's Eight Golden Rules of Interface Design [7]
  VI. UX Planet Principles [8]
 VII. The Startup Principles [9]

VIII.   Principles in the Design of Mobile Medical Apps [10]
IX.   Mobile Health Consumer App Design Aspects [11]
X.   Ergonomics of human-system interaction - Part 110: Principles of dialogue design (ISO 9241-110:2006)

Furthermore, the Food and Drug Administration declares: "Usability is often confused with design, human factors engineering is a better term. Usability is not just chic color and trendy design elements."

Strict and often complex regulations are a major constraint on the digital healthcare market. Regulation is often cited as one of the main reasons for the slow development of digital healthcare solutions. A survey conducted by mHealth App Economics in 2017 showed that 18% of digital healthcare players are reluctant to develop apps due to uncertain regulatory frameworks [1].

The healthcare sector is subject to intensive regulation. Both digital and non-digital healthcare solutions that could pose a risk to patient safety must be approved by an official regulatory body such as the Food and Drug Administration in the United States. Currently, many medical apps are of poor quality and sometimes potentially dangerous [12]. Also, the great potential is not used.

In July 2017, the Food and Drug Administration announced a new approach to the approval of digital healthcare solutions, the Digital Health Innovation Plan. Instead of approving individual digital products, entire companies could be approved, and digital products approved by these pre-selected companies would not have to go through a regulatory process for each of their product approvals. This development is still new, but the Food and Drug Administration appears to be initiating a paradigm shift in the regulation of digital healthcare solutions. This could serve as a blueprint for other countries to follow [1].

At present, however, a medical app still has to undergo comprehensive, time-consuming and cost-intensive certification processes. One factor that must be extensively tested in this context is usability. In the European Union, the standard IEC 62366 Medical devices - Application of usability engineering to medical devices is to serve as support. This standard is closely linked to ISO 14971 Medical Devices - Application of Risk Management to Medical Devices. It follows that usability is primarily seen as a risk factor. According to the Food and Drug Administration, more damage is caused by incorrect operation than by technical errors. In the IEC 62366-1:2007 standard, usability is described as a characteristic of the user product interface that encompasses effectiveness, efficiency, as well as the user's ability to learn and satisfaction. Also, here a usability file is promoted, which covers the following points: Extended purpose including user specification and usage context, core tasks and pre and post conditions and subtasks, usage requirements, user product interface specification including main functions, verification results, validation plan and validation results. Since the new version of the 2015 standard, the standard compliance requirements are very similar to the Food and Drug Administration requirements.

The standard requires that usability be extensively tested and documented. However, the user experience is not considered.

The standard requires the testing of usability. This means that the medical device must perform various tasks in an environment of representative selected test persons from the user group under observation without help, but with a test leader. As Jakob Nielsen points out, testing with potential users is the most effective way to identify usability problems [13]. These tests are documented and evaluated.

IEC 62366-2 assumes that with six testers approx. 80% of the errors are found (recommended for formative tests), with 15 test subjects approx. 90% of the errors (recommended for summative tests). Both the IEC 62366-2 and the Food and Drug Administration agree that the figures can only be read per target group.

The good usability of the products enables users to perform tasks quickly and correctly. The usability measures are effectiveness, efficiency and user satisfaction.

2   Methods

With remote testing, testers can use the application asynchronously in their natural environment according to their needs and the requirements of the app. These activities can be stored by little additional programming effort and sent to the developers without affecting the test subjects.

Depending on the functionality of the app, timestamps can be set at important points in the app. A flowchart is helpful for this, because so it is possible to see the whole procedure of the app. If these are then set in a predefined flow context, it is easy to see where the user's handling problems were. So, the whole activity can be tracked by simple button events and an analysis of the runtime behavior can be created. Each timestamp needs a unique name so that the evaluator knows exactly which button belongs to which timestamp and can place it in the correct sequence [14].

In addition, it is possible to record the entire screen in order to be able to reproduce the behavior in even more detail. Audio recordings can also be documented, if the test persons are animated to think aloud, i.e. to pronounce all thoughts, positive as well as negative, questions, etc., the developers can give the best insight. However, this data must also be evaluated manually, which is difficult to achieve with a large group of testers and requires more time and money due to the additional effort.

Remote testing has the advantage that the testers do not only have to fulfill the given task, but mostly all areas of the application have to be tested automatically including the main and secondary functions, as well as to be defined for certification.

Since the testing is carried out in the everyday life of the users, many testers do not notice any more that they are testing a medical app because the test environment is not present.

In the case of a large group of testers, it is advisable to determine the optimal way to complete a task, the so-called happy path. For this purpose, the buttons that are required for this have to be defined so that they can be automatically compared later with the timestamps or their sequence. In addition, it is possible to define the time range between two buttons. This not only makes it possible to evaluate whether the effective way was found, but also whether it was found quickly.

Further functionalities of the smartphone can also be used, for example to determine the location of use.

Furthermore, no professional trainer is required, as the test persons use and test the app asynchronously according to their needs in their familiar environment. A test leader is only required when the test results are evaluated. However, he or she can also act asynchronously.

However, it can be an advantage that the test persons fill out questionnaires after the test phase has been completed, depending on the requirements of the app and its developers. These can be standardized, such as the System Usability Scale [15] and the User Experience Questionnaire [16], or individually adapted to the requirements of the app and its developers.

The advantages and disadvantages of the usability laboratory and the remote variant are listed in Table 1.

Some of the disadvantages of remote testing can be eliminated with regular online meetings. Here the test coordinator and the respondent have the opportunity to exchange

Table 1. Usability laboratory with remote tests in comparison

Usability laboratory	Remote usability tests
Advantages:	
• Certainty that the test person will carry out the task conscientiously • Direct observation of the entire test situation • More details can be observed	• Size of the tester group can be extended • Larger selection of test subjects • Tester is located in its natural environment, so it feels more comfortable and a more natural result is created • Lower expenses • More usability problems can be detected as more cases and applications are tested with the app • Less strenuous for the test persons, as the test environment is less present • Possibility of automated evaluation of results • Test persons can test the app more freely, according to their needs. This results in much more diversified results • Less costs (resources, space, travel expenses …) • Comfort, better in everyday working life • It is easier to find test persons because they are often more likely to take part in a test in which they do not have to travel • Simplified finding of test persons through recruitment via the Internet • Suitable if the target group is difficult to reach (at different locations) • Not fixed location • Not time-bound • Simplified recruitment of usability experts

(continued)

Table 1. (*continued*)

Disadvantages:	
• Complex recruitment of test persons • Uncomfortable for test persons, as they are in a test situation and in an unfamiliar environment • It is time-consuming to plan the recruitment and the execution of the tests • Expensive (recruitment, provision of usability laboratory and resources), depending on the budget not many users can be checked and developers only meet the required minimum requirements	• No direct observation, one does not directly see the reactions of the user, some problems may remain undiscovered because gestures and facial expressions of the user are missing and therefore the entire emotional reaction is missing • Code of the test app must be slightly adjusted • It is unknown whether the test persons really test the app carefully and seriously • It is more difficult to interact, interview, train and observe the participants • If hardware is to be provided, some logistics are required to distribute it to the participants and collect it again. In the case of pure software applications, regular installation support is required • Confidentiality during screen sharing; it must be ensured that no confidential data of the test person is displayed • Technical problems can occur more frequently. Under certain circumstances help can only be offered after some time

ideas, the test coordinator can ask specific questions to the satisfaction and draw first results and the respondent can convey his or her first impressions and get possible questions about handling answered. This also provides the respondent with an opportunity to perform certain tasks set by the test leader so that the test leader can directly perceive the facial expressions and gestures of the proband. However, there are disadvantages that cannot be avoided in the usability laboratory. The respondent is taken out of his natural environment and thus becomes aware of the test situation. He or she no longer acts as usual. Therefore, the execution of synchronous tasks is only recommended in exceptional cases.

It is also important to mention that various studies have already shown that the results of remote usability are at least comparably good with the results of classic usability tests, such as a usability laboratory [17–19].

The study by Tullis et al. [20] has shown that test subjects are more willing to participate in a remote test than in a laboratory test. In this study 108 people agreed to participate in a remote test, while only eight people could be found for a test in the usability lab. One reason for this is the lower effort a remote test entails compared to a laboratory test for the test subjects [21].

Studies comparing a laboratory test with a remote test show that both synchronous and asynchronous remote usability tests produce quantitative and qualitative comparable results. The number and severity of the found usability problems could not be determined significantly either [17]. Often even more usability problems were detected by a remote test [16]. The impression of the test persons is also of great importance. The remote test situation is usually positively received. In the study by Brush et al. [17], seven out of eight participants found the remote tests more pleasant than the situation in the usability laboratory. Of these eight test persons, four preferred the remote test, but no test person preferred the test in the laboratory.

In order to decide which type of testing is appropriate, a questionnaire was developed:

1. Doesn't the app fall under the MDD or MDR according to its purpose? If so, is the app already certified?
2. Has the app been developed for long-term use?
3. Does the app have more than five main and secondary functions?
4. Are the users people without medical qualifications?
5. Is the app used by private individuals in their private environment?
6. Is there a wide range of users?
7. Are the test persons at different locations, widely distributed?
8. Can the test persons use their own smartphones, or is the use of a private smartphone advantageous?
9. Can the testing be carried out without additional hardware?
10. Isn't the respondent's facial expressions and gestures of decisive importance in the evaluation?

If most of the above questions are answered with "YES", remote testing is recommended. The financial factor is not to be despised, but it is strongly dependent on individual framework factors. In the same way, time can still influence the selection of the test, but here this point has to be considered very individually, too.

With the presented method not only, the usability and the user experience can be tested, the entire compliance can be evaluated. Measurement parameters such as frequency of use, duration of use, completeness, continuity and regularity can be easily collected. In this case the developer can quantify these metrics with a range in order to compare the results of the tests, too. Or he or she does not give a range and interprets the evaluation freely in order to draw his conclusions. This depends strongly on the requirements of the application and developer and the group size of the testers.

It can be assumed that an increase in usability quality will also increase compliance.

3 Results

In order to find weak points and difficulties regarding usability in the mobile app, it was decided to assign timestamps to different buttons. The following questions were defined in advance:

"How long does the user spend in our app?"
"How long does a user need to complete a certain process (e.g. adding food)?"
"When does the user abort a process or delete his entries?"

"Where does the user call up the help function?"

In accordance with these questions, the buttons in the app are provided with timestamps to measure the time intervals between and during the various processes. After the evaluation, the measured time can be used to identify the processes in which the user needs longer, or deletes or aborts them more frequently, and to identify where further usability problems exist and analyze them. An alpha test is then performed to determine standard times and optimum values for comparison with the users and to detect deviations. Furthermore, by measuring the total time the user has spent in the app, compliance can be tested to determine whether the users are all using the app regularly, as prescribed, and conscientiously.

To see where to set timestamps, it is helpful to create a simplified flowchart which shows all main and secondary functions as shown in Fig. 1. In this way, the best points for time stamps can be found easily and individually, so that the best possible evaluation is available.

The diagram should provide a precise overview of what is relevant for processes and what happens in them. The red dashes are actions like add, fill in text fields, select or save settings and so on. The trash can always indicate the point in time at which individual elements are to be deleted in the process. The red X indicates the period in which the process can be aborted and the green question mark indicates the period in which the user has the possibility to call up the help function.

Note that an individual minimum number of timestamps is required for comprehensive results, but too many measurement points can complicate interpretation and possibly even falsify it. This figure is based on the developer's own alpha test to control the process, as shown in the appendix.

The app developed in the DiDiER project (Digitization of Services in the Nutritional Counselling Process) funded by the German Federal Ministry of Education and Research (grant 02K14A150) is used here as an illustrative example. The purpose of this mobile app is to make it easier for the patient to keep a diary by documenting all distorted foods and their symptoms, from which the diagnosis of possible food intolerances and allergies can be made by professional nutritionists [22]. As part of this study, 25 test persons will receive a smartphone including the DiDiER App over the period of their diagnosis (two to six weeks), on which they must record all nutrition-relevant data, such as distorted foods, symptoms, including strength and possible cofactors. For this purpose, the study participants are provided with various smart services, such as a Food Information Service, which also enables the scanning of food barcodes so that all ingredients can be stored directly. The Food Information Service is a collection of existing food databases that are enhanced by various quality optimization algorithms [23]. It is also possible to photograph symptoms and foods, as well as search by text input in the Food Information Service. The developed standards are expected to lead to a significant increase in the quality of nutritional advice for patients and nutritionists.

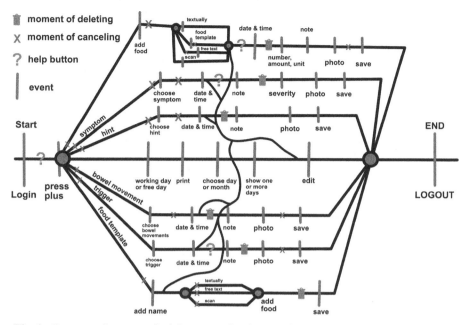

Fig. 1. Sequence diagram to find the appropriate buttons for timestamps (Color figure online)

Currently, the entire system, consisting of patient app and consultant platform, is being tested in a study. The study protocol was reviewed and approved by the Ethics Committee of the Carl von Ossietzky University Oldenburg, Germany.

The questions already presented, as to decide whether remote testing would be appropriate, were answered as follows (Table 2):

Table 2. Answering the questionnaire to decide if remote tests are suitable for the DiDiER App

No.	Question:	Answer:
1.	Doesn't the app fall under the MDD or MDR according to its purpose? If so, is the app already certified?	Yes, the app does not fall under MDD/MDR because of its purpose, so far, the app itself is a pure tool for documentation, therefore no certification is necessary
2.	Has the app been developed for long-term use?	Yes, at the moment the app should be used for a period between two and six weeks. Later the app will be used even longer
3.	Does the app have more than five main and secondary functions?	Yes, the mobile app has several main and secondary functions
4.	Are the users people without medical qualifications?	Yes, the users of the app come from many different backgrounds and do not need medical training

(continued)

Table 2. (*continued*)

No.	Question:	Answer:
5.	Is the app used by private individuals in their private environment?	Yes, it is used by private individuals in everyday life
6.	Is there a wide range of users?	Yes, the users, both during and after the study, should use the app by various users
7.	Are the test persons at different locations, widely distributed?	Yes, the app can be used from anywhere and is not location-bound. However, the test persons are in the vicinity of their nutritionists during the study
8.	Can the test persons use their own smartphones, or is the use of a private smartphone advantageous?	Yes, the app can be used from any smartphone. But during the study, the subjects receive a smartphone
9.	Can the testing be carried out without additional hardware?	Yes, no additional hardware is required
10.	Isn't the respondent's facial expressions and gestures of decisive importance in the evaluation?	Yes, facial expressions and gestures do not play an important role in the evaluation

A timestamp on the login and logout button can be used to determine how long the respective user has been using the application. Since a button event is also saved on the different view options, for example on the calendar views, a statement can then be made as to which view is preferred. Furthermore, a start point and one or two end points (saving the entered data and canceling the entry) have been defined for each sequence. So, it can be tracked exactly how long the tester needs for a sequence, if he or she confirms it or when this task is aborted. Each help button is provided with a tracker so that it is clear where the user needs special help and is unsure how to use it.

The collection of button tracks makes it possible to track the entire usage without any gaps.

At the end of each test phase, the entire data is displayed pseudonymized in tables for evaluation. Different events are grouped so that the evaluation is simplified.

No audio or screen recordings are made during the study. This is not required here.

4 Conclusion and Outlook

In many countries within Europe, the population is accustomed to insurance paying for most health-related matters. It is therefore difficult to get users to pay for a health app. So, developers need to use other ways to cover the costs of development and certification and make a profit. At the moment there is a trend for developers to contact different insurance companies, so that these insurance companies include the app in their offer [1].

This has to be considered for distributors, because they either have to get in contact with many different health insurance companies or convince the user directly. In both cases, more than just certification is often expected. Usability is one of the most important factors, and even more so is the overall user experience. Because if the app is not easy to use, it is not popular to use and the potential increase in quality of life remains unused.

With the presented concept apps can be tested completely and comprehensively regarding their usability. With this easier way, they can identify and reduce possibly risk factors. The test persons can be easily found in remote testing, since no effort and costs are incurred for the journey. Earlier studies have already shown that the results of remote tests and in the usability laboratory are comparable or even more errors are found in remote tests.

Timestamp can be used to collect all relevant information on specific buttons without influencing the test persons. Additional information can be obtained through further possibilities, such as screen- and audio monitoring and consultation hours with experts. The evaluation of the collected data can take place time-independently and can be automated by previously defined happy path.

The test method is currently used in the study for testing the DiDiER App. The developed questionnaire demonstrates that the DiDiER App is suitable for this purpose. Usability results are expected by the end of 2019. The data to be evaluated will then also be examined for compliance and compared with the previously defined compliance area. The creation of the automated evaluation with the help of the happy path is one of the next steps.

If the results are as positive as currently expected, the presented concept will be adapted to further apps in the health sector and further investigated, for example with regard to the effectiveness of the smartphone application.

It is expected that the new remote tests will lead to an enormous increase in quality and a decrease in risk, even though the medical app has already been certified according to the EU directive. The IEC 62304 Medical device software - Software life-cycle processes (IEC 62304:2006 + A1:2015) also requires permanent validation.

Acknowledgment. This research was done within the framework of the DiDiER project, which is funded by the German Federal Ministry of Education and Research (grant 02K14A150). Different institutes are working together on this joint project. Particularly the German Allergy and Asthma Association (DAAB) as application partner and executor of the study and EUROKEY GmbH Saarbrücken, which took over many parts of the development of the app, are to be mentioned here.

The cooperation between the University of Applied Sciences Kaiserslautern and Carl von Ossietzky University was extremely positive and beneficial.

Appendix

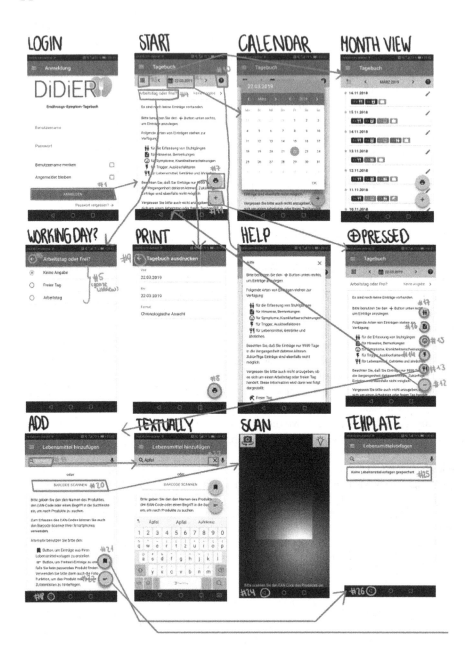

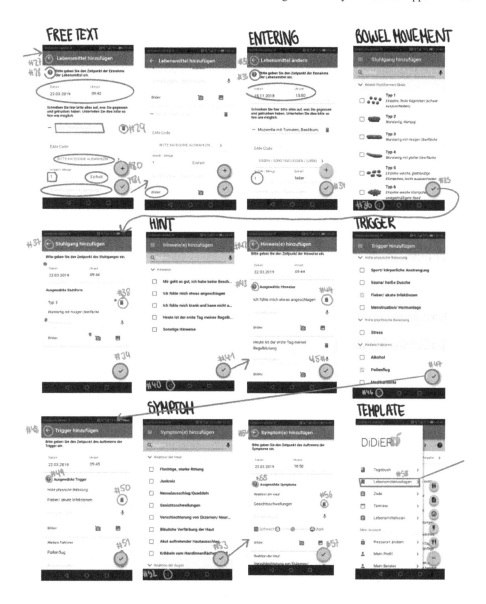

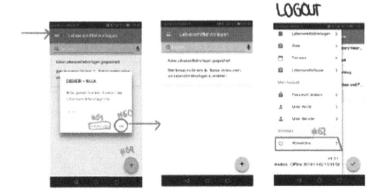

References

1. Research 2 Guidance mHealth App Economics 2017/2018
2. Healthcare Information and Management Systems Society Promoting Usability in Healthcare Organizations: Initial Steps and Progress Towards a Healthcare Usability Maturity Model
3. Healthcare Information and Management Systems Usability Evaluation Guide for Clinicians Practice: https://www.himss.org/himss-emr-usability-evaluation-guide-clinicians-practices-9-essential-principles-software-usability. Accessed 14 May 2019
4. IOS Design Principles. https://developer.apple.com/design/human-interface-guidelines/ios/overview/themes/. Accessed 14 May 2019
5. Android Design Principles. https://www.designprinciplesftw.com/collections/android-design-principles. Accessed 14 May 2019
6. Stoyan, S.R., Hides, L., Kavanagh, D.J., Zelenko, O., Tjondronegoro, D., Mani, M.: Mobile app rating scale: a new tool for assessing the quality of health mobile apps. JMIR Mhealth Uhealth 2015 Jan-Mar, **3**(1), E 27, p. 1
7. Ben Sheiderman's Eight Golden Rules of Interface Design https://faculty.washington.edu/jtenenbg/courses/360/f04/sessions/schneidermanGoldenRules.html. Accessed 14 May 2019
8. UX Planet: Mobile UX Design: Key Principles https://uxplanet.org/mobile-ux-design-key-principles-dee1a632f9e6. Accessed 14 May 2019
9. The Startup, Mobile App Design Principles: 13 Rules for Creating Apps that Stick https://medium.com/swlh/infographics-mobile-app-design-principles-13-rules-for-creating-apps-that-stick-f607959692be. Accessed 14 May 2019
10. Lienhard, K.R., Legner C.: Principles in Design of Mobile Medical Apps: Guidance for Those who Care. University of Lausanne, Switzerland
11. MLSDev: Healthcare Mobile App Development: Types, Trends, & Features https://mlsdev.com/blog/healthcare-mobile-app-development. Accessed 14 May 2019
12. Albrecht, U.V.: Chances and Risks of Mobile Health (Chancen und Risiken von Gesundheits-Apps) (2016) Hannover, Germany (2016)
13. Nielsen, J.: Usability Engineering. Academic Press, Boston (1995)
14. Brooke, J.: SUS - a quick and dirty usability scale. United Kingdom (1986)
15. Sauer, J., Muenzberg, A., Hein, A., Roesch, N.: Simplify testing of mobile medical applications by using timestamps for remote, automated evaluation. In: 2019 15th International Conference on Wireless and Mobile Computing, Networking and Communications (WI Mob) (2019)

16. Laugwirtz, B., Held, T., Schrepp, M.: Construction and evaluation of a user experience questionnaire. In: HCI Usability Education, Work, pp. 63–76 (2008)
17. Brush, B.A.J., Ames, M., Davis, J.: A comparison of remote and local usability studies for an expert interface. In: CHI Vienna, Austria, pp. 1179–1182 (2004)
18. Thompson, K.E., Rozanski, E.P., Haake, A.R.: Here, there, anywhere: remote usability-testing that works. In: SIGITE 2004, pp. 132–137. ACM, USA (2004)
19. Hartson, H.R., Castillo, J.C., Kelson, J., Neale, W.C.: Remote evaluations: the network as an extension of the usability laboratory. In: CHI 1996, pp. 228–235 (1996)
20. Tullis, T., Fleischman, S., McNulity, M., Cinanchette, C., Bergel, M.: An empirical comparison of lab and remote usability-testing on web sites. In: Usability Professionals Association Conference (2002)
21. Dumas, J.C.: Usability evaluation from your desktop. In: Association for Information Systems (AIS) SIGCHI Newsletter, November 2003, pp. 6–8 (2003)
22. Elfert, P., Eichelberg, M., Tröger, J., Britz, J., Alexandersson, J., et al.: DiDiER digitized services in dietry counselling for people with increased health risk related to malnutrition and food allergies. In: IEEE Symposium on Computers and Communications (ISCC), pp. 100–104. IEEE (2017)
23. Muenzberg, A., Sauer, J., Hein, A., Roesch, N.: The use of ETL and data profiling to integrate data and improve quality in food databases. In: 2018 14th International Conference on Wireless and Mobile Computing, Networking and Communications (WI Mob), pp. 231–238 (2018). https://doi.org/10.1109/wimob.2018.8589081

Mobile Application for Celiac Disease Patients' Wellness and Support

Sara Altamirano$^{(\boxtimes)}$, Gudrun Thorsteinsdottir, and Verónica Burriel

Utrecht University, Heidelberglaan 8, 3584 CS Utrecht, The Netherlands
{s.e.altamiranoortega,g.thorsteinsdottir}@students.uu.nl, v.burriel@uu.nl

Abstract. Celiac disease affects an estimated 1% of the population. The only existing treatment is a strict gluten-free diet but there are myriad aspects of managing the disease that affect the lifestyle of both the CD patient and those close to them. The goal of this study was to design, develop and test a prototype of a mobile application to promote wellness and support for individuals with CD. The proposed application's aim is to serve as a platform for CD patients and members from their social circle, to help with sharing general and specific information about four lifestyle aspects: social, emotional, food, and wellness. The application aids with the management of a gluten-free diet from the social circle perspective for the specific CD patient. Perceptions towards the usability of the application were gathered from 22 participants and analyzed via a USE questionnaire. The results from the survey reported overall satisfaction of the prototype and useful insights were gathered for subsequent versions. The general expected benefit of this evidence-based application is improved quality of life for the CD patient due to their social circle being well informed about the management of the disease and its potential complications.

Keywords: Mobile application · mHealth · Celiac disease · Medical informatics · Gluten-Free

1 Introduction

Autoimmune diseases (AID) include a wide variety of illnesses targeting different parts of the human body. The American Autoimmune Related Disease Association (AARDA) has classified more than 100 AID, making it the third most common type of disease in the United States. The AARDA identifies AID as a major health problem affecting up to 50 million individuals in the United States alone, which translates to an alarming 15% of the population. Some AID are within the top 10 leading causes of death among women aged 65 and older, and 75% of Americans with AID are women. According to the AARDA website, AID are responsible for more than 100 billion US dollars annually in direct healthcare costs and most AID patients see four doctors over three years before a correct diagnosis [8].

© ICST Institute for Computer Sciences, Social Informatics and Telecommunications Engineering 2020
Published by Springer Nature Switzerland AG 2020. All Rights Reserved
G. M. P. O'Hare et al. (Eds.): MobiHealth 2019, LNICST 320, pp. 18–35, 2020.
https://doi.org/10.1007/978-3-030-49289-2_2

Many autoimmune diseases seem to vary in incidence by region or ethnicity. For instance, Southern European and Asian countries have a lower incidence of type 1 diabetes and multiple sclerosis than do Northern European countries. This variation may be caused by the irregular prevalence in specific ethnic groups of a gene associated to a particular AID. Likewise, dissimilarities in diet or in the existence of a triggering pathogen or chemical agent due to geographic factors may affect the frequency of an AID [22]. Regardless of the public health scale of the problem, the unknown aetiology of AID, the complexities involved in diagnostics, the increased costs, and the unavailability of cures, scientific research has focused on a small portion of more than 100 known AID [12].

Celiac Disease (CD) is an AID that requires effective self-management in adherence to a strict gluten-free diet (GFD), which is the only existing treatment for the disease. The list of symptoms that CD patients have is extensive and varies from childhood to adulthood. Some of the symptoms that are commonly experienced by children are abdominal pain and stunted growth issues. Moreover, symptoms that adults can experience are diarrhea, fatigue, anemia and reduced bone disease, among many others [27]. The proportion of people with CD varies among regions in the world. The reported prevalence of CD in South and North America was 0.4%–0.5% whereas the value for Asia was 0.6%. However, the prevalence in Europe and Oceania was slightly higher at 0.8%.

One of the authors of this study has CD and understands the importance of technological support for the management of the condition. As with any chronic disease, support is a team effort in conjunction with the social circle of the patient. With CD, the patients find themselves having to explain their condition numerous times, and providing the same CD information repeatedly. Therefore, a one-stop platform that centralizes accurate and readily-available information, personalized to each CD patient and their social circle, is of utmost importance. With feedback from other CD patients and analysis of well-reputed CD websites, we designed and developed a prototype of a mobile application to promote wellness and support for patients suffering from CD. A total of 22 CD patients and members from their social circle tested the initial prototype of the mHealth application and responded to a survey after the trial. The survey acquired perceptions towards the features of the app and usability of the design. The prototype contains general CD information due to the broad spectrum of CD symptoms. However, in future versions, the app will include information personalized to each patient. The patients will, therefore, be able to share individual pre-approved food and restaurants with their social circle, along with preferences and information about the disease and other psychological disturbances that accompany the disease, for each specific case.

The remaining sections of the study are as follows: Sect. 2 entails information about CD and how social support can aid the patient managing the disease thus explaining the problem statement and the need for the mHealth app. Related mobile applications for gluten intolerant people and CD patients are described in Sect. 3. In Sect. 4, the design of the application is visualized and explained in detail. The results from the survey are reported and analyzed in Sect. 5. Finally, Sect. 6 details the findings along with potential benefits, limitations of this study, and future work.

2   Problem Statement

In countries like the United States, the United Kingdom, and Germany, approximately 20% of the population has been reported to experience adverse reactions to foods such as wheat, nuts, fruits, and milk [13]. Historically, wheat-related disorders have been identified as CD and wheat allergy or non-celiac gluten sensitivity [23], referred as gluten intolerance in this study. Gluten-related conditions vary significantly in aetiology, but adherence to the GFD is of utmost importance for CD patients due to gluten reactivity involving autoimmune mechanisms [28].

Celiac disease is a systemic autoimmune disorder activated by gluten in genetically-predisposed individuals and affects an estimated 0.5 to 1.0% of the population worldwide [19]. Gluten is a protein found in cereals such as wheat, rye, and barley. CD is characterized by an extensive range of symptoms, a specific serum auto-antibody response, and variable damage to the small intestinal tract. Diagnosing CD can be difficult because some of the symptoms overlap with myriad other diseases, such as irritable bowel syndrome, chronic fatigue syndrome and depression. Since CD is hereditary, it is recommended that family members get tested as well. The longer the individual remains undiagnosed and untreated, the greater the chances of developing complications [15].

The treatment for CD is a lifelong GFD. However, some people do not improve on this diet and face additional health complications due to their deteriorating health. The adherence to this strict dietary regime varies among patients and is the main cause of persistent symptoms [15,18]. Therefore, it is advised to develop effective strategies to help patients follow a strict GFD, manage their various symptoms, and deal with all the implications of CD [16]. Participation of a close support group for the CD patient has been associated with higher quality of life scores, especially when face-to-face interaction may improve long-term quality of life and health outcomes [25]. Therefore, we recognize the need for a mobile application that helps CD patients manage their specific condition with support from their immediate social circle. We leave aside the search functionality through a catalog of gluten-free (GF) foods, because the majority of mobile health (mHealth) applications on the market today for CD patients are focused on finding GF food.

Following a strict GFD has a significant negative impact on quality of life in social settings for CD patients. Particularly related to social aspects such as traveling, eating out, and family life. Lee et al. [24] reported that CD patients, even though they know it will cause damage, typically cheat on their GFD because: 46.3% think the diet limits their social life, 55.3% perceive the diet as embarrassing, 24.9% say dining out is too difficult, 30.8% say the diet is socially isolating, and 33.3% report family and friends do not understand the need to follow the diet. Social support is therefore crucial for adherence to the GFD. Some solutions suggested by Lee et al. [24] are accommodation by family and friends, school and community support, group support, and others in their circle following a GFD.

3   Literature Review

The identified related work are mHealth applications that allow patients to self-regulate their health and diet in real time. Most applications aid in understanding the nutritional content of food consumed and focus on regulating lifestyle choices and diet. Within those applications, there are additional functionalities for identifying GF food for gluten intolerant individuals or CD patients [17, 21, 29]. However, there are CD specialized applications available on the market which contain more functionalities to monitor symptoms and the disease itself, such as *MyHealthyGut* [16] and *Eat! Gluten-Free* [2]. Additionally, a mobile tool for automated text messaging was identified in the literature, it aims at improving CD patient engagement and ultimately the quality of life [20].

3.1   mHealth Applications for Gluten-Free Diet

The Gluten-Free Living Association recommends several user-friendly mHealth applications which aid gluten intolerant individuals adhering to a GFD. Whether it is to find a GF product or restaurant or even if the GF requirements need to be communicated in a different language, these applications are a mean to assist in daily life [29]. Nonetheless, extra precautions need to be taken by the CD patient to ensure the foods are not only GF but also safe for individuals with CD due to cross-contamination in the kitchen. The vast majority of the reported mHealth applications in the section can be found in the list of recommendations from the association. Additionally, identified scientific literature is provided for two of the applications. In Table 1, the identified mHealth applications for gluten intolerance and CD are listed along with a short description of each application.

The *Find Me Gluten Free* application is for individuals that have gluten intolerance of any kind and patients with CD. The application contains information and reviews from members of the GF community of approved restaurants, grocery stores and cafes [3]. *AllergyEats* is a similar application that locates allergy-friendly restaurants in the United States and users can read reviews about the recommended restaurants and make their decisions accordingly [1].

The barcode-scanning technology is common in mHealth applications for understanding in a quick and easy way whether the product contains gluten and other nutritional values that are of interest for patients with CD and other gluten sensitivities. Applications that operate with this technology and recommended by Gluten-Free Living association are *The Gluten Free Scanner* [7], *Sift Food Labels* [11], *ShopWell Diet* [10] and *Is that Gluten Free?* [5].

Dunford et al. [17] describe the *FoodSwitch* application that uses barcode-scanning technology. The app operates with a large database of branded food which includes information on energy, protein, sugar and fiber. It provides users with nutritional information of packaged food in an easy language and suggests healthier alternative products if applicable. The initial launch of the application proved to be highly successful and in response to that the GlutenSwitch functionality was implemented later on. With the added functionality, people could receive recommendations and information on GF food, targeted mainly to CD patients and gluten intolerant individuals [17].

Handel [21] reviewed several mHealth applications of good quality that provide "information, strategies, and tracking capabilities related to patient self-management, health and wellness approaches". The mHealth application *Is That Gluten Free?* was one of these good quality applications that was discussed in the article [21] and recommended by the Gluten-Free Living Association as mentioned earlier [29]. The selection was based on several quality criteria such as ease of use, scope of information, recommendations and professional expertise. *Is That Gluten Free?* is an application that includes a large amount of verified GF products targeted for CD patients and other gluten intolerant individuals. The database includes comments from the manufacturers of the GF products and information regarding cross-contamination [21].

Education in mHealth applications is also of importance for individuals struggling with food intolerance, allergies, digestive-related problems, and CD. The main purpose of the *mySymptoms Food Diary* application is to educate about various diseases and discover patterns that relate consumption of food and symptoms. The users can not only track the food but also medication, exercise and emotions. Additionally, the application has a multi-user platform, meaning that every family member or other members in the social circle can have their own personalized page and share between one another [9].

3.2   mHealth Applications Specialized for Celiac Disease

The Celiac Disease Foundation is a leading disease advocacy group for CD in the United States. The foundation introduced an mHealth application in 2015, *Eat! Gluten-Free*, specialized for CD patients. The application contains a large digital hub of GF products along with pictures, recipes and details about the manufacturers. Additionally, CD patients are provided with the latest news and research concerning their disease [2].

Dowd et al. [16] developed a theory-based mHealth application, *MyHealthyGut*, for individuals to effectively deal with CD through self-management and subsequently improve their gut health. Perception and desired functions were gathered from CD patients and healthcare professionals through questionnaires and focus groups. Ninety percent of the participants reported a need for an app to help them manage celiac disease and that the most determining factors for using the app were "ease of use, available functions, nutritious GF recipes and cost". Additionally, participants considered the functionalities tracking the GFD and symptoms, supplements for healthier gut and cooking instructions, to be valuable for managing the disease and increase their quality of life.

Table 1. Available mHealth applications for gluten intolerance and CD patients.

Category	Name of application	Description	Price	Source
Dining out	Find Me Gluten Free	Locates GF restaurants, bars, grocery stores, cafes, etc. Users can additionally find information about the menus and contact information	Free	[3]
	AllergyEats	Users can find allergy-friendly restaurants in the US and search based on their personal food restrictions	Free	[1]
	Gluten-Free Restaurant Cards	The application contains 40 card images from CeliacTravel.com. Those cards can be shown to the staff of the restaurants and can be found in many languages	Free	[6]
Grocery Shopping	Fooducate Healthy Weight Loss & Calorie Counter	With the use of Barcode scanning technology, the user can find easily accessible nutritional information about products in the grocery store	Free, (gluten functionality needs to be purchased)	[4]
	The Gluten Free Scanner	Users can scan in products and each product that is scanned gets graded based on its nutritional value	$3.99	[7]
	Is that Gluten Free?	Large database of verified GF products and information about the manufacturers	$7.99	[5]
	Sift Food Labels	Barcode scanning technology and user-given easy, broken down information about the nutritional value	Free	[11]
	ShopWell Diet, Allergy Scanner	Barcode scanner with large, database. Additionally, to gluten the app provides allergy alert for example peanuts and soy	Free	[10]
	FoodSwitch	Bar-scanning technology and the GlutenSwitch functionality can be found within the application that is specifically for the GFD	Free	[17]
Gluten-Free Education	mySymptoms Food Diary	Track food that is consumed, symptoms and bowel movements for CD patients and food intolerance patients	Free	[9]

3.3   Automated Text Messaging Tool for CD Patients

The effectiveness of *Text Message Intervention (TEACH)* as a pragmatic approach for engaging CD patients was studied among adolescents in a randomized trial. The purpose of the tool was to aid younger patients suffering from CD due to the fact that they are more likely to not follow the strict GFD compared to other groups. The tool sends automated text messages and its intention is to educate and increase the engagement among young adults. The reported results from the study indicated a significant improvement in patient activation and quality of life for the adolescents in the TEACH intervention group [20].

3.4   Deficiencies of mHealth Applications

Some deficiencies were identified among mHealth applications for CD disease and gluten intolerance. The focus of the proposed mHealth application of this study is CD *patients* whereas the vast majority of the applications focus on gluten intolerance and CD. As was reported by Sapone et al. [28] the two conditions vary greatly, where CD is the "only clinical form of gluten reactivity involving autoimmune mechanisms." The adherence to a strict GFD is therefore ever more important for the CD patient. The *mySymptoms Food Diary* is the only identified application that provides multi-user functionality [29], which demonstrates the need for an mHealth application where CD patients can share lists of GF food and restaurants they trust and other important information about CD with their social circle. This can improve their overall quality of life and adherence to the GFD [24]. Lastly, psychological disturbances, such as anxiety and depression, have been associated with CD [14]. None of the identified mHealth applications address mental health of CD patients. The proposed application of this study includes information and common symptoms of mental health illnesses that CD patients might experience after being diagnosed with the disease, the goal with subsequent prototypes is to customize this information for the specific CD patient using the app.

4   Methods

The goal of the app is to serve as a platform for interaction between the CD patient and their social circle, namely the target users of the application. The app is to be used as a centralized place to exchange relevant information and gain understanding needed for social interactions, but more importantly, to give the patient a sense of safety and belonging. As reported by Lee et al. [24], social support is crucial for the CD patient in terms of accommodations by family and friends. That support can ultimately improve the patient's quality of life [25].

4.1   Design of the Prototype

The prototype was designed, built and deployed with the JustInMind[1] toolkit. This is a free, all-in-one prototyping tool for web and mobile apps. The toolkit provides a comprehensive library of UI components, objects and controls for Android and iOS mobile prototypes. With this tool, the developer can build a simple wireframe and interactive prototypes.

The initial prototype consists of 21 screens divided into four main sections: *Social, Wellness, Food* and *Emotional*. See Fig. 1 for the thank you screen for testing the prototype, the main menu of the app and the main screens of the aforementioned four sections. A sample screen from each of the four sections of the app can be seen in Fig. 2.

---

[1] https://www.justinmind.com/.

To design these four sections, we interviewed a CD patient, gathered feedback through the *celiac.com* website, and did an analysis of the sections included in well-reputed websites such as *beyondceliac.org*, *gluten.org*, and *celiac.org*. The CD patient expressed that they would like an app that has information about "our symptoms, a food section and traveling tips!" On the *celiac.com* forum, we received insights on having a food list such as:

> "Many of us have various food intolerance issues and have a whole list of foods we can not have, because I hate having to practically repeat my list to the family. Like a catalog. So family knows which prepackaged products we like and they can bring. Family traditions often involve bringing something over food wise. If they have the ability to know what they can bring, I think it could offer a way to deepen interactions and get the family involved."

Lastly, from the three main well-reputed websites mentioned above, we were able to identify the most common topics they cover (other than finding GF foods, which is not the focus of the app), which are: symptoms, testing and diagnosis, living with CD, community, concerns, GFD, recipes, food safety (cross-contamination), diet and nutrition, health and wellness, lifestyle, restaurants, children with CD, living GF, meals, dining GF, and social eating. We incorporated most of these topics in our first prototype. Keeping in mind that the main goal of the app is social circle support, it is important to acknowledge that the target group are CD patients alongside their social circle.

The Four Sections of the Prototype. The first section of the app is the *Social* section. It contains four subsections: *Celiac 101, Socializing, Dating,* and *Traveling.* The *Celiac 101* section is designed to provide a snapshot of CD by supplying statistics about the condition. Moreover, this subsection explains that CD is a chronic, genetic disorder that affects the CD patient's lifestyle. The second subsection, *Socializing,* explains the dynamics of dining out and gives a list of questions to ask when eating at restaurants; it also gives advice on what to do, such as always carrying snacks. The third subsection, *Dating,* covers dating by giving tips and ideas for sharing information with potential and current partners, such as which questions to ask, communicating, and planning ahead. The last subsection, *Traveling,* gives traveling tips and advice since finding GF options can be difficult in a foreign country with a foreign language.

The next section of the app, *Food,* covers dietary aspects, by means of four subsections: *Restaurants, Grocery List, What To Watch For* (cross-contamination), and *Quick Guide.* The *Restaurants* subsection has a list of restaurants approved by the CD patient, because of experience or preference, making it easy and stress-free to decide where to eat when dining out, with a Google Maps component. The *Grocery List* is similar to the restaurant list because it features a customized grocery list that helps both the CD patient when shopping for groceries, as well as friends and family when trying to decide which groceries to buy for a social gathering. The third subsection, *What to Watch For,* features a list of common sources of cross-contamination, which can

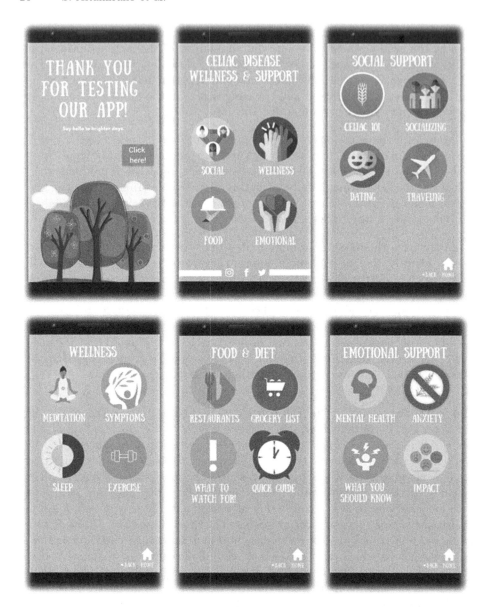

Fig. 1. Thank you screen, main menu and four sections of the mobile app: Social, Wellness, Food, Emotional

be very hard to manage because there are many sources and ways in which food and environment can become contaminated with gluten and make the CD patient ill. The last subsection offers a *Quick Guide* to easily distinguish GF foods from unsafe foods, answering the question: "What *can* you eat?"

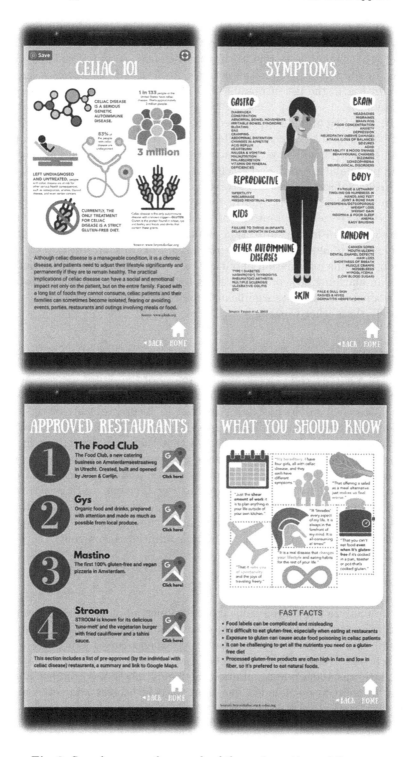

Fig. 2. Sample screens from each of the main sections of the app

General information about how good sleeping habits are maintained, increasing well-being with practices such as meditation, the varied symptoms of CD and the benefits of exercise are provided in the *Wellness* section of the application, by means of the following four subsections: *Meditation, Symptoms, Sleep*, and *Exercise*. In Fig. 2, the list of possible CD symptoms are shown as designed in the prototype.

Lastly, the *Emotional* support section brings up the importance of being aware of how mental health can be affected once diagnosed with CD. Symptoms (that the patient should pay close attention to) are listed, such as "crying a lot for no particular reason" and "feeling worthless or extremely guilty", in the *Mental Health* subsection. Special attention is put towards education on general anxiety in the subsection *Anxiety* in the application, due to the numerous CD patients who experience symptoms of anxiety disorder after being diagnosed. Fast facts are given in the subsection *What You Should Know*, see Fig. 2, such as *it is hereditary* and *it robs you of spontaneity of traveling freely*. The *Impact* subsection contains information about how CD can impact the CD patient. For example, an alarming 80% of CD patients believe CD is a burden in their lives or that women with CD are significantly more likely to miscarry or give birth prematurely than other women.

4.2 Method

By means of a survey, the perception of usability of the prototype was gathered from the app target: CD patients and their family and friends, along with which functionalities they would modify or include in future versions of the mobile app. There were two types of participants: informed CD patients and informed social circle. The participants were notified that they could withdraw from the survey at any time and remain anonymous. The survey was adapted from the USE Questionnaire [26] and measured participants' usability perception towards four categories: *Usefulness, Ease of use, Ease of Learning* and *Satisfaction*, on a five point Likert scale. Additionally, the survey acquired information about overall satisfaction of the four main sections of the app, open-ended questions about the sections and subsections, as well as additional comments.

5 Results

In order to analyze the results from the USE Questionnaire, averages were calculated for the scores per the following categories: *Usefulness, Ease of Use, Ease of Learning* and *Satisfaction*. The results were then scaled to 100% from a five point Likert scale, ranging from Strongly Disagree to Strongly Agree. The overall response rate was 100% due to all questions being marked as *required*, with the exception of the two open-ended questions for which eight and seven answers were received respectively. A total of 22 people participated in the testing of the prototype and answering the survey. The results per category were as follows:

Usefulness. The overall perception of the *Usefulness* of the application was positive amongst the participants, ranging from 3.73 to 4.73 in the five point Likert scale, see Fig. 3. The lowest score (3.73) was reported in "The app does everything I expected it to do", this is well reflected in the various suggestions provided by the participants for more functionalities that ought to be included in future versions of the application, such as "recipes" and "restaurant cards".

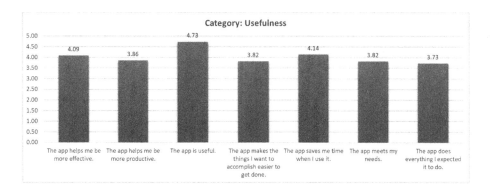

Fig. 3. Category Usefulness results

Ease of Use. In the category *Ease of Use*, the participants found the application easy to understand and manipulate. However, the majority of the participants reported the flexibility and recovering from mistakes in the application as "Neutral". See Fig. 4 for the reported numbers for each question in the category.

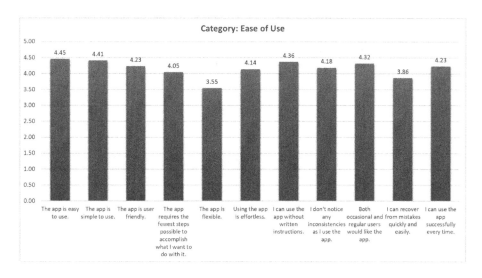

Fig. 4. Category Ease of Use results

Ease of Learning. The reported ability to learn ranged from 4.23 to 4.55 in terms of how quickly and easily the participants learned to use the application, see Fig. 5.

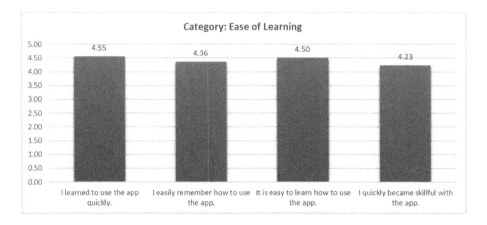

Fig. 5. Category Ease of Learning results

Satisfaction. The participants reported overall *satisfaction* of the design, ranging from 3.68 to 4.55 in various subcategories, see Fig. 6 for all reported values. The participants indicated that they "felt they would need the app" and they "would recommend it to a friend", where both subcategories were reported as 4.55 (Agree).

The results from the four categories of the USE questionnaire report overall positive perceptions towards the usability of the application, indicating that CD patients are willing to share with their social circle the general information about the disease and thereby decreasing the social anxiety that comes with the feeling of exclusion. Additionally, the social circle is willing to actively participate in the

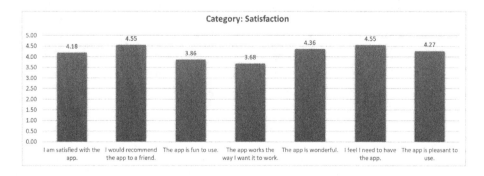

Fig. 6. Category Satisfaction results

management of wellness and support for CD patients, recognizing the important role their involvement plays in a CD patient's improved quality of life.

The average result per category can be seen in Table 2. The reported values for the four categories were somewhat similar, from 4.02 to 4.41. The *Satisfaction* category reported the highest perception (4.41) amongst the participants, however, the regard to the *usefulness* of the design was reported the lowest (4.02) of the four.

Additionally, questions on overall satisfaction rating of the four app sections were gathered and the reported median for the all the categories were 4, see Table 3. It is important to mention that the *Wellness* section had four out of 22 responses marked as 2 on the five point Likert scale, meaning that they were *dissatisfied* with this section.

Table 2. Summary of results per category from USE Questionnaire using Likert scale

Category	Average score	Scaled to 100	Likert scale
Usefulness	4.02	80.33	Agree
Ease of Learning	4.16	83.18	Agree
Satisfaction	4.41	88.18	Agree
Ease of Use	4.21	84.16	Agree

From analyzing the answers to the open-ended questions that were included in the survey, categories were identified via clustering by affinity of topic, Fig. 7 presents a word cloud summarizing the findings. The open-ended questions were optional, thus we consider respondents of these questions as "key users" or users that demonstrated an increased interest in development of the app. From the suggestions by the key users, the following were determined as the most important benefits they expect from the app: appealing user interface, gluten-free restaurants list, lower stress from explaining the GFD, family stories/testimonials, buying GF items, help with different languages, GF recipes, medical information, fast performance, and interactive/customizable design.

Table 3. Median scores of overall satisfaction of four app sections - results from USE Questionnaire

App section	Median score	Likert scale
Social	4	Agree
Wellness	4	Agree
Food	4	Agree
Emotional	4	Agree

Regarding the user interface, respondents said: "nice construction", "fantastic", "very cool", "great design"; one respondent pointed out that the text was "small". Regarding GF shopping, one respondent made the following statement, "I would add a section of other items that contain gluten, such as makeup, toiletries, etc. I would also add a recipe section, as I find it's one of the most challenging aspects of being celiac: what to eat on a daily basis." Lastly, another respondent added, "This would help with going on vacation, without having stress to find an explanation anywhere on the internet."

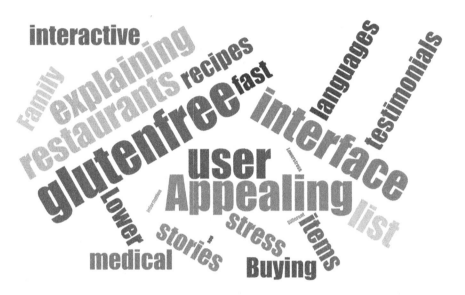

Fig. 7. Word cloud summarizing the findings from open-ended questions.

6   Discussion

6.1   Findings

The majority of the respondents perceived the usability of the application as useful, easy to learn, satisfying and easy to use. The reported average scores in the previously mentioned categories ranged from 4.02 to 4.41 (Agree), on a five point Likert scale, see Table 2, Which indicates a positive attitude of the interaction of the app and its' potential for future releases. Additionally, participants were satisfied with the four sections of the application: *Social, Wellness, Food* and *Emotional*, where the reported median scores were 4 (Agree) for all categories, see Table 3. The overall perception of the application was well-conceived where participants reported the design as appealing and user friendly.

Like Handel [21], who based the selection of quality mHealth applications on several criteria such as ease of use and aesthetically pleasing applications, the reported findings also indicate that the proposed application can be considered of high quality due to high scores of the perceived usability.

Finally, some suggestions for future development of the applications were provided from the respondents such as diversity of languages, a recipe section, a testimonials section, and a list of non-food items containing gluten.

6.2   Potential Benefits

The potential benefits of the proposed application for CD patients, which in turn could improve the patients quality of life, are:

- Potentially decreasing limitations in personal and social life, such as traveling and participating in celebrations.
- Possibly providing better GFD support and knowledge from social circle, such as having GF and celiac-safe options for CD patients at all social gatherings.
- Likely decreasing anxiety related to the fear of falling ill from food consumption and inconvenience of finding GF options when dining out.
- Enabling the GFD to be less socially isolating and more inclusive by providing appropriate and accessible information easily and quickly to the social circle.
- Supplying enhanced understanding of the overall impact of the condition from family and friends, not just in terms of physical health but also mental health and lifestyle choices.

6.3   Limitations

Failing to find enough suitable subjects willing to test the app prototype is a limitation in this study. Therefore, the sample size was small. There were two types of participants for the survey: 1) informed CD patients and 2) informed social circle. The target group for participating in the study were CD patients who are aware of their symptoms and have experience managing their condition through lifestyle changes and following a strict GFD. The social circle of these particular CD patients has to be willing to be helpful and understand how important social support and overall wellness is for the CD patient. If they are not aware of this factor, then the mobile application will not seem useful to them. The latter can be an important limitation to this study because these type of subjects are difficult to find in large numbers. Creating enough incentives for users to frequently use the app could be another limitation, but more testing needs to be performed to determine user loyalty.

6.4   Future Work

Scientific publications on mHealth applications for CD patients are scarce and only one study was identified in the literature that described an application for managing CD exclusively [16]. Consequently, there are multiple opportunities to perform research on the topic. Potential future work and future versions of the prototype include expanding the range of target users of the application. The application has great potential of helping other patients with food intolerance issues and who are interested in managing their diet for medical reasons because sharing it with their social circle would positively impact their quality of life. Additionally, the application can be modified for adhering to the needs of children in future versions. Finally, valuable data was gathered from the survey, where the participants provided suggestions for potential features for future versions of the application. Remarks mentioning a more interactive design and personalization are paramount because these are core benefits the app will offer in the final version and a competitive advantage, contrasting with other mHealth apps. Additionally, further prototypes could be adapted and used for other long-term conditions that require similar strict diet management such as food intolerance and allergies, i.e. fish, peanuts, tree nuts, milk, eggs, shellfish, wheat, soybeans, etc.

Acknowledgments. The authors would like to thank Dr. P.W. (Paweł) Woźniak from the Faculty of Science at Utrecht University for his help with the analysis of the results, and Dr. T.J. (Trenton) Hagar from the Faculty of Humanities at Utrecht University for his help with the grammatical structure of the article. Additionally, the authors would like to thank the CD patients and their friends and family members who were willing to dedicate time to testing the app prototype and answering the survey.

References

1. Allergy Eats. https://www.allergyeats.com/. Accessed 17 Mar 2019
2. Celiac Disease Foundation. https://celiac.org/about-the-foundation/featured-news/2015/06/celiac-disease-foundation-launches-gluten-free-allergy-free-marketplace-app. Accessed 18 Mar 2019
3. Find Me Gluten Free. https://www.findmeglutenfree.com/. Accessed 17 Mar 2019
4. Fooducate Healthy Weight Loss Calorie Counter. https://www.fooducate.com/. Accessed 18 Mar 2019
5. Garden Bay Software. http://www.gardenbaysoftware.com/. Accessed 18 Mar 2019
6. Gluten-free restaurant cards. http://www.celiactravel.com/. Accessed 18 Mar 2019
7. Gluten Free Scanner. https://scanglutenfree.com/. Accessed 18 Mar 2019
8. AARDA Homepage. https://www.aarda.org. Accessed 10 Mar 2019
9. mySymptoms Food Diary. https://skygazerlabs.com/wp/. Accessed 18 Mar 2019
10. Shopwell Diet. http://www.shopwell.com/mobileapp. Accessed 18 Mar 2019
11. Sift Food Labels. http://siftfoodlabels.com/. Accessed 18 Mar 2019
12. Autoimmune diseases - modern diseases. In: Autoimmune Diseases - Modern Diseases Proceedings: Brussels, 25 September 2017. European Parliament, Brussels, Belgium (2017). http://www.europarl.europa.eu/committees/en/supporting-analyses-search.html
13. Bischoff, S., Crowe, S.E.: Gastrointestinal food allergy: new insights into pathophysiology and clinical perspectives. Gastroenterology **128**(4), 1089–1113 (2005)
14. Carta, M.G., Hardoy, M.C., Boi, M.F., Mariotti, S., Carpiniello, B., Usai, P.: Association between panic disorder, major depressive disorder and celiac disease: a possible role of thyroid autoimmunity. J. Psychosomatic Res. **53**(3), 789–793 (2002)
15. Cassell, D., Rose, N.: The Encyclopedia of Autoimmune Diseases. Infobase Publishing, New York (2014)
16. Dowd, A., Jackson, C., Tang, K.T., Nielsen, D., Clarkin, D.H., Culos-Reed, S.N.: MyHealthyGut: development of a theory-based self-regulatory app to effectively manage celiac disease. Mhealth **4**, 19 (2018)

17. Dunford, E., et al.: FoodSwitch: a mobile phone app to enable consumers to make healthier food choices and crowdsourcing of national food composition data. JMIR mHealth uHealth **2**(3), e37 (2014)
18. Green, P.H., Cellier, C.: Celiac disease. New Engl. J. Med. **357**(17), 1731–1743 (2007)
19. Gujral, N., Freeman, H., Thomson, A.: Celiac disease: prevalence, diagnosis, pathogenesis and treatment. World J. Gastroenterol. WJG **18**(42), 6036 (2012)
20. Haas, K., Martin, A., Park, K.: Text message intervention (TEACH) improves quality of life and patient activation in celiac disease: a randomized clinical trial. J. Pediatr. **185**, 62–67 (2017)
21. Handel, M.J.: mHealth—using apps for health and wellness. EXPLORE J. Sci. Heal. **7**(4), 256–261 (2011)
22. Hsieh, F.H.: Primer to the immune response. Ann. Allergy Asthma Immunol. **113**(3), 333 (2014)
23. Lebwohl, B., et al.: Gluten introduction, breastfeeding, and celiac disease: back to the drawing board. Am. J. Gastroenterol. **111**(1), 12 (2016)
24. Lee, A., Ng, D., Diamond, B., Ciaccio, E., Green, P.: Living with coeliac disease: survey results from the USA. J. Hum. Nutr. Dietet. **25**(3), 233–238 (2012)
25. Lee, A., Wolf, R., Contento, I., Verdeli, H., Green, P.: Coeliac disease: the association between quality of life and social support network participation. J. Hum. Nutr. Diet. **29**(3), 383–390 (2016)
26. Lund, A.M.: Measuring usability with the USE Questionnaire. Usability Interface **8**(2), 3–6 (2001)
27. Reilly, N.R., Green, P.H.R.: Presentation of celiac disease in children and adults. In: Rampertab, S.D., Mullin, G.E. (eds.) Celiac Disease. CG, pp. 95–105. Springer, New York (2014). https://doi.org/10.1007/978-1-4614-8560-5_8
28. Sapone, A., et al.: Differential mucosal IL-17 expression in two gliadin-induced disorders: gluten sensitivity and the autoimmune enteropathy celiac disease. Int. Arch. Allergy Imm. **152**(1), 75–80 (2010)
29. Stanley, M.: Top 10 gluten-free apps. https://www.glutenfreeliving.com/gluten-free-foods/shopping-gluten-free/top-10-gluten-free-apps. Accessed 17 Mar 2019

Real-Time Continuous Monitoring of Cerebral Edema Based on a Flexible Conformal Coil Sensor

Jingbo Chen[1], Gen Li[2], Mingsheng Chen[1], Jun Yang[1], and Mingxin Qin[1,2(✉)]

[1] Department of Biomedical Engineering and Medical Imaging, Army Medical University,
Chongqing 400038, China
qmingxin@tmmu.edu.cn
[2] School of Pharmacy and Bioengineering,
Chongqing University of Technology, Chongqing 400054, China

Abstract. Objective: Cerebral edema, as a common secondary disease after stroke, can result in brain hernia and even death, effectively monitoring the process of cerebral edema do benefit the prognosis of stroke patients. While current methods have their inherent drawbacks, we utilized a novel frequency shift (FS) method to reflect the severity of cerebral edema. Method: In this paper, 12 rabbits (10 rabbits for experimental group and 2 rabbits for control group) were enrolled in the 24 h monitoring experiment. Those rabbits underwent monitoring utilizing a novel flexible conformal coil sensor, for which the FS induced by changed equivalent impedance of brain was extracted as the evaluation index. Findings: The results showed that this novel coil sensor can effectively monitor the process of cerebral edema. This innovative method has great potential in clinical usage which can assist medical staff conducting timely treatment in terms of its early warning capability.

Keywords: Cerebral edema · Frequency shift · Coil sensor · Electromagnetic induction · Real-time monitoring

1 Introduction

Cerebral edema is a common secondary disease after stroke disease (Savitsky et al. 2016), which has a negative impact on the rehabilitation and prognosis of patients. Patients with severe cerebral edema may even cause brain hernia and death. Therefore, the monitoring of cerebral edema is necessary and good intervention helps to improve the prognosis. At present, cerebral edema monitoring for clinical patients mainly includes ICP method and CT/MRI imaging (Ristic et al. 2015). Yet ICP is an invasive way and those imaging instruments require extra transit and diagnostic time. Literally, a novel non-invasive monitoring method are desperately needed. The microwave method utilizing sensors such as patch antenna and the electromagnetic induction method using coil sensors have been widely studied (Qureshi et al. 2016; Yan et al. 2017; Chen et al. 2017). In this paper, we designed a novel flexible conformal coil sensor to monitor the process of cerebral

G. M. P. O'Hare et al. (Eds.): MobiHealth 2019, LNICST 320, pp. 36–39, 2020.
https://doi.org/10.1007/978-3-030-49289-2_3

edema in rabbits by electromagnetic induction. The results showed that this sensor can effectively monitor the development of cerebral edema and the FS signal is positively correlated with the severity of cerebral edema.

2 Methodology

The biological tissues in brain have different dielectric properties where the permitivities and conductivities of different biological tissues (such as gray matter, white matter, blood, etc.) are different at a specific frequency (González and Rubinsky 2006). When brain lesions occur, the cranial contents' distribution and metabolism change, thereby changing the intracranial average permitivity and conductivity (Sun et al. 2014; Yan et al. 2017; Chen et al. 2017).

In order to detect changes in intracranial dielectric properties caused by cerebral edema lesions, a newly designed flexible conformal coil sensor was used to detect the equivalent impedance change according to the two-port network test principle (Griffith et al. 2018). The system consists of the novel coil sensor, a vector network analyzer (VNA, Agilent E5061B, USA), and a gas anesthesia machine, as shown in Fig. 1. The frequency range of the VNA is 1–100 MHz and the sensor was attached directly above the head of the rabbits. The frequency shift (FS) of the sensor's resonance frequency is extracted, which is caused by the disturbance of the physiological changes of the rabbit.

12 New Zealand white rabbits were enrolled in this experiment (experimental group: n = 10, control group: n = 2). In experimental group, cerebral edema model was established by epidural freezing method via liquid nitrogen freezing (Kawai et al. 2003). In this scenario, the severity of cerebral edema gradually deepens with time (Li et al. 2017). Rabbits in control group received same procedure except freezing. After procedure, all rabbits were monitored for 24 h with the novel coil sensor and the sampling rate was 12 times per hour.

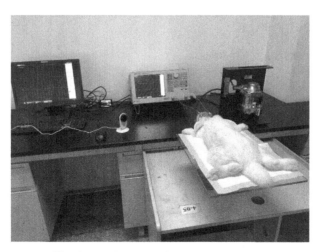

Fig. 1. Physical map of the detection system

3   Results

Figure 2 shows the FS data in the experimental group and the control group (mean ± SD). It can be found that the trends were significantly different between the FS signal in those two groups. In the experimental group, FS showed an upward trend with aggravated cerebral edema, reaching 1.08 ± 0.25 MHz at 24th h. In contrast, the FS in control group slightly increased and then fluctuated around 0.18 MHz (0.18 ± 0.01 MHz), in which the slight drift may be caused by the surgery on the scalpe. The data of the experimental group and the control group showed significant difference from the 5th h (t-test, $p < 0.05$), indicating that FS can effectively monitor the pathological changes of cerebral edema.

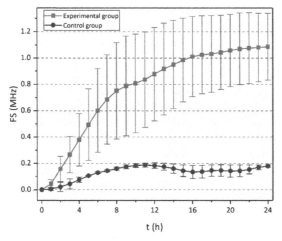

Fig. 2. Results of FS in experimental group & control group

4   Conclusions

Based on the principle of two-port network test, this paper uses a new flexible conformal coil sensor to detect changes in brain dielectric properties caused by cerebral edema. The results showed that this method can effectively monitor the pathological changes of cerebral edema. Compared with control group, experimental group's FS could show significant difference at early stage (2th h after procedure). This indicated that FS can be used as a novel non-invasive monitoring indicator to assist the medical staff giving timely adjustment and implement of the treatment program. Still, this novel sensor for cerebral edema monitoring still needs optimization of the parameters so as to elevate the reliability and sensitivity. Eventually, we hope to improve its early monitoring ability and improve its effectiveness.

References

Chen, M., Qingguang, Y., Sun, J., Jin, G., Qin, M.: Investigating the relationship between cerebrospinal fluid and magnetic induction phase shift in rabbit intracerebral hematoma expansion monitoring by MRI. Sci. Rep. **7**(1), 11186 (2017)

González, C.A., Rubinsky, B.: The detection of brain oedema with frequency-dependent phase shift electromagnetic induction. Physiol. Meas. **27**(6), 539–552 (2006)

Griffith, J., et al.: Non-invasive electromagnetic skin patch sensor to measure intracranial fluid-volume shifts. Sensors **18**(4), 1022 (2018)

Kawai, N., Kawanishi, M., Okada, M., Matsumoto, Y., Nagao, S.: Treatment of cold injury-induced brain edema with a nonspecific matrix metalloproteinase inhibitor MMI270 in rats. J. Neurotrauma **20**(7), 649–657 (2003)

Li, G., Ma, K., Sun, J., Jin, G., Qin, M., Feng, H.: Twenty-four-hour real-time continuous monitoring of cerebral edema in rabbits based on a noninvasive and noncontact system of magnetic induction. Sensors **17**(3), 537 (2017)

Qureshi, A.M., Mustansar, Z., Maqsood, A.: Analysis of microwave scattering from a realistic human head model for brain stroke detection using electromagnetic impedance tomography. Prog. Electromagn. Res. **52**, 45–56 (2016)

Ristic, A., Sutter, R., Steiner, L.A.: Current neuromonitoring techniques in critical care. J. Neuroanaesth. Crit. Care **2**(02), 097–103 (2015)

Savitsky, B., Givon, A., Rozenfeld, M., Radomislensky, I., Peleg, K.: Traumatic brain injury: it is all about definition. Brain Inj. **30**(10), 1194–1200 (2016)

Sun, J., et al.: Detection of acute cerebral hemorrhage in rabbits by magnetic induction. Braz. J. Med. Biol. Res. **47**(2), 144–150 (2014)

Yan, Q., Jin, G., Ma, K., Qin, M., Zhuang, W., Sun, J.: Magnetic inductive phase shift: a new method to differentiate hemorrhagic stroke from ischemic stroke on rabbit. Biomed. Eng. Online **16**, 63 (2017)

Remote Patient Monitoring

Evaluating End-User Perception Towards a Cardiac Self-care Monitoring Process

Gabriella Casalino, Giovanna Castellano, Vincenzo Pasquadibisceglie, and Gianluca Zaza(⊠)

Computer Science Department, Università degli Studi di Bari Aldo Moro, Bari, Italy
{gabriella.casalino,giovanna.castellano,vincenzo.pasquadibisceglie,
gianluca.zaza}@uniba.it

Abstract. This study examined the perception of end-users regarding the monitoring process offered by an innovative cardiac self-care system. The main goal was to assess the efficacy of the process implemented by a smart device designed to support people for real-time monitoring of cardio-vascular parameters in everyday life, thereby encouraging patients to be more proactive in heath management. Most participants showed positive response about the potential benefits of the proposed self-care solution and were willing to adopt the system despite some concerns related to trust and privacy.

Keywords: Ambient assist living · Personal healthcare · Pervasive monitoring · Remote diagnosis

1 Introduction

More than half of all deaths across the European Region are caused by Cardio-vascular disease (CVD). In 2017, the European Parliament Heart Group identified CVD as the major cause of death, killing over 2 million people each year in Europe alone[1]. In principle, CVD patients can lead a normal life as long as they are continuously monitored and alerted to the emergency services in case of abnormal situation. Hence the regular monitoring of vital signs, such as heart rate, is the basis to detect a risk level of cardiovascular disease [1].

In recent years the development of self-care monitoring solutions have shifted the monitoring process from the traditional event-driven mode (i.e., when a specific change in patient condition leads to a medical intervention, such as admission to hospital) to a new scenario where the patients use personal self-care devices to monitor continuously their vital parameters directly at home, through smart-home technologies [2–4]. The use of self-monitoring systems can provide assistance without limiting or disturbing the patient's daily routine, giving greater comfort and well-being. Moreover, this enables the patient to be

---

[1] European Parliament Heart Group (EHN) (2017) Cardiovascular Disease Statistics. http://www.ehnheart.org/cdv-statistics.html (March 14, 2019).

© ICST Institute for Computer Sciences, Social Informatics and Telecommunications Engineering 2020
Published by Springer Nature Switzerland AG 2020. All Rights Reserved
G. M. P. O'Hare et al. (Eds.): MobiHealth 2019, LNICST 320, pp. 43–59, 2020.
https://doi.org/10.1007/978-3-030-49289-2_4

more proactive in heath management, and allows the healthcare providers to make more informed decisions on the basis of real-time data [5].

Many mobile platforms currently support software enabling self-management of cardiovascular disease and capable of collecting cardiovascular data [2]. However, cardiovascular disease most commonly affects older adults, and these individuals have the greatest barriers to mobile healthcare solutions [6]. Hence more engaging self-care solutions that avoid mobile devices should be designed in order to provide the necessary level of support for patients of different ages thus creating a significant behavioral change in population.

Along with this new proactive paradigm for personal healthcare, in [7] we have recently proposed an intelligent monitoring system based on a smart mirror for contact-less estimation of main cardiovascular parameters as well as for the prediction of cardiovascular disease. The underlying idea is to allow the patient to monitor his cardiac status at home, with perfect integration in his daily routine and avoiding the use of additional (mobile) devices. The only effort required to the patient is a very natural action, i.e. looking at himself in front of a mirror for 1 min. The proposed solution is a cheap mirror-based device that is very easy to use, hence it is suitable not only for personal use but also for telemedicine applications.

So far we have tested the efficacy of the smart mirror in terms of accurate measurement of vital signs and reliable assessment of cardiovascular risk. Now, we want to further develop understanding of the benefits and functionalities of our solution that end-users deem as either desirable, undesirable, or inadequate. To this aim, in this paper we present the results of a preliminary study about perception of end-users (health people, cardiopathic patients and caregivers) towards the self-care monitoring process accomplished through the proposed healthcare system.

2   Related Works

The study of the users' needs and perceptions is fundamental to understand their willingness to accept or reject a new technology. The factors that could affect the user acceptance of a new technology have been detected and formalized in several models and frameworks [8], such as the Technology Acceptance Model (TAM) [9], or its evolution the Unified Theory of Acceptance and Use of Technology (UTAUT) [10], that have been widely used in a variety of contexts.

In the healthcare field, more than in others, the users' acceptance and trust of the new technologies is of primary importance. We need to take into account the human characteristics and the social background to avoid a mismatch between the users' expectations and the services available [11].

Several works focus on the users' perception of the new technologies in healthcare. Electronic medical records (EMR) systems have been recently adopted in different part of the world. Interest of the researchers has been the study of opinion by both the practitioners and the patients [12–16].

The users' concerns about security and privacy related to healthcare services affect their risk perception and attitudes toward using IoT-based medical devices

[17,18]. Particularly in [19] the authors focus on users' perception of biometric authentication technologies.

Safety and acceptability are critical issues when people interact with robots in healthcare [20]. Kim et al. compare the users' reactions to different kind of robotic arms and fingers' touch, whilst Ahn et al. gathered young people's perceptions about healthcare service robots for old people [21]. Pal et al. propose a theoretical framework to detect the core factors affecting the elderly users' acceptance of smart home services for healthcare [11]. They conducted an empirical evaluation across four Asian countries to test the framework. Agrell et al. focused on patients' perceptions of home telecare [22]. Febriani et al. designed a smart health chair for car driver's seat, that is able to monitor health vital signs. In their study they analyze the usability and the user satisfaction in interacting with the smart health chair [23].

Health care administrators look at technological innovative solutions to improve the servic quality. Several works discuss the acceptance of information technology in the context of Health Information Management (HIM) [24–26].

Mobile health (mHealth) services are a new frontier for tele-medicine. Zhang et al. investigate the factors that influence individuals' acceptance of mHealth services [27]. Similarly Velez et al. propose a mobile health application for Rural Ghanaian Midwives and study its users' acceptance [28]. Elloumi et al. studied patient and caregiver's perception regarding pervasive cardiac healthcare technology [29].

All the above mentioned works show that a critical issue in designing new healthcare solutions is to assess their acceptability relying on the users' perceptions towards benefits and risks. For this reason, once developed a first prototype of our self-care system [7] we tried to analyze the end-users' attitude and perceptions about the innovative monitoring process introduced by the proposed solution. The rest of the paper is devoted to briefly describe the developed self-care system and to present the results of our study about end-user perceptions.

3   The Proposed Self-care Monitoring System

The proposed self-care system is an intelligent mirror designed to detect some vital parameters without the use of contact sensors [30]. The mirror is equipped with a camera that captures the video frames of the patient who is looking at himself in the mirror. Each frame is processed in real time to extract the remote photoplethysmography signal [31] that measures the change of cardiovascular tissue coming from some regions of the face, in our case the forehead. In fact, the impulse of cardio-vascular wave that flows through the body periodically, stretches the vessel walls, with consequent fluctuations in blood volume. These fluctuations modulate the absorbency of light passing through a given volume of tissue, so it is possible to evaluate the variation of light during a normal cardiac cycle. These changes originate a waveform that resembles the changes in the pulsatile arterial blood in the tissue [32]. Hence by processing the photoplethysmographic signal we can estimate values of cardio-vascular parameters, namely heart rate, breathing rate, and blood oxygen saturation.

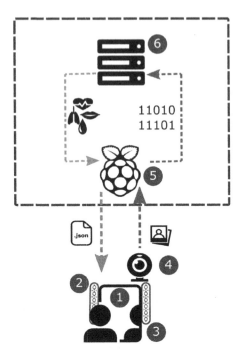

Fig. 1. Hardware architecture.

Our solution differs from other existing contact-less solutions to monitor vital parameters since it integrates a decision-making component that supports medical diagnosis of cardiovascular disease. This component is based on fuzzy IF-THEN rules that were defined with the help of a physician. Starting from these rules the system is able to infer a level of cardiovascular risk starting from the vital parameters acquired by the smart mirror [33]. The output of the fuzzy rule-based system represents an immediate feedback for the patient about his health status, as well as valid support for clinicians in the diagnosis of possible cardiovascular diseases.

Moreover, the use of the device to monitor vital parameters every day enables the collection of a large amount of data about the health status of patients. These data can be checked by the physician who can analyze the accumulated information in a timely manner and provide additional feedback.

3.1   HW Architecture

The device has been designed to be low-cost, immediate to use and easy to be integrated in any home environment. It includes few low-cost basic hardware components (Fig. 1). It is made of a see-through mirror ① with a 12"12" 3 mm thick acrylic film that is partially reflective and partially transparent. The peculiarity of this mirror is that the light can pass equally in both directions, however when one side of the mirror is brightly lit and the other one is kept dark, the darker side becomes difficult to see from the brightly lit side because it is masked by the much brighter reflection of the lit side. Behind the mirror is a monitor that allows users to display information. An illuminated environment ensures a higher quality in the process of detection of vital parameters. To improve the lighting conditions in the environment two strips of LED lights ② ③ have been integrated into the sides of the frame. Each strip includes 18 LED lights having these characteristics: 12 V, 6.0 W, 0.5 A and 120 beam angle. A HD camera ④ is assembled with the see-through mirror to record high-quality video frames. We used the Microsoft LifeCam (3.44" length, 1.57" width) provided with autofocus. A HD 1080p sensor enables acquisition of high quality images. The system is composed of a client/server architecture. The client is a Raspberry pi board ⑤ with CPU Quad Core 1.2 GHz Broadcom BCM2837 64bit, 4 USB ports, 1 GB RAM, Micro SD for the boot of the operating system and data storage. In the current prototypical version of the system, the server ⑥ is a desktop computer equipped with CPU Intel(R) Core(TM) i5–5200 2.20 GHz 64 bit, 4 GB RAM and 500 GB hard disk.

3.2   SW Architecture

The proposed system includes a front-end module that manages the graphical interface and the user-system interaction, and a back-end that processes data coming from the front-end and outputs the results.

The front-end was developed using the engine template Jinja2 that allows creation of HTML or XML files that are sent to the client via HTTP. Using the scripting languages we capture the video frames from the camera and compose the POST request to send data to the Web Service. The Web Service provides the result in JSON format.

The back-end is a Web Service implemented in Flask which is a micro web framework compatible with Python 3.6. Flask is based on the toolkit Werkzeug and the template engine Jinja2, both based on the BSD (Berkeley Software Distribution) open source license. The tool Werkzeug provides several utilities for WSGI (Web Server Gateway Interface) applications and a transmission protocol that establishes and describes communications between servers and web applications. The Client/Server communication is developed using the Ajax scripting language that, combined with the HTML language, enables the exchange of data in background between the browser and the Web Service.

3.3   Application Scenarios

The proposed mirror-based system is intended to be used in the field of personal healthcare (Fig. 2). It was designed as smart device to be installed mainly in a home environment, especially in rooms that are typically equipped with a mirror (bathroom, living room, bedroom). A possible scenario in home environment is the following. Emma is a middle-age lady who is affected by hypertension. For

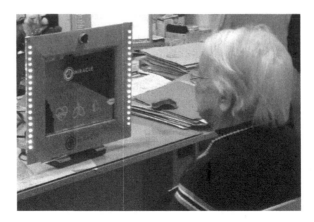

Fig. 2. Application scenario of the proposed healthcare device

this reason she needs to monitor her vital parameters regularly. Every morning, once woken up, she goes to the bathroom to carry out daily actions such as brushing her teeth or combing her hair. While making these natural actions Emma can monitor her vital signs by just looking at herself in the mirror, with no need of additional devices. The possibility to check the personal health status through a simple gesture like looking at oneself in a mirror is especially comfortable for elderly people who may have difficulty to self-monitor their vital parameters through the use of contact devices such as the pulse oximeter, or through mobile devices such as smartphones.

The proposed smart mirror could be well employed in public environments such as pharmacies where other monitoring and prevention services such as weight control are frequently offered. Using the smart mirror every customer entering in the pharmacy could easily and quickly check his health status by looking in the mirror, with no need of any contact device.

4   Evaluating End-User Perception

In this section we report the results of a preliminary study on end-user perception about the developed system. Our focus was primarily in identifying the concerns and attitudes that patients of different ages might have of the concept, as well as exploring potential barriers to acceptance, such as different computer skills and technology awareness. Broadly, the aim of the study is to generate useful feedback for the subsequent deployment of the system.

We defined six main research questions about the factors that could affect the users' acceptance of a our new healthcare technology:

A) What are the social and demographic factors that influence the user's acceptance?
B) Do users perceive the benefits of the self-care monitoring system?

C) Do users see any risk or privacy violation in using the system?
D) Is the system easy to use?
E) Are the users willing to actually employ the system?
F) Do users find the system really innovative?

These points were detailed in a questionnaire that was submitted to each participant at the end of the test session. In each test we used the smart mirror to detect the vital parameters (heart rate, breath rate and blood oxygen saturation) while the subject was sitting in front of the mirror for 1 min. Each subject was required to mirror himself, resting in state of spontaneous breathing. Besides collecting the answers to the submitted questions after test, we also collected general information about the overall reaction and feeling of each user. To this aim the conductor who supported the users during the test took notes on the opinions expressed by some users.

4.1 Social and Demographic Factors

The study involved 30 users, including 21 males and 9 females. The prevalence of male subjects is justified by the fact that, according to different studies [34, 35] men are more likely to be at risk for heart attack much earlier in life than women. The sample covered different age groups: young, adult, middle-aged and elderly participants were involved in the study, with ages ranging from 21 to 81 years old. The level of education varied according to the age, but most of the users (27/30) had a high education level and some of them (21/30) were graduate or undergraduate students. Beside the demographic factors, we collected information about the lifestyle (smoke, alcohol, sport) of users in order to find possible correlations between the attention to health and the positive perception towards the self-care process. We observe that most of the subjects lead a healthy lifestyle: 25/30 do not smoke, 24/30 do not drink or moderately drink and 18/30 practice sport. Furthermore, we wanted to evaluate whether subjects with cardiovascular problems, or with cardiac problems in their family history, are more sensitive to adopt the self-care monitoring system. Few participants (7/30) had cardiovascular problems, whilst half of the sample (15/30) had at least one relative who suffered from it. It is interesting to note that participants were not always able to discover if they had a history of cardiac conditions in their family or they did not seek for such information. Table 1 summarizes the distribution of social and demographic factors among the considered sample.

4.2 Benefits

To evaluate the users' perception about the benefits that the self-care system could bring in the all day life, we considered the following three questions:

q-b1 *Do you think that using this system can lead to a reduction in health care costs?*

q-b2 *In your opinion, does the use of this system strengthen the concept of prevention?*

Table 1. Social and demographic factors

Factors		Frequency
Gender	Male	21
	Female	9
Age	21–30	15
	31–40	5
	41–60	8
	61+	2
Education	Primary school	1
	Secondary school	2
	High school	6
	University	14
	Ph.D	7
Smoke	No	25
	Less than 5 time per day	2
	Between 5 and 10 time per day	0
	More than 10 time per day	3
Drink alchool	No	12
	One per week	12
	Twice per week	6
	More than 4 time per week	0
Practice sport	No	12
	Less than 3 times per week	8
	3 times per week	7
	More than 3 time per week	3
Cardiovascular Problems	Yes	7
	No	23
Family history Cardiac problems	Yes	15
	No	15

q-b3 *Do you feel that monitoring your state of health on day-to-day can bring benefits?*

When asked these questions, the majority of patients (28/30) felt that the technology could lead to a reduction in healthcare costs because the daily health monitoring could help the prevention of cardiovascular diseases (29/30) and as a consequence could improve their well-being (28/30). These findings are illustrated in Fig. 3. It is clear that almost all the users perceive the benefits of using the self-care system in terms of all the three research variables, i.e. health cost reduction, prevention increasing and daily monitoring.

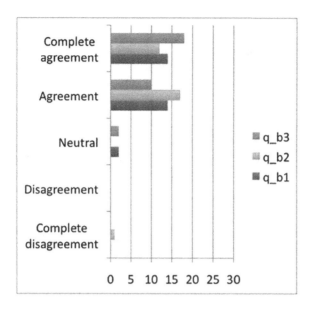

Fig. 3. Distribution of the users' answers to questions related to benefits.

We further analyzed these results in terms of age and gender of the users. We observed that the majority of the male subjects (15/21) perceives the use of the monitoring system as a benefit, but they do not completely agree with the questions. Actually 2 male subjects gave a neutral answer to question q-b1, thus showing some doubts about the possibility to reduce healthcare costs. Actually they were all young men who had never had serious personal healthcare problems and hence they probably were not able to fully appreciate the economic advantage of using a self-care system with respect to standard checkup procedures. Arguably for the same reason, 2 young male subjects expressed a neutral answer to question q-b3. Conversely, the female subjects gave all agreements answers thus showing to appreciate the benefits of a self-care monitoring solution. Only one middle-age female subject was in complete disagreement on question q-b2. This could be probably due to misunderstanding of the question.

On the overall, these results demonstrate an open-minded and positive attitude to the self-care concept. This is supported by the following comments drawn from some transcripts during the test:

"I don't have much time for regular checkups. Sometimes getting a doctor's appointment is very difficult. If you can monitor your parameters at home that would be great."

"I suffer from cardiovascular diseases and I am forced to check my parameters every day through the pulse oximeter, but this brings me pain in my finger. It would be great to have a device that measures my values without hurting or touching me."

4.3   Risks and Privacy

Another objective of this study is to understand the perceived security when using the medical device. Two main topics were identified, privacy violation and risk perception. On the basis of these topics, the following questions were formulated:

q-r1 *Do you think that the use of the system could affect your privacy?*
q-r2 *Do you perceive the use of the system as risky?*
q-r3 *Do you think that the automatic forwarding of your vital parameters to your doctor may involve risks or privacy violation?*

The distribution of collected answers is shown in Fig. 4. As it can be seen, most of the examined subjects consider the self-care system to be fairly safe, hence they do not think that it could be risky in terms of privacy (agreement answers to q-r1 were 17/30). However, it is worth to note that many neutral answers were received, demonstrating that most users were in doubt about the guarantee of privacy. In particular, during the real-time tests we observed that the web camera integrated into the mirror gave rise to a number of concerns, such as:

"Will the web-cam record my video continuously?".
"Is it possible that someone uses the cam for spying me?".
"Who ensure me that the webcam data would not be sent to unauthorized parties?"

Conversely, almost all participants did not see any risk in using the system (complete disagreement answers to q-r2 were 26/30). In spite of that, some doubts about the system were collected during the test:

"You should not exclusively rely on the output of the software".
"Wrong results could panic the patients."
"An automatic monitoring system could lead to a self medication, eliminating the benefits of prevention. Automatic sending of data to the physician could avoid this risk."

Finally, the totality of the patients thought that the automatic sending of the data to their physician does not involve risks (disagreement answers to q-r3 were 30/30). In fact, some participants highlighted the following advantages:

"Great! My doctor will immediately control my state of health."
"I will be able to avoid long queues in the waiting room."

Finally, from the analysis of age and gender, we observed that surprisingly, male adults trust more in the system than male younger subjects.

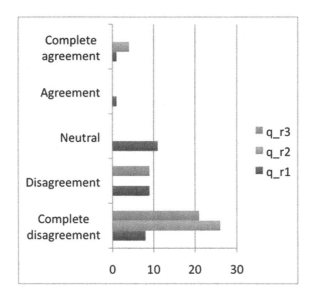

Fig. 4. Distribution of the users' answers to questions related to risks.

4.4 Usability

To evaluate how much the system is ease-of-use, these questions were formulated:

q-u1 *Did you find the interaction with the system easy to use?*
q-u2 *Do you positively rate your experience with the monitoring system?*
q-u3 *Did you find the interaction with the system comfortable and not invasive?*

The results illustrated in Fig. 5 clearly show that almost all users consider the system easy to use. Actually, the majority of the subjects (26/30) provided agreement answers to question q-u1. Users also expressed their opinion on the use of the device and many of them stated that they found the system very easy to use. During the tests we witnessed that the participants easily followed the given instructions and there were no problems during the measurement phase. Only four subjects evaluated difficult the use of the system, but this was due to the fact that during the test session a finger pulsoximeter was used to acuire standard values to be compared to the values measured by the mirror-based system. The pulsoximeter was wrongly considered as a part of the monitoring system, and therefore the whole system was considered unconfortable. Only after compiling the questionnaire these subjects discovered that the pulsoximeter was used only for comparison.

The overall user experience with the system was positive for almost all the participants. Indeed (26/30) subjects gave agreement answers to question q-u2.

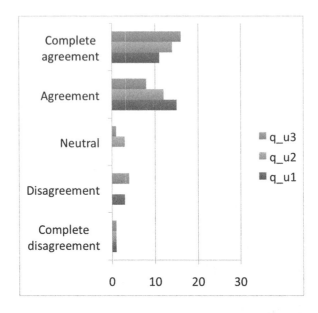

Fig. 5. Distribution of the users' answers to questions related to usability.

Finally, almost all the users (24/30) declared that they found the system comfortable by giving agreement answer to question q-u3. Some of them were even surprised by the speed with which the system returns the measured parameters. Their main comments were the following:

"I thought it would take more time to detect my vital signs."
"Already finished! I thought it would take longer!"

Moreover, as it could be expected, younger subjects, and those with higher education were more confident in using the new technology than the others.

4.5   Acceptance

Finally, we evaluated how much users would be willing to adopt the system at home and also how much they would be willing to spend for such a device. To this aim, the following questions were submitted:

q-a1 *Would you adopt the self-care system in your home environment?* [YES/NO]

q-a2 *How much would you be willing to spend on this device?* [less than 400€, 400€, more than 400€]

We estimated 400€ as reference price taking into account both the cost of HW equipment (see-through mirror, monitor, HD camera, strips of LED lights and Raspberry pi board) and the cost of the know-how for software development and engineering of the entire system.

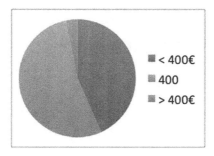

Fig. 6. Distribution of answers to question q-a2.

All the 30 participants answered YES to question q-a1 thus stating a global willing to adopt the system in home environment. Moreover almost half of participants (16/30) consider 400€ to be an appropriate price for the system. The remaining (13/30) subjects would spend less and only (1/30) subjects would be willing to spend more than 400€, as shown in Fig. 6.

4.6 Innovation

The final research variable of our study was the innovation of the system perceived by users. A single direct question was submitted in this case, namely: *Do you think that the mirror-based system is a really innovative solution?*

All the subjects answered positively to this questions, since they were all impressed by the novelty of the proposed monitoring technology. Actually during the tests many participant were amazed by the mirror-based device. Even if most of the users usually interact with electronic devices, they could not conceive how a simple mirror could evaluate vital signs without any contact with the skin. All the users were very surprised about the potential of the mirror-based device. Moreover, at the end of the test, many users claimed to be happy to have discovered that there was a new way of measuring parameters, which they did not know at all before.

5 Discussion

Overall, participants in this study showed a positive attitude toward the use of the new self-care monitoring process. Figure 7 summarizes the average perception of users in regards to the three main factors (benefits, risk and usability) expressed as an average agreement score given for each factor. To compute the average agreement score, we assigned a score to each answer as follows:

– Complete Agreement: 5
– Agreement: 4

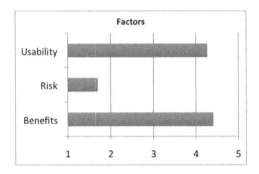

Fig. 7. Averaged perception of users about the main considered factors.

- Neutral: 3
- Disagreement: 2
- Complete Disagreement: 1

It can be seen that a high score was achieved in regards to the potential benefits of the self-care monitoring process. In general positive responses were related to the benefits of continuous, real-time monitoring of a range of parameters related to health condition and the possibility to receive quick feedback in case of potential problems. As concerns usability, the high average score confirms that the mirror-based solution was correctly designed to be easy-to-use, comfortable and not invasive at all. Users see in the mirror an object of daily use, and therefore they find very natural to interact with the mirror-based monitoring device.

A low score was obtained for the negative factor of risks, still indicating an overall positive perception by users'. Actually only some users expressed doubts related to trust and privacy. As concerns the trust, users were immediately convinced about the reliability of the system since the measurements made by the device were comparable to the measurements of the pulse-oximeter used during tests. However they trusted less the response of the intelligent component of the system that suggests a level of cardio-vascular disease according to the estimated parameters. Indeed some users were not completely aware about the decision-support nature of the system that is obviously intended only as a support to the clinician. By no means it is intended to substitute the final decision of the medical expert. Furthermore, aspects of risk or lack of privacy were highlighted by some users for the presence of the web cam and the internet connection. However, most users were not particularly concerned by these aspects since they were aware that these issues are indispensable in any smart connected device.

6 Conclusions

Proactive healthcare systems are aimed to provide users with healthcare solutions to be used directly at home. In this work we have presented a study about end-users' perception toward an innovative solution specifically designed for proactive monitoring of the cardiac status. It is a mirror-based device capable to measure vital parameters in a contact-less fashion. The results of this study showed that there is a general positive feeling towards our self-care monitoring solution, both among young and old people. Despite the encouraging positive results, a deeper analysis should be carried out in order to better explore all the factors that may hamper the acceptance of the self-care monitoring process introduced by the smart mirror. Further work is in progress to collect more data about users' perception so as to provide a solid groundwork describing relationships that people tend to develop with our technology. This will be fundamental to foresee the potential success of our new solution before its actual adoption. To conclude, we believe that this work may also contribute to spread and reinforce the idea of a proactive healthcare model representing patients as being more actively involved in the managing of their healthcare.

Acknowledgements. This study is partially supported by Ministero dell'Istruzione, dell'Università e della Ricerca (MIUR) under grant PON ARS01_01116 "TALIsMAn". The authors are members of the INdAM Research group GNCS.

References

1. Cook, S., Togni, M., Schaub, M.C., Wenaweser, P., Hess, O.M.: High heart rate: a cardiovascular risk factor? Eur. Heart J. **27**(20), 2387–2393 (2006)
2. Lupton, D.: The digitally engaged patient: self-monitoring and self-care in the digital health era. Socl Theory Health **11**(3), 256–270 (2013)
3. Swan, M.: Health 2050: the realization of personalized medicine through crowdsourcing, the quantified self, and the participatory biocitizen. J. Person. Med. **2**(3), 93–118 (2012)
4. Diaz, M., Ferrer, M.A., Impedovo, D., Pirlo, G., Vessio, G.: Dynamically enhanced static handwriting representation for Parkinson's disease detection. Pattern Recogn. Lett. **128**, 204–210 (2019)
5. Margiotta, N., Avitabile, G., Coviello, G.: A wearable wireless system for gait analysis for early diagnosis of Alzheimer and Parkinson disease. In: 2016 5th International Conference on Electronic Devices, Systems and Applications (ICEDSA), December 2016, pp. 1–4 (2016)
6. Searcy, R.P., et al.: Mobile health technologies for older adults with cardiovascular disease: current evidence and future directions. Current Geriatrics reports, pp. 1–12 (2019)
7. Casalino, G., Castellano, G., Pasquadibisceglie, V., Zaza, G.: Contact-less real-time monitoring of cardiovascular risk using video imaging and fuzzy inference rules. Information **10**(1), 9 (2019)
8. Taherdoost, H.: A review of technology acceptance and adoption models and theories. Procedia Manuf. **22**, 960–967 (2018)
9. Davis, F.D.: User acceptance of information technology: system characteristics, user perceptions and behavioral impacts. Int. J. Man Mach. Stud. **38**(3), 475–487 (1993)
10. Venkatesh, V., Morris, M.G., Davis, G.B., Davis, F.D.: User acceptance of information technology: toward a unified view. MIS Q. **27**, 425–478 (2003)

11. Pal, D., Funilkul, S., Charoenkitkarn, N., Kanthamanon, P.: Internet-of-Things and smart homes for elderly healthcare: an end user perspective. IEEE Access **6**, 10 483–10 496 (2018)

12. Handy, J., Hunter, I., Whiddett, R.: User acceptance of inter-organizational electronic medical records. Health Inform. J. **7**(2), 103–107 (2001)

13. dos Santos, E.S., Martins, H.G.: Usability and impact of electronic health records for primary care units in portugal. In: 6th Iberian Conference on Information Systems and Technologies (CISTI 2011), June 2011, pp. 1–3 (2011)

14. Vathanophas, V., Pacharapha, T.: Information technology acceptance in healthcare service: the study of Electronic Medical Record (EMR) in Thailand, pp. 1–5. IEEE (2010)

15. Scheepers, R., Scheepers, H., Ngwenyama, O.K.: Contextual influences on user satisfaction with mobile computing: findings from two healthcare organizations. Eur. J. Inf. Syst. **15**(3), 261–268 (2006)

16. Weeger, A., Gewald, H.: Acceptance and use of electronic medical records: an exploratory study of hospital physicians' salient beliefs about hit systems. Health Syst. **4**(1), 64–81 (2015)

17. Alraja, M.N., Farooque, M.M.J., Khashab, B.: The effect of security, privacy, familiarity and trust on users' attitudes towards the use of iot-based healthcare: the mediation role of riskperception. IEEE Access **7**, 111341–111354 (2019)

18. Wilkowska, W., Ziefle, M.: Perception of privacy and security for acceptance of e-health technologies: exploratory analysis for diverse user groups. In: 2011 5th International Conference on Pervasive Computing Technologies for Healthcare (PervasiveHealth) and Workshops, pp. 593–600. IEEE (2011)

19. Rodrigues, P., Santos, H.: Health users' perception of biometric authentication technologies. In: Proceedings of the 26th IEEE International Symposium on Computer-Based Medical Systems, pp. 320–325. IEEE (2013)

20. Kim, D.H., et al.: User perceptions of soft robot arms and fingers for healthcare. In: 2016 25th IEEE International Symposium on Robot and Human Interactive Communication (RO-MAN), pp. 1150–1155. IEEE (2016)

21. Ahn, H.S., Lee, M.H., Broadbent, E., MacDonald, B.A.: Gathering healthcare service robot requirements from young people's perceptions of an older care robot. In: 2017 First IEEE International Conference on Robotic Computing (IRC), pp. 22–27. IEEE (2017)

22. Agrell, H., Dahlberg, S., Jerant, A.F.: Patients' perceptions regarding home telecare. Telemed. J. e-Health **6**(4), 409–415 (2000)

23. Febriani, R., Wuryandari, A.I., Mardiono, T.: Design interaction of smart health chair approach the usability aspect on shesop health care. In: 2015 4th International Conference on Interactive Digital Media (ICIDM), December 2015, pp. 1–6 (2015)

24. Abdekhoda, M., Ahmadi, M., Dehnad, A., Hosseini, A.: Information technology acceptance in health information management. Methods Inf. Med. **53**(01), 14–20 (2014)

25. Rodger, J.A., Pendharkar, P.C., Paper, D.J.: End-user perceptions of quality and information technology in health care. J. High Technol. Manag. Res. **7**(2), 133–147 (1996)

26. Malato, L.A., Kim, S.: End-user perceptions of a computerized medication system: is there resistance to change? J. Health Hum. Serv. Adm. **27**(1), 34–55 (2004)

27. Zhang, X., Han, X., Dang, Y., Meng, F., Guo, X., Lin, J.: User acceptance of mobile health services from users' perspectives: the tole of self-efficacy and response-efficacy in technology acceptance. Inform. Health Soc. Care **42**(2), 194–206 (2017)

28. Vélez, O., Okyere, P.B., Kanter, A.S., Bakken, S.: A usability study of a mobile health application for rural Ghanaian midwives. J. Midwifery Womens Health **59**(2), 184–191 (2014)
29. Dhukaram, A.V., Baber, C., Elloumi, L., van Beijnum, B.-J., De Stefanis, P.: End-user perception towards pervasive cardiac healthcare services: benefits, acceptance, adoption, risks, security, privacy and trust. In: 2011 5th International Conference on Pervasive Computing Technologies for Healthcare (PervasiveHealth) and Workshops, pp. 478–484. IEEE (2011)
30. Pasquadibisceglie, V., Zaza, G., Castellano, G.: A personal health care system for contact-less estimation of cardiovascular parameters. In: 2018 AEIT International Annual Conference, pp. 1–6. IEEE (2018)
31. Challoner, A.: Photoelectric plethysmography for estimating cutaneous blood flow. Non-invasive Physiol. Meas. **1**, 125–151 (1979)
32. Allen, J.: Photoplethysmography and its application in clinical physiological measurement. Physiol. Meas. **28**(3), R1 (2007)
33. Casalino, G., Castellano, G., Castiello, C., Pasquadibisceglie, V., Zaza, G.: A fuzzy rule-based decision support system for cardiovascular risk assessment. In: Fullér, R., Giove, S., Masulli, F. (eds.) WILF 2018. LNCS (LNAI), vol. 11291, pp. 97–108. Springer, Cham (2019). https://doi.org/10.1007/978-3-030-12544-8_8
34. Weidner, G.: Why do men get more heart disease than women? an international perspective. J. Am. Coll. Health **48**(6), 291–294 (2000)
35. Schwarzer, R., Rieckmann, N.: Social support, cardiovascular disease, and mortality. In: Heart Disease: Environment, Stress, and Gender. NATO Science Series, Series I: Life and Behavioural Sciences, vol. 327, pp. 185–197 (2002)

Walking Pace Induction Application Based on the BPM and RhythmValue of Music

Atsushi Otsubo[1(✉)], Hirohiko Suwa[1,2], Yutaka Arakawa[3,4],
and Keiichi Yasumoto[1]

[1] Nara Institute of Science and Technology, Ikoma, Nara 630-0192, Japan
otsubo.atsushi.nv4@is.naist.jp
[2] RIKEN, Wako, Saitama 351-0198, Japan
[3] Kyushu University, Fukuoka 819-0395, Japan
[4] JST PRESTO, Tokyo, Japan
http://ubi-lab.naist.jp/

Abstract. Walking has been attracting attention as an important means for prevention and improvement of lifestyle diseases, such as high blood pressure and diabetes. However, walking at a continuous pace with high load can be challenging, and health benefits cannot be expected when walking with low load. A walking pace support system is necessary in order to achieve effective walking. Hence, we are developing Beat-Sync, a smartphone application that realizes the induction of a natural and accurate walking pace by the rhythm of music. This application can select songs from a user's music library. However, some songs, such as songs with a fast (slow) rhythm or complex beats, are not suitable for walking pace induction. In the present paper, we consider the speed and clarity of music rhythm to be an important factor in selecting a song that is suitable for walking pace induction and make an index and clarify its effect on walking pace induction. In the present study, BPM is used as an index of rhythm speed, and RhythmValue (RV) is proposed as an index of rhythm clarity. In order to verify the effectiveness of the index, we conducted walking pace induction experiments using 30 songs with different speeds and clarities (two sets of 15 songs) with 14 participants. As a result, the experiments confirmed that the proposed index can distinguish songs that are suitable or unsuitable for walking pace induction and can select songs that are suitable for walking pace induction.

Keywords: Music · Walking pace induction · BPM · RhythmValue · Smartphone application

1 Introduction

In recent years, walking activity has been highlighted as a major solution to prevent lifestyle diseases, such as high blood pressure and diabetes [13]. However,

G. M. P. O'Hare et al. (Eds.): MobiHealth 2019, LNICST 320, pp. 60–74, 2020.
https://doi.org/10.1007/978-3-030-49289-2_5

walking at a continuous pace with high load can be challenging, and health benefits cannot be expected when walking with low load [4]. It is important to walk the correct route at the right pace in order to improve an individual's health.

A number of walking support systems have been developed to solve this problem [7,9,16]. In a previous study, we developed a walking support system based on heart rate prediction [7,16]. This system suggests a walking route and pace for each walker according to his/her request (target calorie usage, walking time, etc.) and conditions (gender, age, exercise habit, etc.). However, the system only provides suggestions, such as "Please walk at 5.2 km/h." Therefore, it is difficult for the user to adjust to the walking pace. It is necessary to have a support method for the user to adjust to the walking pace presented by the system. Several studies have already developed walking pace adjustment systems [9,11,19,20]. In order to adjust walking pace, there is a method of advising increased or decreased walking speed through a screen and/or voice of a smartphone, but this method cannot accurately adjust the speed of the walker to the target speed. Moreover, in this method, walkers need to watch their smartphones while walking, which may lead to accidents.

Therefore, we decided to use music to induce walking pace in a natural, accurate, and fun manner. Several studies have shown that music affects body movement [1,3,5,6,8,14,15,18]. Fraisse and Noorden et al. reported that people tend to prefer to match their body movements to music [1,18]. Hence, we are developing an application called BeatSync [12] (Fig. 2), which realizes natural and accurate walking pace induction by adjusting the walking pace to the rhythm of music. This application can select a song from the user's music library. However, there are some songs that are not suitable for walking pace induction. For example, when a song's rhythm is too fast (slow) or complex, it will be difficult to adjust the walking pace of the user to the pace of the music. For the induction of the walking pace, it is necessary to select a song of appropriate rhythm speed and clarity.

In the present paper, we consider the speed and clarity of the rhythm of the song are major factors affecting walking pace induction. Therefore, BPM is used as an index of rhythm speed, and RhythmValue (RV) is proposed as an index of rhythm clarity. Hence, we consider that the selection of songs that are suitable for walking pace induction becomes possible by these two indexes. In order to investigate the effectiveness of the indexes, a walking pace induction experiment was conducted using 30 songs with different speeds and clarities (two sets of 15 songs) with 14 participants. As a result, it was confirmed that a song suitable for walking pace induction could be selected by the proposed index. Concretely, it was confirmed that for a BPM of 90–120, walking pace induction is possible regardless of RV, and, at other BPM values, the range in which walking pace induction is possible narrowed as RV decreases.

2 Previous Research

This section describes applications and research about walking support systems.

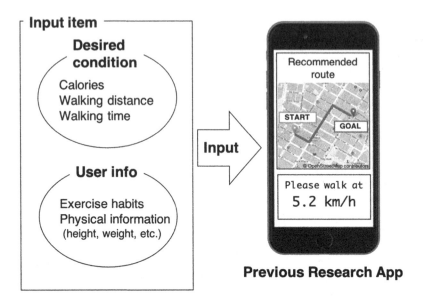

Fig. 1. Previous research application (created by the author based on [7]).

2.1 Existing Walking Support Systems

RunKeeper[1] and iSmoothRun[2] are currently used as walking support applications. In these applications, the heart rate meter and the smartphone are connected by Bluetooth, and the heart rate is displayed on the smartphone. Therefore, if the heart rate becomes too high, the walking speed can be reduced in order to lower the heart rate. However, in these systems, when a heart rate meter is not attached, it is not possible to confirm the heart rate. Furthermore, even when a heart rate meter is attached to the user, the present heart rate is displayed, but the future heart rate cannot be predicted. Therefore, the Runkeeper app can only decrease the walking pace when the heart rate becomes too high.

On the other hand, we are developing a walking support system based on heart rate prediction using smartphones [7,16]. This application predicts the heart rate while walking using walking pace, road gradient, and user information (height, weight, exercise habits, etc.) and shows the walking route and walking pace that are suitable for conditions such as time limit, target calorie usage, and maximum heart rate (Fig. 1). However, realizing an interface to accurately adjust the user's walking pace has been problematic. Hence, it is necessary to induce a walking pace through some method.

---

[1] Runkeeper https://runkeeper.com/.

[2] iSmoothRun http://www.ismoothrun.com/.

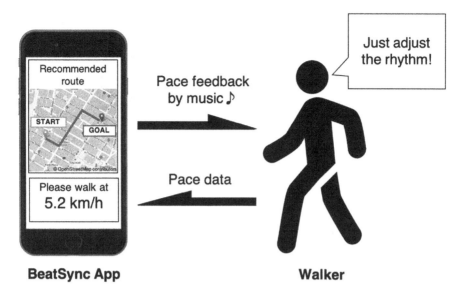

Fig. 2. Image of the BeatSync application.

2.2 Walking Pace Induction System

Watanabe et al. developed a walking pace induction system using a shoe-shaped interface [19]. They clarified that constant-walking-pace induction is possible by generating vibrations in the instep of the foot using a shoe-type device and changing the pace of these vibrations. However, this method requires special devices and is not widely adopted.

MPTrain [11] and the IM4Sports music system [20] can be induced to the target walking pace by following the rhythm of the music. These are systems that select the song of the optimum speed in proportion to the heart rate and goal before the music ends and choose the next song. However, in order to change the song itself, the induction was either delayed, or many songs had to be retained.

Tajadura-Jimenez et al. reported that modified walking sounds change one's own perceived body weight and affects the user's walking pattern [17]. Walk-In Music [9] uses this effect and generates music based on the walking pace and induces the walking pace. Walk-In Music has the advantage whereby there is no need to prepare songs. However, the generated music is composed of monotonous drum sounds, and so is not preferable to the user. Nagashima reported that boredom and habituation to monotonous rhythms reduce the attentiveness of participants [10]. We considered that it is important to use the user's preferred song rather than monotonous sounds, such as a drum, to induce the walking pace.

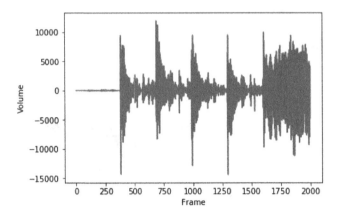

Fig. 3. Volume component for each frame of the song (first 2,000 frames).

Therefore, we proposed a method by which to induce a walking pace using only a single (or a few) song(s) by controlling the reproduction of the speed of music, which can be easily used by everyone [12] (Fig. 2). Concretely, an application capable of inducing a walking pace with a limited number of songs by using the "Superpowered" library with less deterioration of tone quality, even by changing the reproduction speed of music (time stretching processing), was developed for smartphones usable by everyone. As a result of the walking induction experiment using song data prepared in advance by six participants using this application, the walking pace of all participants could be adjusted in the range of 102 to 120 steps per minute. However, in this experiment, it seemed easy to adjust the walking pace to the rhythm of a song, because the musical piece was close to the walking pace of the examinee and the beats were clear. In the real environment, it is preferable to use a song that the user likes, but the speed and clarity of the rhythm are different for all songs. Hence, it is not always easy to adjust the walking pace to the music.

Therefore, in the present study, the speed and clarity of rhythm are made to be an index and are used as parameters for song recommendation. The number of beats per minute (BPM) is an index that indicates the speed of the rhythm. However, there is no index for the clarity of rhythm. Therefore, we index the clarity of song rhythm (degree of clarity of the periodic beat) as the Rhythm-Value (RV). By indexing, the system can choose a suitable song for walking pace induction.

3   Proposed Index

This section describes how to index the speed and clarity of the rhythm of a song.

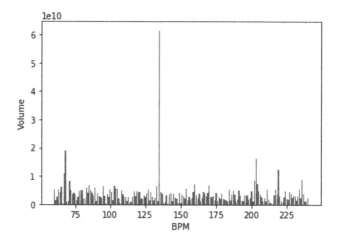

Fig. 4. Volume component for each BPM (BPM 60–240).

3.1   Indexing the Speed of Rhythm: uBPM

Regarding the speed of the rhythm of a song, there is an index called BPM, which indicates the number of beats per minute. Many songs have a specific BPM that can be obtained by analyzing the frequency of audio waveform data of songs. In the present paper, a song's specific BPM is described as the unique BPM (uBPM). Here, uBPM is calculated as follows:

- Step 1-1: Divide a song's waveform data into frames. The volume (effective value) of each frame is then obtained (Fig. 3).
- Step 1-2: Calculate the volume increment between adjacent frames.
- Step 1-3: Calculate the volume component for each BPM by analyzing the frequency component of the volume increase (Fig. 4).
- Step 1-4: The BPM with the largest volume component is defined as uBPM.

In Step 1-1, in order to reduce the calculation amount, the song's waveform data is divided into frames (one frame includes 512 samples, approximately 0.01 s), and the volume (effective value) of each frame is obtained. In Step 1-2, the volume increment between adjacent frames is calculated. This is because most of musical instruments have the common feature that the volume increases rapidly at the moment of sound emission. On the other hand, the appearance of the volume decreases differently depending on the type of instrument. In Step 1-3, the volume increment is analyzed by analyzing the frequency component in order to determine the volume component for each BPM. Since the uBPM of many songs is within the range of 60–240, the volume component is calculated for each BPM in this range. In Step 1-4, the BPM of the largest volume component of BPM 60–240 is selected as the uBPM. The waveform shown in Figs. 3 and 4 is the analysis result of "original smile" by SMAP, a J-POP song.

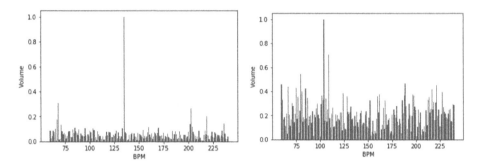

Fig. 5. Volume component for each BPM of songs with clear rhythms (left) and songs with complex rhythms (right). Left: SMAP Original Smile (J-POP), RV: 94, Right: Beethoven's 5th Symphony, RV: 79.

3.2 Indexing the Clarity of Rhythm: RV

Currently, since the clarity of the rhythm has no index, we devise a method to index the clarity. The rhythm of music consists of the size of the periodic volume (beat strength), and it is easy to walk when the rhythm of song is clear.

Summary of Indexing. Between songs with clear and complex rhythms, a difference appears in the volume component for each BPM of the song obtained in the previous section in Step 1-3. Figure 5 shows the volume component per BPM in songs with clear or complex rhythms. The volume components of each BPM are normalized to be 1 at the maximum in order to index different songs by the same standard. In songs with clear rhythm, the volume component of uBPM becomes much larger than other BPM volume components (Fig. 5 left). In contrast, in songs with complex rhythms, the volume components of BPMs other than the uBPM become large (Fig. 5 right). In the present study, we use this tendency as an indicator of the clarity of rhythm. RhythmValue (RV) is defined as the clarity of the rhythm indexed by 0–100. The closer RV is to 100, the clearer the rhythm is. The closer RV is to 0, the less clear the rhythm is.

Process of Indexing. To calculate RV, we first determine the volume components for each BPM beforehand (Steps 1-1 to 1-3 of the previous section), then apply the process of indexing, Steps 2-1 to 2-3 shown below.

- Step 2-1: Normalize each BPM volume component to a maximum of 1.
- Step 2-2: Calculate the average of the normalized volume components (VOL_a) excluding uBPM.
- Step 2-3: Output values up to 0–100 using Eq. (1) below.

$$RV = (1 - VOL_a) \times 100 \tag{1}$$

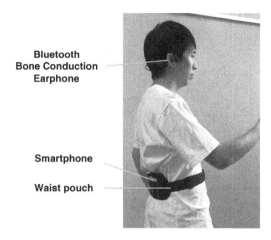

Fig. 6. Experimental situation.

In Step 2-1, in order to make it possible to compare songs with different sound levels, the volume components for each BPM obtained are normalized to be 1 at maximum (Fig. 5). In Step 2-2, calculate the average of the volume components (VOL_a) excluding uBPM. Since the volume components are normalized in Step 2-1, the magnitude of volume components other than uBPM can be expressed in the form normalized by 1 at maximum by calculating the average value. VOL_a approaches 0 if the rhythm of the song is clear and approaches 1 if the rhythm is complex. In Step 2-3, Eq. (1) is used to give index values of up to 0–100.

4   Evaluation Experiment

Evaluation experiments are conducted to confirm the effectiveness of uBPM and RV and their effects on the induction of walking pace. This section describes the experiments and experimental applications.

4.1   Summary of the Experiment

The purpose of this experiment is to clarify the effect of differences in uBPM and RV on the induction range of walking pace. If the uBPM and RV of a song with a large walking pace induction range can be specified, these values can be used for song selection in the walking pace induction. An experiment was carried out with 14 participants (men and women) in their 20's in a flat place without a slope. A walking pace induction experiment (5 to 15 min) and a survey (1 min) were conducted using one song. This experiment was approved by the Ethics Review Committee (Approval Number 2018-I-8) at Nara Institute of Science and Technology. In order to express the differences among songs, 15 categories were created based on uBPM (five categories) and RV (three categories) (Table 1). Two songs are selected for each category, and a total of 30 songs are used (Table 2).

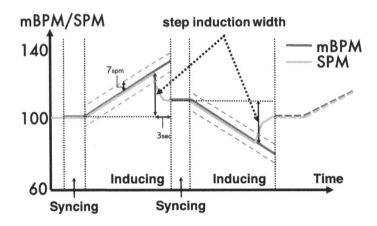

Fig. 7. Image of walking pace induction.

The experiment took a long time (150–450 min) because it was necessary to repeat the set of the walking pace induction experiment and the survey for 30 songs. Since walking for a long time may cause exhaustion, the maximum number of songs per day was limited to six (up to 90 min), and sessions were divided into several days according to the participant's convenience. The contents of the experiment were explained to the participants before the experiment, and the application for the validation, Bluetooth bone-conduction earphones, and waist pouches were distributed (Fig. 6). A Bluetooth bone-conduction earphone was used to ensure safety by enabling people to listen to ambient sounds while walking and listening to music. In addition, a waist pouch was distributed to enable people to walk empty handed and to cope with unexpected accidents such as falls.

4.2   Details of Walking Induction Experiment

The playing speed of music is dynamically changed during the walking pace induction experiment. In the present paper, the BPM of the music being played is described as mBPM (Music BPM)[3]. Figure 7 shows an image of walking pace induction. First, mBPM is played according to the walking pace (steps per minute: SPM), and then the paces of the song and the walking speed are synchronized (Fig. 7 Synchronizing). The number of steps per minute (SPM) is then induced by slowly varying mBPM (Fig. 7 Inducing). In this experiment, 1 mBPM is changed every two seconds. The induction ends when the walking pace does not follow the pace of the music (more than seven differences between mBPM and SPM) for more than three seconds continuously. The difference in mBPM from the beginning of induction to the point at which it becomes impossible to follow is defined as the step induction width. The upper and lower limits

---

[3] mBPM can be different from uBPM since the music playback speed can be changed.

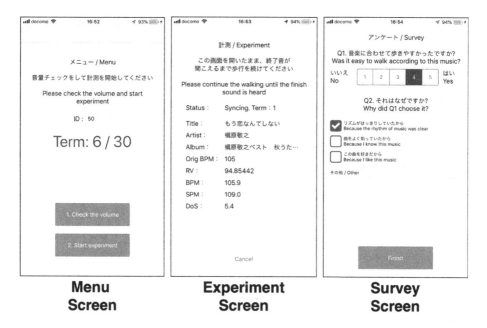

Fig. 8. Screenshot of the application used for the experiment.

of the inducible walking pace are different depending on the user, but it is possible to simply compare the inducible range of the walking pace by using step induction width.

We considered that the clearer the rhythm, the easier it is to adjust to the rhythm of the song, and the wider the step induction width is. Furthermore, in the survey carried out at the end of each set, it was confirmed that it was easy to walk with music, as well as the reason thereof.

4.3 Details of the Survey

The participants answered the survey after each walking pace induction experiment (Fig. 8 Right). The survey was based on whether it was easy to walk with the music, as well as the reason thereof. The survey items are as follows.

Table 1. uBPM and RV categories.

RV	uBPM				
	60–90	90–120	120–150	150–180	180–210
Less than 80	A	D	G	J	M
80–90	B	E	H	K	N
90–100	C	F	I	L	O

Table 2. Songs used in the present study.

Song name	uBPM	RV	Category	Song name	uBPM	RV	Category	Song name	uBPM	RV	Category
Song-1	74	74	A	Song-11	164	82	K	Song-21	106	94	F
Song-2	78	86	B	Song-12	166	95	L	Song-22	136	79	G
Song-3	74	93	C	Song-13	199	71	M	Song-23	130	82	H
Song-4	106	67	D	Song-14	190	88	N	Song-24	135	94	I
Song-5	106	86	E	Song-15	194	96	O	Song-25	177	79	J
Song-6	105	95	F	Song-16	74	79	A	Song-26	160	88	K
Song-7	135	71	G	Song-17	74	89	B	Song-27	170	92	L
Song-8	130	88	H	Song-18	75	93	C	Song-28	186	75	M
Song-9	135	93	I	Song-19	100	76	D	Song-29	200	82	N
Song-10	156	79	J	Song-20	100	88	E	Song-30	194	94	O

– Was it easy to walk with music?
  - Five levels: 1 to 5 (1: Difficult to walk, 5: Easy to walk)
– Q2 Reason for selecting Q1.
  - A1 The rhythm was clear
  - A2 I know this song well
  - A3 I like this song
  - A4 The rhythm was not clear
  - A5 I didn't know this song well
  - A6 I don't like this song
  - A7 Other (free description)

If the answer to Q1 is 4 or 5, the selectable answers to Q2 will be A1, A2 and A3. Furthermore, when the participant chooses 1 or 2 as an answer to Q1, A4, A5 or A6 become selectable. If the answer to Q1 is 3, A1–A6 can not be selected. Then, A7 is always descriptive.

4.4 Experimental Application

The developed verification application is equipped with the function of walking pace synchronization, induction, induction finish decision, and a survey for carrying out the experiment of the previous section (Fig. 8). The application was developed as an iOS app and implemented in the Swift programming language. For the playback of music and change of the mBPM, the Superpowered library (see Footnote 2), which can only change the reproduction speed while maintaining the sound height (pitch) without damaging tone quality, as far as possible, is used. The user's walking pace (SPM) is detected in real time using acceleration. During the walking pace induction experiment, mBPM and SPM are recorded every second. For each set of experiments, the application works as follows. When the application is started, a menu screen (Fig. 8 Left) is displayed first. Users tap "Start Experiment" to go to the experiment screen (Fig. 8 Center). When walking starts in this state, a walking pace induction experiment is started. When the walking pace induction experiment ends, the survey screen (Fig. 8 Right) is displayed. After responding to the survey, the menu screen (Fig. 8 Left) is displayed again.

5   Results

This section describes the experiment results and discusses the proposed index.

5.1   Walking Experiment Results and Discussion

Although there was difference in individual results, the difference in the step induction width was generated by the difference between uBPM and RV of the songs. Table 3 shows the average step induction width of all participants tabulated for the uBPM and RV of each song. In all uBPM categories, the step induction width increases as RV increases. For example, when the uBPM category is 60–90 and the RV category is less than 80 or 90–100, the step induction widths are 13.89 and 20.21, respectively. Furthermore, in all RV categories, when the uBPM category is 90–120, the step induction widths become the largest. As shown in Table 3, in each uBPM category, the step induction width increases as the value of RV increases. Since RV represents the clarity of the beat of the song, we considered that the higher the value of RV, the easier it was to walk with the rhythm of song. Moreover, in any RV category, the category of uBPM 90–120 has the largest step induction width. Ishizaki et al. reported that the listener feels uncomfortable when the playback speed of the music is changed greatly [2]. Therefore, the maximum step induction width was observed when the category of uBPM was 90–120, which is closest to the general walking pace of around SPM100. In addition, as the uBPM category moves away from 90–120, which is close to the walking pace, i.e., as the playback speed greatly changes from the original speed of the song, the effect of RV appears remarkably. Compared with songs having clear rhythms, songs having complex rhythms with small RV were found to be difficult to induce the walking pace when the playback speed was changed.

Therefore, when these results are applied to BeatSync app, songs will be recommended a priory from the RV category 90–100 and uBPM category 90–120 according to Table 3, and then the surrounding categories are recommended. Moreover, it is also feasible to use a new index, which is calculated by multiplication of RV and uBPM for the song recommendation.

5.2   Survey Results and Discussion

Table 4 shows the results of the survey (Q1). Similar to the results shown in Table 3, we found that the closer the uBPM category is to 90–120, the easier walking in rhythm is. When uBPM and SPM are close to each other, there was little sense of incongruity and walking to the rhythm of music was easier, because the reproduction speed of music does not change greatly from the speed particular to the song. Therefore, when the uBPM category is 90–120, it is easy to walk in rhythm, regardless of RV. In categories other than uBPM category 90–120, the effect of RV is remarkable. When the RV category was 90–100, the uBPM category was 60–180, and the answer (answer is over 3) for which music was easier to walk was obtained. However, when the RV category was less than

Table 3. Average (Standard Deviations) of the step induction width for 14 participants.

RV	uBPM				
	60–90	90–120	120–150	150–180	180–210
Less than 80	13.89 (7.51)	21.27 (11.65)	18.46 (9.02)	16.79 (12.73)	14.01 (7.08)
80–90	15.16 (7.36)	21.86 (14.03)	19.79 (12.06)	19.58 (10.34)	16.63 (7.41)
90–100	20.21 (13.60)	23.20 (17.69)	20.22 (9.72)	19.79 (12.45)	19.57 (9.50)

Table 4. Average (Standard Deviations) of Survey Q1 (Ease of walking with rhythm of music) [1: Difficult to walk - 5: Easy to walk].

RV	uBPM				
	60–90	90–120	120–150	150–180	180–210
Less than 80	3.00 (1.05)	3.86 (0.89)	2.68 (1.19)	2.36 (1.13)	2.21 (1.10)
80–90	3.43 (1.07)	4.00 (1.05)	3.29 (1.27)	3.04 (1.29)	2.61 (1.23)
90–100	3.86 (0.89)	3.96 (1.00)	3.79 (1.07)	3.46 (1.26)	2.89 (1.13)

80, the response that it was easy to walk with music was obtained only for a limited range, where the uBPM category was 60–120. Table 5 shows the results of Q2 (Reason for Q1) of the survey. In Q2, the reason for Q1 was selected from specified items. Table 5 shows the item, the number of items selected, and the results of average the step induction width of the all participants and all songs for the selected item. A difference of approximately 5.7 steps appears on the step induction width depending on whether the song is known or unknown. In other words, the range of steps that can be induced by a known song is larger than that of an unknown song. It seems to be easy to walk in accordance with music, because the rhythm of the song is grasped in advance. However, in this experiment, the effect of the song preference on the step induction width was not observed.

Table 5. Results of Survey Q2 (reason for choosing Q1).

Item (reason of Q1)	Number of selections (out of 420)	Average step induction width
The rhythm was clear	164	20.4
I know this song well	91	21.2
I like this song	23	21.9
The rhythm was not clear	95	15.7
I didn't know this song well	75	15.5
I don't like this song	6	22.7
Average of all songs	–	18.7

6   Conclusion

We have developed a walking support application called BeatSync, which runs on a smartphone, with the aim of inducing walking pace naturally and accurately to a target by focusing on the rhythm of music. This application uses song data stored in the smartphone, however these songs depend on the individual, so there are songs that are suitable or not suitable for walking pace induction. Then, in the present paper, we considered that the speed and clarity of the rhythm of the song greatly affected the walking pace induction, and made an index using these characteristics. Specifically, we used BPM as an index of the rhythm's speed and proposed the RhythmValue (RV) as a new index of the rhythm's clarity. Furthermore, a walking experiment and survey were carried out with 14 participants using two sets of 15 songs (total 30 songs) with different BPMs and RVs. The results of these experiments confirmed that the proposed index can discriminate songs that are suitable or unsuitable for walking pace induction and can select songs that are suitable for walking pace induction. Concretely, it was confirmed that for a BPM of 90–120, walking pace induction was possible regardless of RV, and, at other BPM values, the range in which the walking pace induction was possibly narrowed as RV decreased.

Acknowledgments. The present study was supported in part by JSPS KAKENHI Grant Number JP16H01721 and JST PRESTO Grant Number 16817861.

References

1. Fraisse, P.: Rhythm and tempo. Psychol. Music **1**, 149–180 (1982)
2. Ishizaki, H., Hoashi, K., Takishima, Y.: E-035 a study on measurement function of user comfortness according to song tempo change for DJ mixing. Forum Inf. Technol. **8**(2), 335–336 (2009)
3. Large, E.W.: On synchronizing movements to music. Hum. Mov. Sci. **19**(4), 527–566 (2000)
4. Laursen, A.H., Kristiansen, O.P., Marott, J.L., Schnohr, P., Prescott, E.: Intensity versus duration of physical activity: implications for the metabolic syndrome. A prospective cohort study. BMJ Open **2**(5), e001711 (2012)
5. Leman, M.: Embodied Music Cognition and Mediation Technology. MIT Press, Cambridge (2008)
6. MacDougall, H.G., Moore, S.T.: Marching to the beat of the same drummer: the spontaneous tempo of human locomotion. J. Appl. Physiol. **99**(3), 1164–1173 (2005)
7. Maenaka, S., Suwa, H., Arakawa, Y., Yasumoto, K.: Heart rate prediction for easy walking route planning. SICE J. Control Meas. Syst. Integr. **11**(4), 284–291 (2018)
8. Moelants, D.: Preferred tempo reconsidered. In: Proceedings of the 7th International Conference on Music Perception and Cognition, Sydney, vol. 2002, pp. 1–4 (2002)
9. Murata, H., Bouzarte, Y., Kanebako, J., Minamizawa, K.: Walk-in music: walking experience with synchronized music and its effect of pseudo-gravity. In: Adjunct Publication of the 30th Annual ACM Symposium on User Interface Software and Technology, UIST 2017, pp. 177–179. ACM, New York (2017)

10. Nagashima, Y.: Drawing-in effect on perception of beats in multimedia. J. Soc. Art Sci. **3**(1), 108–148 (2004)
11. Oliver, N., Flores-Mangas, F.: MPTrain: a mobile, music and physiology-based personal trainer. In: Proceedings of the 8th Conference on Human-Computer Interaction with Mobile Devices and Services, MobileHCI 2006, pp. 21–28. ACM (2006)
12. Otsubo, A., Suwa, H., Arakawa, Y., Yasumoto, K.: BeatSync: walking pace control through beat synchronization between music and walking. In: IEEE International Conference on Pervasive Computing and Communications Workshops, PerCom Workshops 2019, Kyoto, Japan, 11–15 March 2019, pp. 367–369 (2019)
13. Piercy, K.L., et al.: The physical activity guidelines for Americans. JAMA **320**(19), 2020–2028 (2018)
14. Repp, B.H.: Musical synchronization. In: Music, Motor Control, and the Brain, pp. 55–76 (2006)
15. Styns, F., Van Noorden, L., Moelants, D., Leman, M.: Walking on music. Hum. Mov. Sci. **26**(5), 769–785 (2007)
16. Sumida, M., Mizumoto, T., Yasumoto, K.: Estimating heart rate variation during walking with smartphone. In: Proceedings of the 2013 ACM International Joint Conference on Pervasive and Ubiquitous Computing, UbiComp 2013, pp. 245–254 (2013)
17. Tajadura-Jiménez, A., Basia, M., Deroy, O., Fairhurst, M., Marquardt, N., Bianchi-Berthouze, N.: As light as your footsteps: Altering walking sounds to change perceived body weight, emotional state and gait. In: Proceedings of the 33rd Annual ACM Conference on Human Factors in Computing Systems, CHI 2015, Seoul, Republic of Korea, pp. 2943–2952. ACM (2015)
18. Van Noorden, L., Moelants, D.: Resonance in the perception of musical pulse. J. New Music Res. **28**(1), 43–66 (1999)
19. Watanabe, J., Ando, H., Asahara, Y., Sugimoto, M., Maeda, T.: Walk navigation system by shoe-shaped interface for inducing a walking cycle. IPSJ J. **46**(5), 1354–1362 (2005)
20. Wijnalda, G., Pauws, S., Vignoli, F., Stuckenschmidt, H.: A personalized music system for motivation in sport performance. IEEE Pervasive Comput. **4**(3), 26–32 (2005)

User-Oriented Interface for Monitoring Affective Diseases in Patients with Bipolar Disorder Using Mobile Devices

Salvador Prefasi-Gomar[1] , Teresa Magal-Royo[1](✉) , Elisa Gallach-Solano[2],
Pilar Sierra San Miguel[3] , Humberto Echevarria Mateu[2],
and Nieves Martínez-Alzamora[1]

[1] Universitat Politécnica de Valencia, Camino de Vera s/n, Valencia 46022, Spain
salvaprefasi@gmail.com, tmagal@degi.upv.es, nalzamor@eio.upv.es
[2] University and Polytechnic Hospital La Fe. Spain, Avenida Fernando Abril Martorell, 106,
Valencia, Spain
gallach.eli@gmail.com
[3] University and Polytechnic Hospital La Fe. University of Valencia. Spain, Avenida Fernando
Abril Martorell, 106, Valencia, Spain
sierra_pil@gva.es

Abstract. Nowadays the design of interfaces on mobile devices in the field of mental health is being studied to be applied in the functional criteria related to usability and user experience (UX). This article presents a methodological and conceptual development of an innovative telematics application oriented to control and management relapse prevention in bipolar disorder patients created by the Psychiatry and Clinical Psychology Unit of La Fe Hospital and the Polytechnic University of Valencia. Application called e-therapy aims to control affective diseases in bipolar disorder through the use of computer-assisted tests related to depression and mania among others. Its development and design took into account aspects of functionality and visual usability aimed at people with affective diseases related to mental health. Therapists, psychologists and doctors can monitor and verify patient's mood in real time as well as detect changes in their vital and affective trajectory that allows early intervention and relapse prevention.

Keywords: Mental health · Bipolar disorder · mHealth · Relapse prevention · Affective diseases · User experience

1 Introduction

In 2015, the Global Observatory for Health defined mHealth as the use of mobile and wireless devices for medical practice and as support for public health. The World Health Organization, WHO developed in 2009 a global survey about mHealth in 112 countries concluding several aspects that have been premonitory today and are still working on them:

G. M. P. O'Hare et al. (Eds.): MobiHealth 2019, LNICST 320, pp. 75–85, 2020.
https://doi.org/10.1007/978-3-030-49289-2_6

- The emergence of mHealth is undergoing significant changes in many private and public health environments. Its implies national health policies must include in their governmental Public health programs projects, future research related to the strategic implementation of new applications based on large scale mHealth environments.
- Some of the barriers found in the implementation of mHealth are related to the control and evaluation of the effectiveness and profitability of Public mHealth applications.
- Although the level of m-Health activity is growing, the evaluation of such activities in the Member States is still very low (21%).
- Security data and privacy of citizens are factors that require legal and political attention to ensure that users are adequately protected.
- States will continue progress in mHealth implementation if they share or develop global standards and architecture of Information and Communication Technologies.

Mental health sector started to develop interactive applications to helps in patient therapies that improve cognitive functions such as attention, perception, executive functions, etc. have derived mainly in creation of applications capable of controlling, monitoring and evaluating the behaviour and mood of the patient to detect symptoms of relapse and thus avoid them.

Nowadays, interactive online applications on mobile devices can improve aspects of educational and social rehabilitation in patients with mental disorders and more specifically with patients with chronic bipolar disorders. In this way, bipolar disorder patients have a better self-understanding of their disease, which will be able have a positive impact on the way of dealing active and consensual way and motivating the sense of monitoring and control from the patient point of view.

As an important part of the psychoeducation and social interventions that patients with a bipolar disorder need is to detect affective diseases related to mania, depression to avoid relapses, hospitalizations or even suicides.

In this way interactive applications related to bipolar disorder have been combined to create control, monitoring and evaluation applications including measurable aspects within the behaviour and mood of the patient to know in real time.

2   Bipolar Disorder

Bipolar disorder can be defined as a psychiatric pathology whose control parameters are focused on its level of severity, chronicity, inheritance and progressive status. A mental disorder is considered to be severe when it has a prolonged duration and ultimately leads to a social and cognitive functional disability is important to the patient.

Bipolar people experiences a permanent oscillation of mood that leads the person to lose the reference point of their habitual mood and emotional psychotic states occur punctually. Altogether, affects mainly to social and affective environment around him [1]. There are three variables related to bipolar disorder: clinical diagnosis, duration and level of disability according to the illness state [2]:

- Clinical Diagnosis considers a severe mental disorder when there are periodic episodes of psychosis. There is an alteration fact in the ability to relate to the social and/or family environment, there is inappropriate behavior or there is an inappropriate or uncontrolled affectivity.

– Disease durations can be considered as severe or chronic when it lasts two or more years. This causes a progressive cognitive and social deterioration point out by the functional control that has been carried out previously for 6 months. National Institute of Mental Health, NIMH, proposes in this dimension criteria more conditioned by functionality than by duration that include aspects as:

  – Receive psychiatric treatment of a greater intensity than standard patient treatment, at least once.
  – Receive continued residential support and other than hospitalization for a sufficient time to create a significant disruption of the person's life situation.
  – Disability of some kind understood as a personal, family, social and labour dysfunction is generated with a moderate to severe intensity over time.

– Bipolar disorder produces a mood regulation and affectivity are altered and moods appear low (depressive episode), exalted (manic episode) or mixture of both (mixed episodes), beyond normal (longer duration or intensity). States among which affective disorders are distributed are [3]:

  – Depression. End or lower state (mood inhibition).
  – Mania. Upper end state (mood exaltation).
  – Euthymic state or normal state.

3 Bipolar Disorder and Social Integration

People with severe and long-term mental disorders like bipolar disorders needs to build a meaningful social and personal life despite suffering serious limitations [4]. Bipolar disorder produces an important change in social and cognitive patient's functionality, especially in their well-being. These changes produce episodes (manic or depressive) with intermediate periods of normal emotional stability or euthymia.

An important aspect that is generated collaterally to the detection and premature relapse prevention in bipolar disorder is the vital change that occurs in the closest environment of the bipolar person that directly affects the family. The need to remain socially and emotionally connected to the environment despite affective disease becomes a key point for patient stability and follow-up. Self-control and awareness about the mental problem helps to therapies, doctors, family and friends becomes an anchor point so as not to be treated as a disabled person and therefore marginalized by society.

According to Appleby, mental health services tend to go beyond traditional clinical care and help patients reintegrate into society, redefining recovery to incorporate quality of life: a job, a decent place to live, friendships and a social life [5].

Social Recovery that many therapists encourage, serves to ensure that bipolar disorder patient normalize his/her social, family and professional environment despite the illness. Social cognition through affective diseases evidences management can provide mechanisms that allow to interact better in certain contexts. With patient's self-reports, therapist can detect any change in their behaviour or in their mood to avoid relapses. There is a strong correlation between social activity and affective control of the patients in a mental illness. For example, patients with mania are much more communicative than usual, and can make more calls or send more messages. In the same way, patients with depression leave home less, send fewer messages or the duration of their calls are much shorter.

Mobile-assisted therapies in mental health applications should help to control social integration of bipolar patient from an effective monitoring of the public health system. In fact, online applications to create self-reports allows real-time communication with the patient including status information through a series of questions related to their mood, social relationships, consumption of medicines, etc. in real time. In this way, doctor or therapist can create behavioural profiles and trends for a controlled follow-up.

Self-report is an essential tool in psychiatric research of relapse prevention with Bipolar Disorder patients. Self-assessment, control and mood monitoring tools, combined with user-centered health care systems motivate patient feels closer to their doctors due to the immediate response in case of relapse [6]. In fact, this tools are instruments that help patients with Bipolar Disorder to better understand their disease and motivate their empowerment. It allow teach patients to recognize the early signs of recurrence of episodes affective, and allow the individualized mood characterization [7].

There are applications available for monitoring and control of Bipolar Disorder which require the active participation of the patient [8, 9]. New technological approach for mood self-control of patients with a Bipolar Disorder is managed through Ecological momentary assessment, EMA [10]. Use EMA techniques through mobile devices allows individual's status information to be collected in real time, during a given period and with a low level of intrusion into the patient's daily life [11]. The use of such devices for patient monitoring and control, allows a collection data automatically generated daily (for example, number of text messages, number of phone calls, GPS data, voice functions, etc....), which reflect behavioural activities that may be related to psychopathology and that would not be easily accessible in any other way [12].

4   User Experience (UX) in Mental Health Interactive Applications

User experience (UX) in digital world focuses on internal and external recognition processes of everything that happens to a user when interacting with a mobile application or with a website, including all experiences or evidences that user perceives and feels while using it.

User experience, UX is the result of the interaction evidences among the user, the digital product and the device, influenced by personal, social, environmental, cultural factors for instance that influence the perception of the digital product. The experience is formalized at the user's cognitive level as a positive or negative perception where digital interaction is one of the most important parts that influence the design of the application.

User experience is defined by the International Organization for Standardization (ISO), in ISO 9241-210 as:

"The perceptions and responses of a person that result from the anticipated use or use of a product, system or service..." [13].

Preece indicated that the user experience comprises a set of evidential quality criteria [14] that include three types of criteria; the classic usability criteria such as efficiency, control capacity or learning capacity; the heuristic criteria oriented to stimulation, fun, novelty, emotions [15, 16] and finally the functional criteria based on the aesthetic and visual graphic design of the application [17].

The origin of the methodologies aimed at evaluating the user experience arose in the twentieth century in the field of digital marketing and related to brand perception in digital environments such as the Internet, as an intangible but evaluable aspect, by the user when accessing a specific website or digital application for the purchase of products or services online [18].

Today, patients with a mental illness find that online web environments can limit their capabilities. The use of the internet is considered a very demanding activity from the cognitive point of view that requires not only a good knowledge and understanding of the characteristics of the web, but also the ability to analyse, synthesize, quickly evaluate and apply the information presented, while avoiding the inconsequential details (announcements) and unreliable information, so abundant in digital world [19].

Several cognitive aspects, including attention, perception, memory and executive functioning are often affected in people with a mental illness. These deficiencies may be linked to difficulties in the use of the Web, for example, when searching the Web, changing tasks, retaining and retrieving information, and ignoring distractions to focus attention.

People with mental disorders have received little attention from web accessibility research and user experience. Thus, an exhaustive review of the literature related to the barriers that people with mental illness face when using the web or applications for mobile devices is necessary to ensure that it is inclusive for this type of group. The available knowledge will help professionals to make informed decisions about the removal of barriers that affect people with a mental illness in general, and with bipolar disorder in particular. And if this is not possible, instead facilitation measures can be provided to accommodate this population group.

Emotional aspects play a fundamental role in the user's interaction with an interactive product, because emotional states affect cognitive processes that influence the user's relationship with the application. Psychology provides essential elements to understand and therefore be able to generate empathy. Thought influences the attention, perception and interpretation of any experience.

5   Conceptualization and Design of an Application for Monitoring Affective Status of a Patient with Bipolar Disorder, E-Therapy

Mobile applications in Mental Health offer the possibility of collecting a significant amount of patient information, which should be used, not only to improve and assess their social integration, mood and health, but also to control and even prevent Mental illness in general [20]. Aspects to consider in the design and implementation of applications related to Mental Health focuses on:

– Creating periodic self-reports by the patient.

- Analyse guidelines and states of affective diseases by automatic sampling of patient data.
- Affective diseases recognition through patient behaviour patterns.
- Visualization and graphic interpretation of the data obtained from the patient.
- Communication and therapeutic feedback among patient, doctor and/or therapist.

E-Therapy application developed by the Unit of Psychiatry and Clinical Psychology of the Hospital La Fe and the Polytechnic University of Valencia allows relapse prevention through affective disorders control in patients with bipolar diseases type I and II. At the present a new mobile application of PC version of e-Therapy allows patients to be an active part of early crisis detection. Through a mobile phone application, you will be able to control patient's emotional state and detect early symptoms to promote early intervention. E-therapy allows the management of the following functionalities:

- The self-report.
Information provided by the patient through self-report is essential for the treatment of most mental disorders. Self-report is mainly designed based on the technology available on the mobile device, (speed, interactivity, touch screen, voice recognition, etc. ...).

- Automatic sampling of patient data.
Since behaviour is a central factor in mental disorder and the ability to monitoring is crucial. Data on physical behaviour, in terms of activity and mobility, can be sampled through sensors incorporated in the mobile device like accelerometer and location sensors for instance. In addition to automatic physical behaviour sampling, smartphone is also a perfect platform for sampling social behaviour and mood data. Scientifics reviews confirms that there is a strong correlation between social activities and disease status [21].

- Behaviour pattern recognition.
In general, high-level behaviour patterns analysis, activity recognition based on automatic and self-reported data, can be a great value in mental affective disorders treatment.

- Visual and graphic data interpretation obtained from the patient.
There are different approaches to data visualization for control, monitoring and evaluation applications of patients with a Bipolar Disorder based on smartphones. The most basic approach is simply to display the display of raw data, applied in a linear, circular, bar or number chart. This approach is often feasible, since patients are familiar with the visualization of data from paper self-assessment forms.

- Communication and therapeutic feedback.
Since the treatment of mental disorder is based on a combination of pharmacotherapy and psychological treatment, the smartphone can become a therapeutic platform. Adherence to medication is essential in the treatment of mental disorders in general and Bipolar Disorder in particular, since it is often a pre-requisite to stabilize the disease. For this reason, some applications incorporate support for the prescription of medications by the psychiatrist, and to get the patient to adjust to these medical prescriptions. By using an application through a smartphone, the pharmacological treatment can be adjusted in a much

more precise way, because by continuously monitoring the parameters of the disease and compliance with the medication, the doctor can continuously adjust the prescriptions.

Another therapeutic approach that continues to support the use of smartphones and applications in mental illness in general, and in Bipolar Disorder in particular, is to reinforce therapy, basing it on the community and on peer-to-peer support groups. Incorporating a web browser can provide access to many online communities, where patients can share experiences and practical advice.

Direct communication between the patient and his doctor is a fundamental part of the treatment and care of patients with mental illness. Again, the smartphone and its applications become solid tools that allow real-time remote communication through text, images and video. The literature shows that simple SMS used as a reminder for patients with a serious and chronic mental disorder can have a positive impact on treatment [22].

Nowadays e-Therapy is designed to notify patient through messages, once a week, to complete the information requested in the questionnaires. These data are sent to a virtual archive that analyses information automatically and informs the psychotherapist about

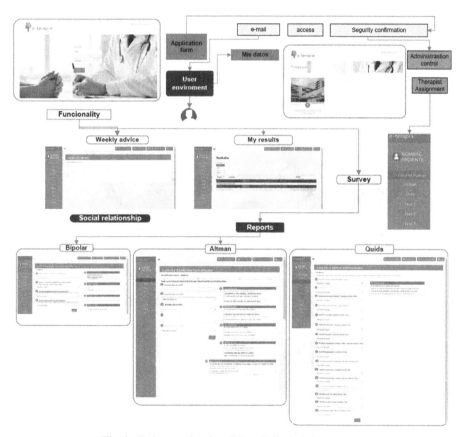

Fig. 1. E-therapy funcionalities (Gallach-Solano 2019)

the risk of relapses of the patient, facilitating that the professional can intervene early, contacting by telephone if he needs it.

Evidences are indicators of aspects such as emotional stability or possible alterations of the patient, and increase the flow of control and communication with the doctor. Currently, it is estimated that about 450 patients with Bipolar Disorders will be able to use the new application (Figs. 1 and 2).

Patients who are using this diseases tool have a number of specific characteristics to be able to be part of this type of therapy:

– Diagnosis of Bipolar I/II Disorder.
– Patient follow-up at the Hospital la Fe.
– Clinical stability and relapse prevention using the application.
– Commitment to psychotherapeutic care and adherence to psychiatric follow-up.
– Owner of a mobile device with Internet access.
– Be familiar with the use of mobile applications.

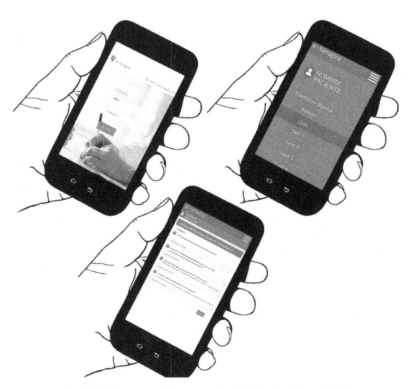

Fig. 2. E-therapy mobile screenshots (Gallach-Solano 2019)

6 Conclusions

MHealth has highlighted the importance of use smartphones becoming an ideal platform to support health care services for patients with a Bipolar Disorder. Information and Communication Technologies, ICT have revolutionized the world in just 20 years. The way of communicating, accessing information and relating to each other has changed, affecting all sectors of today's society, such as economic, educational or health.

Factors such as the emergence of the internet and its increasing use by users, better and faster connectivity between devices and the network, mobile applications for all types of utilities or smart devices more adapted to the daily users' needs are just some of the advances that technology has given us to improve our quality of life in general, and that of people with a serious and chronic mental disorder, in particular.

Health sector has seen an important reef in these advances to adapt them to patient needs in a wide variety of health fields. Mental health applications aimed patient rehabilitation with a serious and chronic mental disorder oriented to affective diseases and relapse prevention control. Patient will be able to maintain cognitive functions (attention, memory, perception, executive functions, etc.), and/or enhance others to replace those affected by the disease. Control, monitoring and assessment tools can manage affective diseases, behavior and mood of the patient detecting relapse symptoms and avoid them. Self-reports are essential tools in psychiatric research, and various graphic instruments of mood are used for self-control in the management and monitoring of depressive and manic symptoms in patients with Bipolar Disorder. Self-assessment, control and mood monitoring tools, combined with user-centered health care systems, have the potential to reach more patients more efficiently, to obtain data on the mood they are in. the patient at all times, and therefore, reduce their suffering, since the patient feels clothed and closer to his doctor due to the immediacy of response in case of relapse.

More than 80% of patients who have tried this application so far, value it very positively, highlighting its usefulness and ease of use. Other advantages that this application represents for the patient, is that it facilitates better monitoring, and easier access to information, and alerts if their therapeutic values are decompensated. In addition, the patient's adherence to pharmacological and psychological treatment is facilitated, thus underlining the commitment to his own recovery.

In addition to the advantages for the user, e-therapy also offers facilities for professional healthcare to control affective diseases patient's follow-up. It can access to the information easily and receive alerts in case that therapeutic evaluation are given outside the range. In this way, the application makes it possible to improve patient monitoring and perform early detections and interventions with the consequent reduction of risks, and significantly improving the patient's quality of life.

References

1. Vieta, E. Colom, F., Martínez-Arán, A.: La enfermedad de las emociones · El trastorno bipolar. Ars Medica. Psiquiatría Ed. (2004)
2. Schinnar, A.P., Rothbard, A.B., Kanter, R., Jung, Y.S.: An empirical literature review of definitions of severe and persistent mental illness. Am. J. Psychiatry **147**(12), 1602–1608 (1990)

3. Durán García, R., Guerrero Romero, A.J.: Trastornos del estado de ánimo. Enfermería en psiquiatría y salud mental. Enfermería 21 DAE Ed. Madrid, Spain (2009). ISBN 978-84-95626-90-5
4. Shepherd, G., Boardman, J., Slade, M.: Making Recovery a Reality. Sainsbury Centre for Mental Health, London (2008). https://www.centreformentalhealth.org.uk/publications/making-recovery-reality. Accessed 21 Aug 2019
5. Appleby, L.: Breaking down barriers: the clinical case for change. Department of Health: London (2007). http://www.dh.gov.uk. Accessed 21 Aug 2019
6. Arnrich, B., Mayora, O., Bardram, J., Tröster, G.: Pervasive healthcare-paving the way for a pervasive, user-centered and preventive healthcare model. J. Meth. Inf. Med. **49**, 67–73 (2010)
7. Faurholt-Jepsen, M., et al.: Smartphone-based self-monitoring in bipolar dis-order: evaluation of usability and feasibility of two systems. Int. J. Bipolar Disord. **7**(1) (2019). https://doi.org/10.1186/s40345-018-0134-8
8. Lal, S., Adair, C.E.: E-mental health: a rapid review of the literature. Psychiatr. Serv. **65**(1), 24–32 (2014). https://doi.org/10.1176/appi.ps.201300009
9. Faurholt-Jepsen, M., Frost, M., Vinberg, M., Christensen, E.M., Bardram, J.E., Kessing, L.V.: Smartphone data as objective measures of bipolar disorder symptoms. Psychiatry Res. **217**(1–2), 124–127 (2014)
10. Shiffman, S., Stone, A.A., Hufford, M.R.: Ecological momentary assessment. Ann. Rev. Clin. Psychol. **4**, 1–32 (2008). https://doi.org/10.1146/annurev.clinpsy.3.022806.091415
11. Torous, J., Firth, J., Mueller, N., Onnela, J.P., Baker, J.T.: Methodology and reporting of mobile health and smartphone application studies for schizophrenia. Harvard Rev Psychiatry **25**(3), 146–154 (2017). https://doi.org/10.1097/hrp.0000000000000133
12. Faurholt-Jepsen, M., Bauer, M., Kessing, L.V.: Smartphone-based objective monitoring in bipolar disorder: status and considerations. Int. J. Bipolar Disord. **6**, 6–13 (2018). https://doi.org/10.1186/s40345-017-0110-8
13. ISO: International Organization for Standardization. ISO 9241-210:2010. Ergonomic of Human-system interaction – Part 210: Human centered design for interactive systems (2010). https://www.iso.org/standard/52075.html. Accessed 21 Aug 2019
14. Preece, J., Royers, Y., Sharp, H.: Interaction Design: Beyond Human-Computer Inter-Action. Wiley, New York (2002). https://arl.human.cornell.edu/879Readings/Interaction%20Design%20-%20Beyond%20Human-Computer%20Interaction.pdf. Accessed 21 Aug 2019
15. Norman, D.: Emotional Design: Why we love (or Hate) everyday things. Basic Book, Boulder Colorado (2003)
16. Hassenzahl, M.: The effect of perceived hedonic quality on products appealing-ness. Int. J. Hum. Comput. Interact. **13**, 479–497 (2001). https://doi.org/10.1207/S15327590IJHC1304_07
17. Tractinsky, N.: Aesthetics and apparent usability: empirical assessing cultural and method-ological issues. In: CHI 1997 Electronic Publications (1997). http://www.acm.org/sigchi/chi97/proceedings/paper/nt.htm. Accessed 21 Aug 2019
18. Ferretto, F.: El papel de la percepción en la experiencia de usuario (2018). https://medium.com/@florferretto/el-papel-de-la-percepción-en-la-experiencia-de-usuario. Accessed 21 Aug 2019
19. Bernard, R., Sabariego, C., Cieza, A.: Barriers and facilitation measures related to people with mental disorders when using the web: a systematic review. J. Med. Internet Res. **18**(6), 157 (2016). https://doi.org/10.2196/jmir.5442
20. Gravenhorst, F., et al.: Mobile phones as medical devices in mental disorder treatment: an overview. Personal Ubiquitous Comput. **19**(2) (2014). https://doi.org/10.1007/s00779-014-0829-5

21. Frost, M., Doryab, A., Faurholt-Jepsen, M., Kessing, L.V., Bardram, J.E.: Supporting disease insight through data analysis: refinements of the MONARCA self-assessment system. In: Proceedings of the ACM International Conference on Pervasive and Ubiquitous Computing, pp. 133–142 (2013)
22. Pijnenborg, G.H.M., Withaar, F.K., Brouwer, W.H., Timmerman, M.E., van den Bosch, R.J., Evans, J.J.: The efficacy of SMS text messages to compensate for the effects of cognitive impairments in schizophrenia. Br. J. Clin. Psychol. **49**(2), 259–274 (2010). https://doi.org/ 10.1348/014466509X467828

The PERFORM Mask: A Psychophysiological sEnsoRs Mask FOr Real-Life Cognitive Monitoring

Danilo Menicucci[1]([⊠]) [iD], Marco Laurino[2] [iD], Elena Marinari[1], Valentina Cesari[1], and Angelo Gemignani[1,2]

[1] Department of Surgical, Medical and Molecular Pathology and Critical Care Medicine, University of Pisa, Pisa, Italy
danilo.menicucci@unipi.it
[2] Institute of Clinical Physiology, National Research Council, Pisa, Italy

Abstract. Everyday life is driven by a wide range of mental processes organized in cognitive, emotional and executive functions. The assessment of these abilities could be improved thanks to the rising of Virtual Reality (VR) technologies, that show a more ecological validity in respect to the artificial laboratory settings. Moreover, mental processes can be investigated via electrophysiological measures, due to the modulation of deep structures controlling the autonomic system, and in turn peripheral organs activity. According to scientific literature, measurements could derive from sensors over periocular area, that is the same area covered by a typical VR headset.

The aim of this paper is to introduce the PERFORM prototype, a wearable mask with embedded sensors able to collect biomedical signals in a non-obtrusive way for the assessment of online cognitive abilities in VR scenarios. We show that PERFORM can collect data related to cardiac pulse, galvanic skin response, movements and face temperature during cognitive tasks in VR. Thanks to the specific electrode placement and the employment of VR scenario, PERFORM will be an ecological tool to assess psychophysiological correlates of online cognitive performances.

Keywords: Cognitive functions · Virtual reality · Psychophysiological signals

1 Introduction

Herein we present the PERFORM prototype, a wearable mask with embedded sensors intended to collect biomedical data in a non-obtrusive way. This mask could be used for assessing real-time cognitive functioning during tasks, putatively performed in virtual reality (VR) environments. The PERFORM prototype would allow studying cognitive functions in naturalistic-like scenarios of VR. The concept of PERFORM prototype is based on previous psychophysiological studies that we summarize in the following. On these bases, we identified the most effective sensor placements to collect signals in a non-obtrusive way for detecting the physiological correlates of cognitive functioning.

G. M. P. O'Hare et al. (Eds.): MobiHealth 2019, LNICST 320, pp. 86–93, 2020.
https://doi.org/10.1007/978-3-030-49289-2_7

1.1 Cognitive Functions: A Brief Overview

Cognition is involved in everything a human being might possibly do; that every psychological phenomenon is a cognitive phenomenon. Cognition refers to all the processes by which the sensory input is transformed, reduced, elaborated, stored, recovered, and used [1]. Cognitive functions comprise a variety of mental processes including attention, memory, decision making, perception and language comprehension: however, cognitive abilities are strongly sustained by executive functioning, driving people to achieve everyday goals [2–4]. Classically, cognitive functioning is assessed in the laboratory with a neurocognitive approach that measure scores and time during the execution of specific tasks; however, investigating parsed and isolated components of cognitive functioning has also limitations [5, 6] since they might not reflect the integrated abilities during real-life in which the focus of attention has to cope with the complexity of real scenarios [7].

1.2 Virtual Reality: An Ecologic Alternative to Laboratory Setting

Virtual reality (VR) is an evolving technology that allows the immersion in and the interaction with near-realistic 3D scenarios [8, 9]; it leads to the development of the "sense of presence" by means of a constant interaction and manipulation of the virtual scenario [10, 11].

Thanks to its characteristics, VR can be used to study cognitive functions in ecologic, naturalistic-like scenarios, allowing overcoming classical limitations of neurocognitive assessment and thus scientific advances in the direction of assessing cognitive abilities such as attention [6], spatial abilities [5, 12], memory [13] and executive functions [14, 15] in real-life [16, 17].

1.3 Central and Peripheral Electrophysiological Markers of Cognitive Functions

Most of the cognitive and executive functions involve brain structures located in the frontal lobe, from which volleys of activity modulate deep structures controlling the autonomic system, the heart rate, the skin blood flow and sweating activity [18].

Compared to cognitive correlates directly from brain activity (via electroencephalography), more robust against movement artifacts [19] and thus more robust for ecologic studies (freely behaving, etc.). Actually, from these signals, the following cognitive correlates can be derived:

– Galvanic Skin Responses (GSR): the changes of the electrical conductance of the skin in response to pulsatile sweat secretion. GSR is a correlate of sympathetic nervous system activity [20];
– Heart Rate (HR): the inverse of the frequency of heartbeats. Changes in HR has been related to cognitive/emotional activations;
– Heart Rate Variability (HRV): indices of HR variability as a function of time of frequency. The indices correlate with the activity of different components of the autonomic nervous system;

– Skin Temperature (T): the face skin temperature is an indirect indicator of a subjective cognitive state. The physiological replication of increasing blood flow to the facial skin is triggered by the autonomic nervous system [21];

On this basis, we conceived a device able to collect in a non-obtrusive way peripheral physiologic signals with correlating the cognitive functioning in VR environment. A suitable solution that we explored was the integration of all the sensors into a single wearable headset, in order to record real-time biomedical signals during cognitive tasks in VR without constraints related to multiple body sites of recording (electrode wiring issue, etc.).

2 Methods

In order to assess real-time cognitive functioning, we chose to record specific psychophysiological parameters (i.e. GSR, HR, T, movement) that are susceptible to cognitive abilities. The choice of the wearable mask in which the sensors are embedded in is intimately linked to the need of recording signals in non-obtrusive way, in order to avoid confound or side effects related to an invasive signals collection. Moreover, the placement of the sensors above the periocular area is highly motivated by the need of projecting a headset to wear during VR task.

2.1 Where to Place Sensors?

The idea is to place the sensors within a wearable headset. We verified the feasibility of the idea on scientific literature that confirmed that sensors placed over periocular area could be valid tool for collecting physiologic peripheral signals:

– Forehead is one of the most reactive body sites to collect GSR, due to its high sweat gland density [22];
– Glabella (the small area between the eyebrows and above the nose) is a valid site to collect pulse signal thanks to the thinning of cranial bone. For this reason, in respect to the gold standard measures (i.e. clinical setting monitoring), it is less invasive [23];
– Forehead, as well as peri-orbital region, represent two face sites for the collection of skin face temperature [24, 25];

2.2 How to Collect Signals?

Despite the great flexibility among the systems currently marketed for the acquisition of biomedical signals, some limitations such as GSR sensor placement, no-dry ECG electrodes, not available sensors to collect the surface temperature in order to perform differential measurements have to be highlighted.

For this reason, we chose a personal computer as signal processing device, while for the hardware platform we decided to use Arduino Nano for the collection of biomedical parameters.

We also developed a tailored software (compatible with Windows 10 O.S.) for data acquisition from PERFORM system. The software is able to real-time visualizing and recording the signals from PERFORM.

In order to design a sensorized headset, signals will be collected by a set of seven dry electrodes placed as describe in the follow:

- four sensors for temperature: two over the forehead and two over the zygomaticus muscle;
- two sensors over the forehead for recording GSR signal;
- one central sensor over the glabella for recording HR signal;
- 3-axial accelerometer placed on the left side of the mask for recording movements;

Locating all the sensors in the periocular space allows integrating them into a wearable mask suitable for the detection of selected parameters during cognitive performance (Fig. 1).

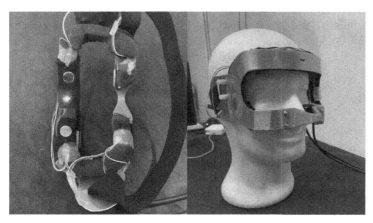

Fig. 1. PERFORM mask prototype: on the left sensor placement in the foam, on the right a front view of the wearable mask.

In the PERFORM prototype, the multiple signals recording has been based on two Arduino Nano 3.x electronic boards, and as biosignals we adopted the following:

- GSR: sensore Grove – GSR (Seeed Technology Co., Ltd.);
- HR: PulseSensor (World Famous Electronics llc);
- Temperature: digital sensors DS18B20 (Maxim Integrated);
- Accelerometer: 3-Axis Analog Accelerometer; Axis Analog Accelerometer (Seeed Technology Co., Ltd);

For bio-signal collection, two Arduino Nano are used:

- Arduino 1 for GSR, Pulse sensors and Accelerometer.
- Arduino 2 for T sensors.

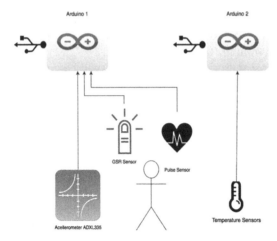

Fig. 2. Schematic description of the PERFORM prototype.

Both Arduino 1 and 2 are wired to a software station via serial communication interface (Fig. 2). This software is conceived for the real-time monitoring of biomedical signals, as well as their processing and storing.

3 Results

The actual prototype of PERFORM can acquire and store the data from sensors ranging from GSR, to heart pulse, movements and skin temperature during the performance of cognitive task. All the sensors are embedded in a foam of a common VR headset. In Fig. 3 the signals (10 s) from different sensors are shown. We are validating PERFORM recording signals while undergoing different cognitive tasks implemented on PEBL

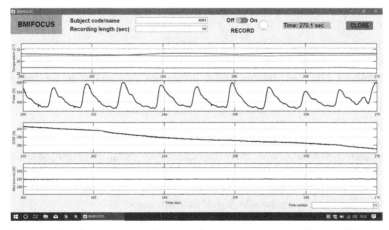

Fig. 3. Ten seconds window of real-time signals from temperature, Pulse, GSR sensors and accelerometers.

software [26]. The cognitive assessment comprises tasks for multicomponent evaluation of: attention (divided, focused, sustained attention); executive functions such as risk taking, decision making, problem solving; visuo-spatial abilities. The sensors will collect signal variations during the task performance associated to the psychophysiological correlates of cognitive functioning. In Fig. 4 an example of one task with the recorded temperature time course is shown.

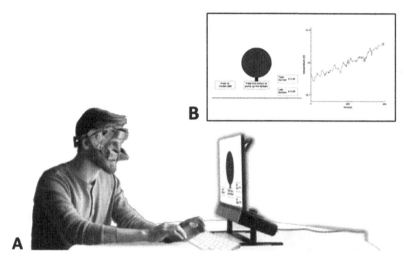

Fig. 4. Panel A. The Balloon Analogue Risk Task (BART) is a cognitive test for measuring risky decision making, i.e. how the potential for reward versus loss is balanced. In the task, the participant is presented with a balloon and earns money by incrementally inflating the balloon, however, at some threshold, the balloon is over inflated and explodes; at this point the participant loses all previously earned money. The participant must decide when to stop inflating and save the earned money. Panel B. Monitoring skin face temperature during the task showed an increasing trend.

4   Conclusion

VR offers an ecological and integrated assessment of cognitive functions. For the electrophysiological assessment of cognitive abilities, the investigation of peripheral activity - GSR, HR, T- is more suitable and ecological than electroencephalography and, herein we demonstrate that all these parameters can be feasibly collected from periocular area. Based on the current lack of ecologic settings for signal collection during cognitive functioning, we present the PERFORM prototype, a wearable mask embedding multiple sensors aimed at collecting biomedical data for assessing real-time cognitive abilities during task in VR. This wearable headset, with GSR, T, Pulse and Movement sensors integrated into the foam of common VR headsets, can be a solution for the "ecologic validity issue" related to classical neuroscientific investigation of cognitive abilities.

Acknowledgments. The research leading to these results was funded by the Project "Brain Machine Interface in space manned missions: amplifying Focused attention for error Counterbalancing" (BMI-FOCUS, Tuscany Region POR CREO 2014/2020). We also thank Davide Cini and Andrea Berton (both at the Institute of Clinical Physiology – CNR Pisa) for the technical assistance.

References

1. Neisser, U.: Cognitive Psychology. Prentice-Hall, Englewood Cliffs (1967)
2. Fuster, J.M.: The prefrontal cortex—an update: time is of the essence. Neuron **30**(2), 319–333 (2001)
3. Anderson, P.: Assessment and development of executive function (EF) during childhood. Child Neuropsychol. **8**(2), 71–82 (2002)
4. Gioia, G.A., Isquith, P.K., Guy, S.C., Kenworthy, L.: Test review behavior rating inventory of executive function. Child Neuropsychol. **6**(3), 235–238 (2000)
5. Parsons, T.D., et al.: Sex differences in mental rotation and spatial rotation in a virtual environment. Neuropsychologia **42**(4), 555–562 (2004)
6. Parsons, T.D., Bowerly, T., Buckwalter, J.G., Rizzo, A.A.: A controlled clinical comparison of attention performance in children with ADHD in a virtual reality classroom compared to standard neuropsychological methods. Child Neuropsychol. **13**(4), 363–381 (2007)
7. Parsons, T.D., Rizzo, A.A.: Initial validation of a virtual environment for assessment of memory functioning: virtual reality cognitive performance assessment test. Cyber Psychol. Behav. **11**(1), 17–25 (2008)
8. Neguţ, A., Matu, S.A., Sava, F.A., David, D.: Virtual reality measures in neuropsychological assessment: a meta-analytic review. Clin. Neuropsychol. **30**(2), 165–184 (2016)
9. Armstrong, C.M., Reger, G.M., Edwards, J., Rizzo, A.A., Courtney, C.G., Parsons, T.D.: Validity of the Virtual Reality Stroop Task (VRST) in active duty military. J. Clin. Exp. Neuropsychol. **35**(2), 113–123 (2013)
10. Elkind, J.S., Rubin, E., Rosenthal, S., Skoff, B., Prather, P.: A simulated reality scenario compared with the computerized Wisconsin Card Sorting Test: an analysis of preliminary results. Cyber Psychol. Behav. **4**(4), 489–496 (2001)
11. Lalonde, G., Henry, M., Drouin-Germain, A., Nolin, P., Beauchamp, M.H.: Assessment of executive function in adolescence: a comparison of traditional and virtual reality tools. J. Neurosci. Methods **219**(1), 76–82 (2013)
12. Wolbers, T., Weiller, C., Büchel, C.: Neural foundations of emerging route knowledge in complex spatial environments. Cogn. Brain. Res. **21**(3), 401–411 (2004)
13. Matheis, R.J., Schultheis, M.T., Tiersky, L.A., DeLuca, J., Millis, S.R., Rizzo, A.: Is learning and memory different in a virtual environment? Clin. Neuropsychologist. **21**(1), 146–161 (2007)
14. Morganti, F.: Virtual interaction in cognitive neuropsychology. Stud. Health Technol. Inform. **99**, 55–70 (2004)
15. Gould, N.F., et al.: Performance on a virtual reality spatial memory navigation task in depressed patients. Am. J. Psychiatry **164**(3), 516–519 (2007)
16. Wilson, B.A.: Ecological validity of neuropsychological assessment: Do neuropsychological indexes predict performance in everyday activities? Appl. Prevent. Psychol. **2**(4), 209–215 (1993)
17. Schultheis, M.T., Himelstein, J., Rizzo, A.A.: Virtual reality and neuropsychology: upgrading the current tools. J. Head Trauma Rehabil. **17**(5), 378–394 (2002)

18. Hogervorst, M.A., Brouwer, A.M., Van Erp, J.B.: Combining and comparing EEG, peripheral physiology and eye-related measures for the assessment of mental workload. Front. Neurosci. **8**, 322 (2014)

19. Reis, P., Hebenstreit, F., Gabsteiger, F., von Tscharner, V., Lochmann, M.: Methodological aspects of EEG and body dynamics measurements during motion. Front. Hum. Neurosci. **8**, 156 (2014)

20. Benedek, M., Kaernbach, C.: A continuous measure of phasic electrodermal activity. J. Neurosci. Methods **190**(1), 80–91 (2010)

21. St-Laurent, L., Prévost, D., and Maldague, X.: Fast and accurate calibration-based thermal/colour sensors registration. In: Quantitative Infrared Thermography (2010)

22. van Dooren, M., Janssen, J.H.: Emotional sweating across the body: comparing 16 different skin conductance measurement locations. Physiol. Behav. **106**(2), 298–304 (2012)

23. Holz, C., Wang, E.J.: Glabella: continuously sensing blood pressure behavior using an unobtrusive wearable device. Proc. ACM Interact. Mob. Wearable Ubiquit. Technol. **1**(3), 58 (2017)

24. Shastri, D., Merla, A., Tsiamyrtzis, P., Pavlidis, I.: Imaging facial signs of neurophysiological responses. IEEE Trans. Biomed. Eng. **56**(2), 477–484 (2009)

25. Abdelrahman, Y., Velloso, E., Dingler, T., Schmidt, A., Vetere, F.: Cognitive heat: exploring the usage of thermal imaging to unobtrusively estimate cognitive load. Proc. ACM Interact. Mob. Wearable Ubiquit. Technol. **1**(3), 33 (2017)

26. Mueller, S.T., Piper, B.J.: The psychology experiment building language (PEBL) and PEBL test battery. J. Neurosci. Methods **222**, 250–259 (2014)

Patient Monitoring and Assessment of ICT Solutions

The Design of a Holistic mHealth Community Library Model and Its Impact on Empowering Rural America

Guy C. Hembroff$^{(\boxtimes)}$, Daniel Boyle, and Timothy Van Wagner

Michigan Technological University, Houghton, MI 49931, USA
{hembroff,dboyle,tavanwag}@mtu.edu

Abstract. Healthcare delivery in rural America poses additional challenges than its urban counterpart. Rural locations more commonly face shortage of physicians, a lack of high-paying jobs with adequate insurance benefits, transportation, health literacy, a stigma with health conditions due to lack of anonymity and difficulties accessing specialty care. Rural communities see higher rates of suicide, heart diseases, respiratory disease, stroke, social isolation, and public health crisis such as the opioid epidemic. More than 46 million Americans, or 15% of the population, live in rural areas within the United States.

Communities play an important role in the health of their residents, as social and economic factors, physical environment, and healthy behaviors make up 80% of an individual's overall health, while clinical care accounts for only 20%. Chronic disease doesn't occur in isolation. Conditions such as diabetes, asthma, heart disease, and obesity are all tied very closely to the environments, culture, and behaviors that surround individuals. Therefore, a significant amount of human health is determined beyond clinical care. For many individuals who are at an elevated risk of developing chronic disease, episodic care that begins and ends inside a hospital or clinic is not adequate to accurately treat the patient.

We propose a holistic mHealth community model for residents to overcome significant barriers of care in rural America by providing an application capable of integrating multiple health and safety data sources through a mobile digital personal health library application. Users are able to securely share their health data with others (e.g. primary care physician, caregiver). Artificial Intelligence (AI) algorithms can strategically connect residents to community resources and provide customized health education aimed at increasing the health literacy, empowerment, and self-management of the user. Communities can use de-identified population health data from this model to improve decision-making and allocation of community resources.

Keywords: Interoperability · Machine learning · Personal health library · Medical privacy and security

© ICST Institute for Computer Sciences, Social Informatics and Telecommunications Engineering 2020
Published by Springer Nature Switzerland AG 2020. All Rights Reserved
G. M. P. O'Hare et al. (Eds.): MobiHealth 2019, LNICST 320, pp. 97–111, 2020.
https://doi.org/10.1007/978-3-030-49289-2_8

1   Introduction

Healthcare delivery in rural America poses additional challenges than its urban counterpart. Rural locations more commonly face shortage of physicians, a lack of high-paying jobs with adequate insurance benefits, transportation, health literacy, a stigma with health conditions due to lack of anonymity and difficulties accessing specialty care [1]. Rural communities see higher rates of suicide, heart diseases, respiratory disease, stroke, social isolation, and public health crisis, such as the opioid epidemic [2]. More than 46 million Americans, or 15% of the population, live in rural areas within the United States [3].

Communities play an important role in the health of their residents, as social and economic factors, physical environment, and healthy behaviors make up 80% of an individual's overall health, while clinical care accounts for only 20% [4]. Chronic disease doesn't occur in isolation. Conditions such as diabetes, asthma, heart disease, and obesity are all tied very closely to the environments, culture, and behaviors that surround individuals [5]. Therefore, as a significant amount of human health is determined beyond clinical care for many individuals who are at an elevated risk of developing chronic disease, episodic care that begins and ends inside a hospital or clinic is not adequate to accurately treat the patient. Advanced technologies aimed to significantly lower these barriers of care provide an opportunity for a substantial positive impact in rural healthcare.

Past work has investigated the association of patient empowerment with improved health [6], and the negative impact of powerlessness [7]. According to work conducted by Shulz and Nakamoto, they found patient empowerment to be desirable due to three variables stemming from traditional thought [8]. First, the increase of personal autonomy in patients regarding decisions made in their health. Second, there is a growing interest in patient empowerment with the view that citizens should participate and take responsibility for their health care in efforts to help control healthcare costs [9]. Third, patient empowerment is advocated as improving health outcomes [10]. The increase in patient empowerment is also linked to increasing one's health literacy, which carries the potential to not only positively affect the individual, but also the community. An example of a lack of health literacy can be seen in the refusal of parents to vaccinate their children against infectious diseases, leading to serious health consequences for not only the child but also the community. By improving the mechanisms in which users feel empowered in managing their health, while simultaneously providing enhanced health literacy knowledge and the communication within the environment in which they live, health outcomes can be improved for individuals and the community population as a whole.

We propose a holistic mHealth community library model to overcome significant barriers of care in rural America by proposing a solution capable of coordinating data for a user's physical health, behavioral health, social and economic factors information, healthy behaviors, and physical environment information. Our proposed model permits users to securely share their health data with others (e.g. primary care physician, caregiver). Communities can use de-identified population health data from this model to improve decision-making and allocation of community resources. The model also serves as an open-source platform to develop tools for accurate assessment of individuals or populations in areas such as disease progression, risk stratification, care management, biosurvelillance, telemedicine, etc. Machine learning algorithms can be developed to accomplish many of these tasks, including to strategically connect residents to community resources and provide customized health education aimed at increasing the health literacy, empowerment, and self-management of the user.

2 Related Work

Over recent years, discussions having been prevalent regarding research and development of patient facing applications with the ability to exchange health information and improve the self-management an individual's health. This ecosystem has seen self-interest and participation from both commercial organizations and academic institutions.

Commercially, an importance has been placed on providing the patient with their own data and its impact to improve health outcomes, literacy, engagement and empowerment. The field continues to attract more developers to this space, including large and well-known commercial companies. Apple Health Records API for example, permits users to aggregate health data where the company has established partnerships with EHR vendors and health providers to allow patients to store their health records collectively [11].

Academically, there exists numerous papers describing the need and theoretical elements of such a model for patients to access their health data and descriptions of the value of incorporating patient generated health data (PGHD) within this system [12–14]. However, we could find no publications that present a holistic mHealth community library model, containing inclusive data surrounding the integration and mapping of health data from multiple sources, identity management provisions, privacy protections, and proposed scalability methods.

3 Background: Integrated Data Source Health Information Exchange and Security

Interoperability, security, and privacy has been widely recognized as an integral requirement for the success of healthcare information exchange. While linking data across various sources within a health system is a challenge, added complexity results when integrating data from multiple systems and devices. Creating an architecture capable of successful interoperability, security, and privacy delivers economic value and more importantly a form of patient safety, as the clinical value of information is enhanced when the best information is available for treating patients [15]. To help ensure a consistency and interoperability of health data, the United States' federal government has taken steps over the past decade to outline requirements and standards in third-party platforms which are critical in the development of proposed models such as ours.

3.1   Interoperability

The Health Information Technology for Economic and Clinical Health (HITECH) Act of 2009 presented incentives for providers to invest in EHRs with a defined minimal set of standards, known as Meaningful Use (MU), in which incentive payments would offset a substantial part of the cost of these systems. As a result, EHR adoption with MU standards exceeds 97% of the United States' hospitals and 74% in physician practices [16]. Stipulations from MU encouraged interoperability between systems along with patient access to their medical records. MU was developed in three stages. The first required patients seen by a provider within a reporting period to have access to an electronic clinical summary in a reasonable amount of time. The second stage required patients to have the ability to view, download, or transmit their health information to a third party. The third and current stage, requires patients to have the ability to connect third-party applications to their medical records through Application Programming Interface (API) technology. APIs are a tool for software appliations to communicate with EHRs and other sources of health data [17]. The 21st Century Cures Act of 2016, extends interoperability further, as it "enables the secure exchange of electronic health information with, and use of electronic health information from, other health information technology without special effort on the part of the use" and provides an explicit API set of requirements for EHRs to obtain certification [18].

As a result of the 21st Centruy Cures Act, Health Level Seven (HL7) released the International Argonaut Project in 2017. The project included major EHR vendors who released industry-developed open APIs built on HL7's latest version called Fast Healthcare Interoperability Resources (FHIR). Shortly after, the U.S. Department of Veterans Administration, along with a consortium of providers and vendors, signed the Open API pledge to expand the set of data resources available to patients, physicians, and care teams through APIs standardized by the HL7 Argonaut Project.

The Office of the National Coordinator (ONC) for Health IT is responsible for EHR certification criteria, which includes requirements for APIs. The ONC's Common Clinical Data Set (CCDS) includes 21 data fields for clinical data, such as demographics, medication lists, lab results, and problem lists [19]. The CCDS does not currently include key data, such as provider notes, imaging, appointment information and cost or payment information.

3.2   Security

Data security and patient privacy requirements for health provider organizations is fairly well-known. While implementation may have more degrees of freedom, the specific laws and regulations, such as HIPAA, are more clear. However, when patients are able to obtain and store their own health information outside of the provider organization, security regulations and monitoring are not as clear. As an example, HIPAA's privacy rule does not include consumer applications, social media, fitness trackers.

With patient's authorized release of their digital health data from the EHRs of provider organizations to third-party applications, the provider organizations relinquish liability to secure, monitor, and audit that data. Many health applications struggle to have consistent security and privacy policies. And some have no policies regarding privacy of data. While this is problematic even in cases where the patient's data is an isolated subset of their health, such as a BlueTooth glucose monitoring application for a diabetic user, this problem gets much worse when patient health data from varying sources is integrated, with the aim of providing a longitudinal record of the patient. Therefore, it is critical, not only for security and privacy, but also for data accuracy, that a robust, secure, and scalable identity management solution is used to ensure security and privacy, monitoring, and auditing of user's data.

4   Model Design and Development

In this section we describe the proposed model, its architecture and its elements of health data exchange, interoperability, security and access. We then provide a discussion regarding the model's replication to other communities within the United States.

4.1   Proposed Methodology in Overcoming Barriers to Care in Rural Health

To help overcome barriers of care we link challenges in rural healthcare to one's health factors. This overlapping of health factors to the challenges of rural health care in Fig. 1, illustrate the importance of providing a platform which can holistically offer health and safety information to the patient and the community.

Data integration, including information regarding a user's health behaviors, physical environment, clinical care, PGHD, and social and economic factors, are key in holistically assessing the user and determining correct course of action. Figure 2 depicts the application's holistic approach to health and safety data integration.

Our model creates a personal health library (PHL) for each resident who downloads and registers with the application. A individual's PHL connects the user to their different data sources of care via secure APIs to retrieve information. For health factors which do not contain previously stored information, such as healthy behaviors and social determinants of health for example, the application requests this information using straight-forward questions. Users are provided the opportunity and are encouraged to update this information as needed.

Participating community health organizations, such as provider organizations, police and fire, food banks, shelters, and local public health departments, are able to keep residents updated on available education and resources, such as free screenings for breast cancer and dental, fire safety and workshops regarding healthy eating on a budget. Participating health and safety organizations are able to review HIPAA compliant de-identified data within this model to better

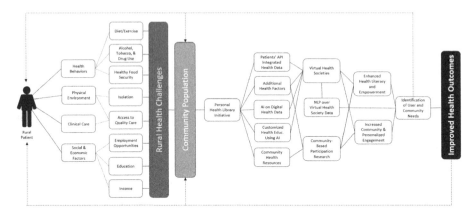

Fig. 1. Rural health challenges and Roadmap to solve these challenges through mHealth community library model

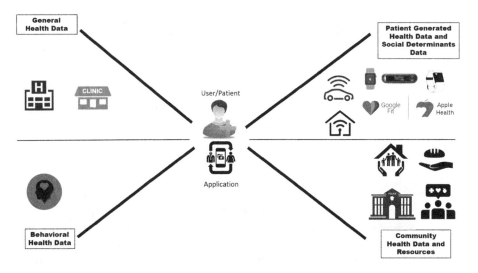

Fig. 2. Coordination of health and safety information for community residents

understand the community population, helping to better utilize their resources and meet the needs of its residents.

AI techniques, such as machine learning, can be used on the collected data to provide insightful information. We have begun developing customized health education algorithms that utilize the National Library of Medicine's MedlinePlus API [20] to provide customized health and safety education reflective of each user's collected data.

4.2   Data Coordination and Interoperability

The open-source mHealth community-centered library application consists of an interoperable backend database server structure to ensure the organization and security of user's health data, and a front-end application server, available as a mobile application and web interface for users to access, share, analyze, and select which data sources they wish to include within their PHL. Figure 3 depicts an example community architecture.

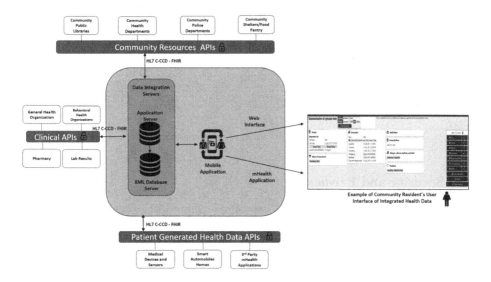

Fig. 3. mHealth community library architecture example

Interoperability exists through within the open-source eXist backend extensible markup language (XML) database mapping mechanism we have developed. Health and safety information received from the APIs or directly from the application's user front-end (e.g. social determinants of health) are placed into the individual's secure table where XML transform algorithms are able to tag each document header to establish accurate mapping of data and ensuring interoperability. Data stemming from the clinical APIs are in the form of Continuity of Care Document(CCD), as most EHRs are required to produce a CCD. An example CCD in raw form can be seen in Fig. 4.

FHIR has emerged as the standard mHealth applications and EHRs are now working to be in compliance with this standard. Scripts were created within the eXist database to map CCD data into the new FHIR standard using guidelines provided by the ONC's CCDS, allowing user's to see an organized, readable, and user-friendly interfaces of their data and providing them the capability to gain much more insight through the development of software tools to accomplish such tasks as customized education, drug to drug alerts, medication adherence reminders, and local community resources available to them.

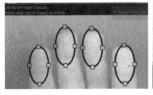

Fig. 4. Example continuity of care document in Raw format

4.3 Security and Privacy

Security and privacy elements have been implemented to protect the confidentiality and integrity of user's data. While authorization and access to the application can be achieved using standard username and strong passwords, there is an option to use biometrics as part of the identify management within the application. The lead author of this paper has developed a biometric solution called Unique Medical Biometric Recognition of Legitimate and Large-scale Authentication (U.M.B.R.E.L.L.A.), which developed an algorithm over touchless fingerprints to produce and secure a unique health identifier (UHID) for each individual [21]. Facial recognition is then used as the second factor of identification. As a result, usernames and passwords are not required but can still be used if needed. Figure 5 demonstrates using UMRELLA's biometric solution within the application for identity management. The UHID for an individual has a the potential to be cross-matched to the internal master patient identifier (MPI) of a healthcare organization, enhancing the accuracy of identifying the correct patient's data, while also increasing the efficiency of exchanging data. It can be used on most devices(e.g. smart phones, tablets, PCs, laptops) with cameras as it is hardware agnostic.

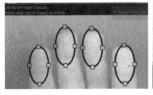
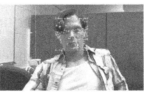

Fig. 5. UMBRELLA's biometric identifcation solution

User information, its privacy, and integrity are managed through attribute-based access control (ABAC), which consists of an authorization policy engine and a RESTful authorization server. The Java API provides an extensible control markup language (XACML) policy decision point (PDP) engine, while the Web API uses an HTTP/REST API and PDP and policy administration points (PAPs) to manage policies and request authorization decisions. Throughout this architecture, access and control is enforced to establish strong user authorization and authentication techniques to achieve security and privacy of user data. To accomplish this, we incorporate elements of open-source AuthZForce into our solution [22].

5   Experimental Setup

To test the model, we established a front-end interface and used the architecture design illustrated in Fig. 3 to assess the application's functionality. We used a variety of servers and virtual machines to simulate both physical and cloud attributes and their respective API connections to the data sources. A view of the application's front-end graphical user interface can be seen in Fig. 6. Bluetooth blood pressure cuffs and smartwatches were used, along with a mhealth mood tracker smartphone application to simulate patient generated health data. Test CCD documents were added to simulate the clinical environment. Users testing the system completed social and economic determinants of health, environmental factors, and health behavior questions upon downloading and logging into the application for the first time. A total of 50 participants were asked to test the system and complete a user satisfaction survey after ten hours of use.

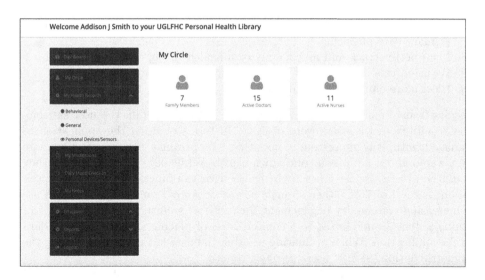

Fig. 6. Application Front-End displaying User's Secure sharing of Health information they wish to share in the MyCircle feature

The population of users testing the system were between the ages of 19 years and 72 years. Ten were primary care physicians, ten were population health quality improvement (QI) personnel, and thirty were students associated with the university where the study was being conducted and used to simulate patients. All participants evaluated the model's application from a *patient's perspective*. Additionally, primary care physicians and population health QI personnel provided feedback regarding their respective roles in the clinical field.

6   Results and Discussion

To determine users' satisfaction with various aspects of this model's application, we asked all 50 respondents, in the role of patients, to indicate their level of agreement or disagreement with each of the following 10 general functionality statements, using the scale Strongly Agree, Agree, Neutral, Disagree, and Strongly Disagree. Below are the patient survey statements used:

1. The mHealth Library Community Model application is easy and intuitive to use.
2. I felt comfortable with choosing from the list of available API connections to link the test application's health data.
3. The method of obtaining a patient's social and economic factors, physical environment, and healthy behaviors data was reasonable.
4. I would feel comfortable with my own health data on this platform.
5. I like having a choice of using biometrics and not having to use usernames and passwords.
6. I feel my data is more secure using biometric authentication and authorization.
7. I would use the share data functionality to share my health data with my primary care physician.
8. I can better track and manage my own health through this application.
9. By using this application, I feel more engaged in community health.
10. I feel more empowered in addressing my health using this application.

Results from the survey are summarized in Table 1. Overall, the user satisfaction results from the users were positive. In terms of using the application to manage health, it is interesting to note that 72% *Strongly Agreed* in feeling more empowered about addressing one's own health. While 62% *Strongly Agreed* they would be able to better track their health with the functionality of this application. A total of 76% either *strongly agreed* or *Agreed* on the application's use of increasing community engagement. In terms of security, a combined 58% of *Strongly Agreed* and *Agreed* to a comfort level of placing their own health data on the application. When evaluating whether the user felt more secure using the biometric option, 88% of users *Strongly Agreed*.

Primary care physicians were asked to complete an additional physician users' satisfaction survey, using the scale Strongly Agree, Agree, Neutral, Disagree, and Strongly Disagree. Below are the physician survey statements used:

1. As a physician, the application is intuitive in letting me see my patients' data.
2. I trust data from other sources.
3. Having data from other health factors, beyond clinical care, is important to holistically diagnose and treat the patient.
4. Patients using this application will be better aware of community health and safety resources available to them.
5. This application will help patients better self-manage their health.

Results from the survey are summarized in Table 2. Primary care physician user satisfaction was overall positive. In the category of using other health factor data (i.e. environmental, social and economic, and healthy behaviors), 80% of physicians *Strong Agreed*. This reinforces the problematic nature of only using clinical care data to diagnose and treat patients. Reflecting on this application's ability for patients to better self-manage their health, 70% *Strongly Agreed* while 20% *Agreed*. An area of concern is the overall trust of data from other sources. 40% of responses were either *Disagree* or *Strongly Disagree*, signaling there is still much work to be done in this domain to provide physicians confidence in using data from other sources.

Table 1. Patient satisfaction survey results by percentages.

Patients' Survey Statements Abbreviated	Strongly Agree % $N = 50$	Agree % $N = 50$	Neutral % $N = 50$	Disagree % $N = 50$	Strongly Disagree % $N = 50$
1. Easy and intuitive	28%	44%	26%	2%	
2. Comfort level connecting data	36%	28%	22%	10%	4%
3. Reasonable time to obtain additional health factors	32%	38%	26%	4%	
4. Comfort level with placing own health data on system	22%	36%	38%	2%	2%
5. Like choice of biometric security	68%	18%	12%		2%
6. Feel biometric option is more secure	88%	8%	4%	2%	
7. Use share option	54%	32%	8%	2%	4%
8. Better track own health	62%	24%	8%	6%	
9. Increased engagement in community health	34%	42%	16%	6%	2%
10. More empowered in addressing my health	72%	24%	2%		2%

Table 2. Physician satisfaction survey results by percentages.

Physicians' Survey Statements Abbreviated	Strongly Agree % N = 10	Agree % N = 10	Neutral % N = 10	Disagree % N = 10	Strongly Disagree % N = 10
1. Appliacation is intuitive	10	70%	10%	10%	
2. Trust data from other sources	20%	30%	10%	20%	20%
3. Patient data beyond clinical care is importent	80%	10%		10%	
4. Improved patient awareness of community health and safety resources	30%	40%	20%		10%
5. Improve patient self-management of health	70%	20%	10%		

Finally, we asked population health QI personnel to complete an additional user satisfaction survey pertaining to the model's evaluation in population health,using the scale Strongly Agree, Agree, Neutral, Disagree, and Strongly Disagree. Below are the population health QI personnel survey statements used:

1. Data from this application provides strong potential to improve community population health monitoring.
2. I would trust data from this application in population health assessment.
3. Data from this application will provide an enhanced mechanism in planning and distributing community health and safety resources.
4. This application's data will improve defining strategic public health initiatives in our community.
5. This application can provide improved methods of communication for public health emergencies.

Survey results reflect a an optimistic outlook on use of the model to improve community population health. QI personnel, like physicians, responded with similar concerns regarding the trust of data from other sources for population health assessment with 20% who *Disagree* and 10% who *Strongly Disagree*. Users reported 70% in the category of *Strongly Agree* the model's use of improving community health and safety initiatives, and 40% of *Strongly Agree* in improving the communication of public health emergencies to citizens (Table 3).

Table 3. Population Health QI Personnel satisfaction survey results by percentages.

Population Health Qls' Survey Statements Abbreviated	Strongly Agree % $N = 10$	Agree % $N = 10$	Neutral % $N = 10$	Disagree % $N = 10$	Strongly Disagree % $N = 10$
1. Improved view of community population health	30%	20%	30%	20%	
2. Trust data for population health assessment	20%	40%	10%	20%	10%
3. Enhanced mechanism for community health and safety	40%	30%	20%	10%	
4. Improve community health and safety initiatives	70%	20%	10%		
5. Improve methods of communicating public health emergencies	40%	30%	20%	10%	

7   Conclusion

In this work we presented the design and testing of a mHealth community library model to assist in overcoming barriers to care in rural America and to empower residents and their community to better manage their health and safety. Innovative methods of data retrieval, interoperability, security and privacy were discussed. Development of the model was done using open-source software, helping this model to be replicated in other communities. Patients, primary care providers, and population health QI personnel reported overall positive experiences using the model's application. Specifically, a high percentage of patients felt empowered to track and manage their health, while also increasing their community engagement. A large percentage of physicians surveyed felt health factor information, beyond clinical care, was important to treating and diagnosing patients and that patients would overall benefit in the self-management of their health. Clinical personnel associated with population health QI were favorable to the application's potential to improve communication of health emergencies and community health and safety initiatives. The highest concern from the survey results was trust of outside data sources.

8   Future Work

Due to the responses regarding trust of health data resulting from other sources, one initiative of future work is to investigate methods which can be used to validate data to the users of the system. Since there remains a significant percentage of the population of both rural and urban environments that do not have access to technology, such as smartphones, computers, or Internet access, this model and its application does not directly help them. As almost 96% of America's population has close proximity to public libraries, which are typically equipped with technology to access a mHealth application such as ours. We feel there is a tremendous opportunity to provide an access point to those who do not have this technology through the public library medium. Our future work, includes working with the National Library of Medicine and public libraries to create an initiative to provide this service to communities across the nation.

References

1. Syed, S.: Traveling towards disease: transportation barriers to health care access. J. Community Health **38**(5), 976–993 (2013)
2. HHS Website Article. https://www.hhs.gov/blog/2017/04/03/public-health-crisis-suicide-and-opioids.html. Accessed 4 Mar 2019
3. US Census Bureau, New census data show differences between urban and rural populations. United States Census Bureau (2016)
4. Braveman, P.: The social determinants of health: it's time to consider the causes of the causes. J. Public Health Rep. **129**(1), 19–31 (2014)
5. Health Analytics Website Article. https://healthitanalytics.com/features/combating-chronic-disease-through-the-social-determinants-of-health. Accessed 13 April 2019
6. Bergsma, L.J.: Empowerment education-the link between media literacy and health promotion. Am. Behavior Sci. **48**, 152–164 (2004)
7. Wallerstein, N.: Powerlessness, empowerment, and health: implications for health promotion programs. Am. J. Health Promot. **6**(3), 197–205 (1992)
8. Schultz, P.: Health literacy and patient empowerment in health communication: the importance of separating conjoined twins. Patient Educ. Counsel. **90**(1), 4–11 (2013)
9. Neuhauser, D.: The coming third health care revolution: personal empowerment. Qual. Manage. Health Care **12**, 171–184 (2003)
10. Edwards, D.: What are the external influences on infomration exchange and shared decision-making in healthcare consultations: a meta-synthesis of the literature. Patient education and counseling 75, 37–52 (2009)
11. Apple Health home page. https://www.apple.com/healthcare/health-records/. Accessed 28 Mar 2019
12. Rajput, Z.: Evaluation of an Android-based mHealth system for population surveillance in developing countries. J. Am. Med. Inform. Assoc. **19**(4), 655–659 (2012)
13. Masys, D.: Giving patients access to their medical records via the internet: the PCASSO experience. J. Am. Med. Inform. Assoc. **9**(2), 181–191 (2002)
14. Reti, S.: Improving personal health records for patient-centered care. J. Am. Med. Inform. Assoc. **17**(2), 192–195 (2010)
15. Walker, J.: The value of health care information exchange and interoperability. J. Health Affairs **24**(1), 5–10 (2005)
16. The Office of the National Coordinator for Health Information Technology. http://dashboard.healthit.gov. Accessed 22 Dec 2018
17. United States Federal Register. http://dashboard.healthit.gov. Accessed 28 Dec 2018

18. Gabay, M.: 21 century cures act. J. Hospital Pharmacy **52**(4), 264–265 (2017)
19. The Office of the National Coordinator for Health Information Technology. https://www.healthit.gov/sites/default/files/draft-uscdi.pdf. Accessed 28 Dec 2018
20. National Library of Medicine Medline. https://medlineplus.gov/. Accessed 5 Jan 2019
21. Hembroff, G.: Improving patient safety, health data accuracy, and remote self-management of health through the establishment of a biometric-based global UHID. Promise New Technol. Age New Health Chall. **42** (2016)
22. AuthZForce. https://authzforce.ow2.org. Accessed 15 Feb 2019

Stop Anxiety: Tackling Anxiety in the Academic Campus Through an mHealth Multidisciplinary User-Centred Approach

David Ferreira[1], Daniela Melo[3], Andreia Santo[3], Pedro Silva[3],
Sandra C. Soares[3,4], and Samuel Silva[1,2(✉)]

[1] DETI – Department of Electronics, Telecommunication and Informatics
Engineering, University of Aveiro, Aveiro, Portugal
sss@ua.pt
[2] IEETA – Institute of Electronics and Informatics Engineering of Aveiro,
University of Aveiro, Aveiro, Portugal
[3] DEP – Department of Education and Psychology, University of Aveiro,
Aveiro, Portugal
[4] William James Center for Research, University of Aveiro, Aveiro, Portugal

Abstract. Anxiety-related disorders have a strong impact on our quality of life. With their epidemiological prevalence, across the population, highly exceeding the capacity for treatment in health facilities, new ways of delivering therapies are needed. The wide availability of mobile technologies, e.g., smartphones, has provided an accessible and ubiquitous platform for delivering psychological therapies and many mobile health (mHealth) systems have been proposed to support users in managing their levels of anxiety. However, many of the available tools provide features without evidence-based support of their adequateness and effectiveness. Furthermore, several tools are designed without specifically considering the users' needs and motivations, resulting in poor adherence or a lack of motivation for systematic use, hindering any positive effects.

Considering the need to more closely focus on the motivations of the target users, this article describes how the efforts of a multidisciplinary team are contributing to support a user-centred approach to design and develop a tool to support anxiety management in the context of an Academic Campus. As a first materialization of this ongoing work, a proof-of-concept application is proposed (StopAnxiety), developed by adopting an iterative approach, and already providing a set of clinician-approved anxiety management techniques.

Keywords: Anxiety · mHealth · Mental health

1 Introduction

The prevalence of mental health disorders across the population has been rising at an alarming rate, having an impact not only in people's lives, but striking a

© ICST Institute for Computer Sciences, Social Informatics and Telecommunications Engineering 2020
Published by Springer Nature Switzerland AG 2020. All Rights Reserved
G. M. P. O'Hare et al. (Eds.): MobiHealth 2019, LNICST 320, pp. 112–126, 2020.
https://doi.org/10.1007/978-3-030-49289-2_9

major hit in worldwide economy. One of the main reasons of this economy burden is the fact that mental health disorders are not an isolated problem, being in many cases, the cause of diseases in other medical areas, such as cardiology [11].

Considering the spectrum of mental health illnesses, anxiety is one of the most common, having a stronger impact on disability and impairment than many chronic medical disorders [12,16,24]. Apart from those that are diagnosed with pathological cases of anxiety, healthy individuals also feel the impact of anxiety on their daily activities, their relationships, and their general mood [5,11,14]. Even though several mental health therapies have already been developed to deal with this issue, many individuals suffering from anxiety disorders do not have access to them, in health facilities, either because they cannot afford it or because of the effects that are inherent to their condition, such as the lack of emotional self-awareness (not allowing them to express what they are feeling since they cannot figure it out by themselves) or the fear of social contexts [12,16]. Nevertheless, even disregarding these considerations, with the growing epidemiological prevalence of anxiety-related disorders, it would not be possible for the health services to provide face-to-face therapy to those in need. Thus, the proposal of methods that could help individuals manage and reduce their own anxiety, in a more independent manner, is of the utmost relevance.

Mobile technologies have provided a promising platform to support people in a wide variety of contexts and mobile Health (mHealth) tools have been proposed to help people in various scenarios, improving their awareness about their condition, providing continuous support, and fostering independent living. In this regard, mHealth approaches for anxiety management have also been proposed. However, while there is a wide range of such tools, most of them are proposed without involving users in their design, providing therapies that lack scientific grounds and evidence of efficacy, and failing to engage users for a long-term use.

To propose novel approaches and methods to tackle these issues, we adopt a multidisciplinary user-centered approach to the design and development of a novel anxiety management system—StopAnxiety—,by working with psychology professionals and potential users and by putting a strong effort in understanding user motivations and in providing evidence-based practises. Without loss of generality, and considering the prominence that anxiety has in the academic context, we consider students and teachers as the targeted audience.

The remainder of this document is organized as follows: Sect. 2 provides a brief overview of current work regarding the proposal of support systems to tackle anxiety; Sect. 3 describes the work carried out to identify the needs and motivations of several users dealing with anxiety, in an Academic Campus; Sect. 4 provides an overview of the accomplished iterative design and development of StopAnxiety, a proof-of-concept mHealth application for anxiety management; finally, Sect. 5 presents overall conclusions and provides several ideas for future work.

2   Mobile Applications for Anxiety Management

With a wide spectrum of available technologies with potential to support anxiety management [9], smartphones have been the main choice due to their high ownership rates (+2 billion owners worldwide), and to the fact that they consist in a portable, ubiquitous and fairly accessible platform [2].

Regarding mental health, several applications have been proposed to provide different levels of support, such as exposure exercises, progressively exposing users to their inner fears, psycho-educational, where the users learn about the existing disorders and how to deal with them, at an early stage, or those suggesting psychological intervention techniques, through which users can manage and reduce their own anxiety levels by performing exercises.

To gather an overall view of the most recent and best considered mobile apps for tackling anxiety, based on community feedback, a review of anxiety management applications was conducted. From the reviewed apps, it was possible to verify that most of them were developed targeting any age, apart from FearFigther [8], WhatsMyM3 [10], Happify and WoeBot [9] that specifically targeted adult individuals. Most of the reviewed apps considered cognitive behavioural therapy principles [1,3,7], one of the most common and best studied forms of psychotherapy, as the base of their proposed interventions. Related to how important the usability factor is, in order to engage the user until the conclusion of the treatment, many features were considered by the reviewed apps, such as in WoeBot [9], where a chatbot is used for the interaction and treatment delivery process, and ThisWayUp, where a comic book style approach is explored. Two positive aspects that were observed, were that all of the reviewed apps, except for AnxietyCoach, were validated in studies regarding their effectiveness, and that all of them proposed therapies that were supported on scientific evidence. However, one of the main problems is that, even though all the apps that were assessed involved a domain expert, in their design and development phase, most of them disregard both the involvement of the patient, and the possibility of communication with the health provider through the application. Additionally, while the reviewed applications are well recognized by the community, adherence continues to be an issue. And the panorama beyond these top applications rapidly gets worse, in a number of aspects, even for those that are commercially available.

Overall, the general conclusion is that even though mHealth applications have an incredible potential for granting additional access to mental health care, there is a significant gap between their commercial availability and the data regarding their efficacy and effectiveness. In this regard, several challenges can be identified:

– **Inappropriate treatments and Lack of Evidence**—One of the most common problems amongst the majority of the commercially available applications for tackling anxiety is the wrong suggestion of treatments, being most of them inappropriate and not even scientifically proven. This is a serious problem that needs to be dealt with since it could actually worsen the health status of the users rather than bring them the health benefits they need [23];

- **Lack of adherence/User engagement**—User engagement is another aspect that should as well be accounted for, since most users that look for these types of applications tend to download them and only use them for a few hours before uninstalling them. This can happen either because they feel that the application does not provide them with the satisfaction of use they desire or the health benefits they need. This way, many users do not use applications long enough to feel the benefits [17];
- **Lack of user involvement in establishing the requirements**—The disregard of the patients in the requirement elicitation phase is something that is very common to happen in the development of anxiety management systems (and mHealth applications, overall), generally due to how important time constrains and commercialization aspects are for the development companies. Unfortunately, this is not an isolated problem since it also has a negative impact in other aspects, such as user engagement and the appropriate proposal of treatments [18].
- **Application efficacy is not clear, and lack of long-term assessment**—Despite the evolution and widespread use of these mHealth apps, there is still a lack of data regarding their efficacy and effectiveness. Many are even released to the market categorized as medical aids, but lack any evidence of their impact [21].

3   Users, Context, and Requirements

The first stage of our work consisted on the identification and characterization of the potential users. To this end, a multidisciplinary team was formed, including psychologists, software, human-computer interaction, and mobile computing engineers, university teachers, and university students.

3.1   Personas

Personas depict fictional characters with the purpose of representing different user types that might use the application, and although they do not actually represent real people, they are based on real data collected from different individuals. These representation profiles can help the developing team to step out of themselves and recognize that different people may have different needs and expectations, allowing the team to focus their attention in what really needs to be designed and further developed, enabling users to properly achieve their own goals [6]. One additional advantage of using Personas, in this process, is that their narrative form helps on multidisciplinary dialogue, improving the outcomes of the discussions [22].

In a first stage, to characterize the users that could benefit from an anxiety management aid, in the academic campus scenario, the team resorted to a brainstorming session, grounded on the anxiety literature, and on the experience of the team elements, regarding anxiety issues in the academic context. The data collected in this session led to the identification of different target groups and

Table 1. Persona of Rute, an undergraduate student.

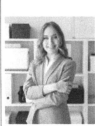

Rute is 20 years old and is currently completing the second year of her degree in Nursing, at the University of Aveiro. She spends much of her time studying for her exams, which is something that always made her very anxious. Although Rute spends a large part of her day trying to study, she often faces blockages that prevent her from progressing, eventually becoming even more anxious than she already is. Despite the adaptation struggles that Rute was faced with, in her first year of college, she still considers that the evaluation periods are the hardest. During her studies, and moments before the start of her exams, Rute normally begins to sweat from her hands, to tremble, and she feels an heavy chest. Sometimes, during the course of her exams, these symptoms are accompanied by blanks, which consequently prevent her from applying the knowledge she knows she has.

Image adapted from pxhere.

Motivation: Rute would like to get the grades that she so hardly worked for by learning how to deal with her anxiety attacks during the course of her exams.

initial versions of Personas were proposed. To further extend these first versions of the Personas, and to validate the initial team considerations, three focus groups were carried out: one with academy students, another with professors, and another with psychologists working with students suffering from anxiety. These discussions enabled a more accurate identification of user motivations and of the main aspects that triggered anxiety issues.

With all the data that was gathered, from both the focus groups and the team brainstorming sessions, five Personas were deemed relevant for a proper characterization of the context of the anxiety management tool to be developed: (a) three primary Personas for different college student profiles (first year students, students in evaluation periods, and students suffering from social anxiety); (b) one primary Persona for a university professor; and (c) one served Persona for a clinical psychologist. From those, and given their extent, only two are provided here, in more detail, for illustrative purposes: the Persona of Rute, an undergraduate student, mostly suffering from anxiety during evaluation periods (Table 1); and Carlos, the Persona of a college teacher (Table 2). Rute is an undergraduate student who is unable to obtain the desired academic performance due to the extreme anxiety she goes through during her evaluation periods. As such, she would like to learn about some possible techniques that would help her remain calm, especially, during times of greater stress. Carlos is a teacher whose main source of anxiety is his inability to manage its own schedule in an efficient way. As such, he would like to have a way to access relaxation techniques so he could relieve the stress of his daily life, and manage his schedule.

Table 2. Persona of Carlos, a University Professor.

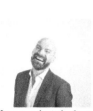

Image adapted from pxhere.

Carlos is a 47 year old college teacher who has taught at the University of Aveiro for 10 years. During his free time he enjoys doing activities, such as spending time with his children, traveling, going to the gym, reading the newspaper, and socializing with his family and friends. Typically, at the end of each day, due to the stress that comes from his work, he arrives home very tired. Carlos feels that he is overwhelmed by an immense amount of work, which occupies most of his time, and he feels his work is not valued enough.

Motivation: Carlos would like to learn about some techniques and procedures that could help him deal with his daily anxiety and stress, particularly in a way that could be available during is daily routines.

3.2   Context Scenarios

Context scenarios can be seen as a way to describe how the envisaged support system can be used to achieve a specific goal, in a certain context, and how it integrates the user's activities and for how long [6]. With this in mind, to perceive the different ways in which the anxiety management tool could be used, several context scenarios were developed. The scenarios were built based on the literature for the different ways to deal with anxiety (e.g., respiratory exercises), covering the contexts reported, by the users, during the focus groups and validated by clinicians to guarantee their validity and appropriateness. Although several context scenarios have been proposed to properly guide the development of the application, given their extent, and for the sake of brevity, only one of them is provided. This scenario represents a situation in which the application detects an increase of Rute's anxiety and proposes the execution of a diaphragmatic breathing exercise.

Rute performs diaphragmatic breathing a few moments before an exam—*The last exam of this semester will start in 15 min. Given the accumulation of tiredness, anxiety and study content that is required for this frequency, the application acknowledges that Rute is very anxious and consequently proposes the execution of a diaphragmatic breathing exercise, a technique that is frequently performed by Rute before any of her frequencies. Before the technique's initiation, the system asks Ruth to sit comfortably, and prepares her for a series of inspiration and expiration cycles. In order to facilitate the realization of this technique, the system emits vibratory signals, given that she is in a crowded and noisy place, so that Rute can feel and understand the transition of each breathing cycle. At the end of each breath, Rute feels more and more relaxed and confident to complete the exam. After the end of this frequency, the student verified that she did not have any brain fade during its course, and that she was capable of answering to all its questions.*

It is important to note that the vibratory alerts were selected instead of the audible ones due to the fact that Rute is in a public space. Also of note are the underlined parts of the scenario, highlighting relevant actions that the system will have to provide, i.e., the requirements.

3.3 Requirements

As a result of all the information gathered about the users, their motivations, and how the system should perform to help them, documented in the scenarios, a first list of requirements was established and is presented in Table 3. For each requirement, a priority level was defined, thus, providing the developers with a grasp on how to select them for the iterative development stages, as explained, ahead, in this document.

It is worth noting that, even after several development iterations, the evaluations that were carried out did not motivate changing any of these initially proposed requirements, but only the way in which they were being accomplished, which further confirmed the validity of the captured user necessities.

Table 3. Requirements subset

Prio.	Subset of elicited requirements
1	1. Implement relaxation techniques
	2. Identify users emotional states
	3. Create safe and highly available users data models
2	4. Allow time scheduling
	5. Present users progress statistics
	6. Adapt application to the user's context
	7. Learn about user preferences
3	8. Allow users to register their thoughts (wav, txt,...)
	9. Provide psychoeducation notifications throughout app usage
	10. Provide psychoeducation section for learning purposes
	11. Enable communication between patients and clinicians
	12. Enable communication among peers

4   Design and Development of StopAnxiety

An iterative User-Centered Design approach was considered for the development of the proposed anxiety management system. Considering the initial subset of requirements, several iterations were performed, and each of the developed prototypes was evaluated by users, resulting in a prototype deemed adequate to undergo first evaluations in more ecological settings. In what follows, we provide a summary of the various iterations carried out, to illustrate how the process evolved, and pay a more detailed attention to the current StopAnxiety version.

4.1   Low-Fidelity Prototype

Paper prototyping is a widely used method in user-centered design approaches, helping developers to prototype systems that meet their user's expectations and needs. Its great advantage is that it allows making quick and cheap changes to the prototype rather than to the system already developed. In light of these considerations, the initial step was to build a paper mockup of the interface layouts that would enable fulfilling the requirements. A few examples are depicted in Fig. 1.

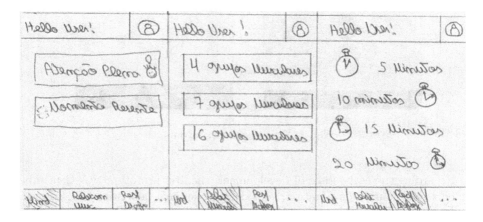

Fig. 1. Paper prototype example

The paper mockup was discussed in a brainstorming session including all elements of the multidisciplinary team, with overall good feedback about the devised approach. One of the suggested modifications concerned how the user's progress in the different activities would be presented. It was suggested that successful completion of exercises would result in advancing their score, but they would not be penalized for those they were not able (or did not want) to complete. So, at most, their stats would remain the same. By doing so, their motivation would not be negatively influenced and their progress would be continuous, although at a slower rate in case of unsuccessful usage.

4.2   First Functional Prototype

The first functional prototype implemented a refined version of the approved paper mockup, leaving out the full implementation of the exercises. The main goal was to have a first iteration of the overall interaction approach for a first usability evaluation. Figure 2 presents some illustrative screen layouts for this initial version.

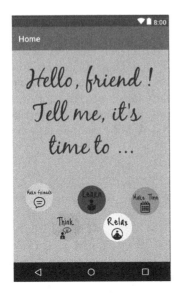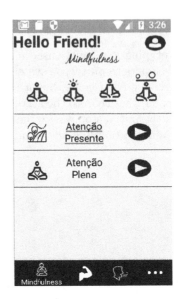

Fig. 2. First illustrative layouts

Regarding the early stage of development, the first prototype was then subjected to an heuristic evaluation, considering Nielsen's heuristics [19], so that potential usability problems could be detected and inform further developments. Five evaluators, three males and two females, aged between 22–24 years old, computer science students, with previous experience in applying heuristic evaluations, analyzed the prototype assessing each violation of the heuristics with a score from 0 (no usability problem) to 4 (major problem preventing the use of the application). Additionally, the evaluators were also asked to suggest possible solutions to solve the detected issues.

Taking into account the identified usability problems, that resulted from this evaluation, the most concerning ones were related to the lack of provided feedback, in cases where input fields were incorrectly filled in or when the user's personal information was updated. The need for additional guiding information was also identified, to allow users to understand some of the system's features. Additionally, it was verified that some core features for dealing with errors and customizing use were missing, such as the possibility of undoing information changes, selecting the alarm type of the techniques, and logging out of the application. In terms of facilitating aspects, it was also deemed useful to have shortcut buttons allowing users to skip guiding information that they already knew.

4.3 Second Functional Prototype

Among the changes considered for the second prototype, the most prominent included the implementation of notifications, with the intent of providing the user with appropriate feedback in each of its action executions, and of new features that were missing, such as logging out of the application or accessing additional information regarding the several existing techniques. Depicted in Fig. 3 are examples that illustrate some of the implemented changes.

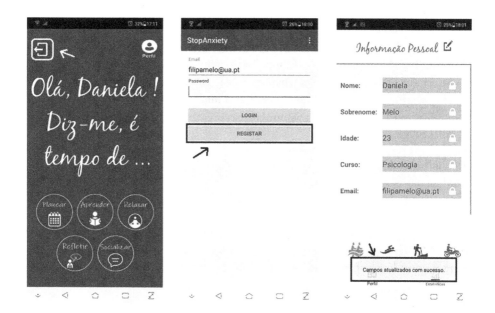

Fig. 3. Implemented changes example

For the second functional prototype, since it already provided a considerable amount of features, the main intent for the evaluation was to discover usability problems made evident while using the application to reach concrete goals. As such, a Think Aloud protocol was applied, asking users to perform specific tasks by using the application, while giving feedback of what they thought and the difficulties they were faced with. For this evaluation, five participants were considered, different from those performing the heuristic evaluation, four males and one female, aged 22–25, all computer engineering students with experience in mobile applications development.

During this session, the participants were asked to perform 10 tasks (see Table 4) and the following variables were measured: the success/unsuccess of the tasks, the time to completion, in seconds, and the number of errors and unforeseen events during their execution. In addition to the proposed tasks, at the end of the evaluation, each participant answered a SUS [4,15] and a PSSUQ [13,20] questionnaire. While there is an overlap between some of the outcomes provided by both questionnaires, we considered that applying both would provide a richer set of information.

Regarding the obtained results, although all the participants were capable of successfully completing the 10 tasks, some difficulties were still encountered.

Table 4. Tasks performed by users during the usability evaluations.

Tasks
1. Register in the application
2. Log in to the app
3. Edit and complete your profile
4. Get more information about the Muscle Relaxation Technique
5. Setup the Diaphragmatic Breathing Technique for a duration of 7 min
6. Select the mute option in the Diaphragmatic Breathing Technique menu
7. Perform the Technique for approximately 1 min
8. Return to the menu of the Diaphragmatic Breathing Technique and perform it with sound
9. Perform the Muscle Relaxation Technique by contracting and relaxing one of the indicated muscle groups
10. Log out of the application

Despite that, the performed SUS and PSSUQ assessments revealed average scores of 75 and 2.176 respectively, which classifies the application as already having a good level of usability, however, still with space for improvements.

4.4   Current Version of Stop Anxiety

Considering the outcomes of the last evaluation, the development of a third version of the prototype ensued. This time, the focus was to further improve usability, and provide a complete implementation of the provided techniques, not only to further validate the application, but also to enable a first assessment of their impact in dealing with anxiety. In what follows, we provide an overall summary of the currently supported set of features.

4.4.1   Main Features

After signing in, the user can access the various features that are present in StopAnxiety from the home screen, where a message is displayed saying "Hi, Daniela! Tell me, it's time to...", followed by the options: "Relax", "Plan", "Learn", "Think", and "Socialize". Note that this way of presenting the user with the different options derives from the fact that we wanted to put the user at the center of the action. It is what he wants that matters, instead of just providing options, such as "Relaxation Exercises", "Schedule Planning", and "Psychoeducation".

Depicted in Fig. 4 are the initial steps that are required for the user to perform in order to successfully access the application.

Regarding the system's main features, when the user chooses to "Relax", several techniques are available for him to perform, such as Mindfulness, Diaphragmatic Breathing, and Progressive Muscular Relaxation. After selecting one of

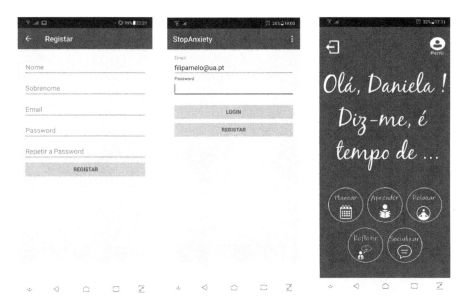

Fig. 4. Required steps for the initial login and the home screen from where the main features can be accessed.

the available techniques, the system provides him with the corresponding technique's procedure, where the user can inform himself before starting its execution. Throughout the technique's progress, the system keeps the user updated with information regarding the steps to perform to successfully complete it. For example, by selecting one of the Progressive Muscle Relaxation Techniques, the system immediately displays its corresponding procedure, using a slideshow, and subsequently provides him with instructions of when and which muscle group needs to be contracted or relaxed. While the muscles and the instructions are presented in the screen, a voice guide is also available for cases when the user simply wants to enjoy its experience without having to look to the screen (Fig. 5).

4.4.2 Evaluation

In order to verify the system's usability improvement after the implementation of the changes that were deemed necessary, for the current version, both the same tasks and evaluation instruments were selected. For this evaluation, five new participants were considered, three females and two males, aged between 21–26 years old, all computer science engineering students. This time, the participants did not have any problems in accomplishing the tasks that were proposed which, since that was not the case in the previous evaluation, might be indicative of an improvement in the usability levels of the application.

In fact, average values of 90.5 and 1.608 were obtained for the SUS and PSSUQ scales, respectively, which demonstrates a notorious improvement compared to the values of 75 and 2.176 from the previous usability evaluation. It

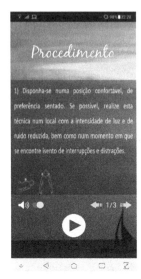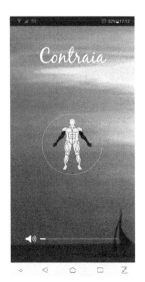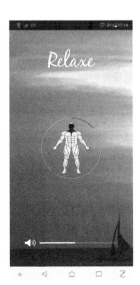

Fig. 5. Progressive Muscle Relaxation Technique. From left to right: the instructions screen, the instruction to contract the muscles in the arms, and instruction to relax the head and neck muscles.

should be noted that the obtained results categorize the assessed application as having a quite satisfactory level of usability, allowing its users to have a highly intuitive and pleasant navigation process.

With the achievement of these results, the current version is deemed ready for an evaluation regarding the impact that the available techniques have in the users anxiety levels.

5   Conclusions and Future Work

This article presents first results of a multidisciplinary user-centered effort to propose support tools for anxiety management. To this end, there was a need to consider methodologies that allowed a more efficient and effective multidisciplinary teamwork and a complete specification of user's needs, motivations and scenarios of use. As such, tools like Personas and Context Scenarios were used, to both foster an easier communication between the team members, and enable an appropriate elicitation of the requirements that served as the foundation to the correct development of the anxiety management system.

Considering the particular case of anxiety management in the academic campus, a proof-of-concept application was developed, adopting an iterative User-Centered Design and development approach, which ensured that the resulting system met the goals and needs of the target users. The resulting application incorporates several evidence-based techniques, such as, Mindfulness, Diaphragmatic Breathing and Progressive Muscular Relaxation. Nevertheless, at this time, we are designing an experimental protocol to assess the actual impact of the anxiety management techniques provided by StopAnxiety in tackling anxiety.

Regarding further evolution of StopAnxiety, a few notable aspects should deserve prompt attention. It would be important to provide a time management feature that suggests schedules adapted to the tasks and biological rhythms of the users, since this is an issue that was transversely identified, during the focus groups, as being one of the main promoters of anxiety in both students and teachers. It would also be highly beneficial to evolve the psychoeducation section, allowing users to learn about the main symptoms of the existing conditions and teaching them how to deal with them, at an early stage, possibly preventing them from developing into real disorders. And, naturally, the user emotional state and context (e.g., time of day, task, location) can be a valuable set of information to adapt the application's response to the user, enabling, for instance, a prompt action when an anxious state is imminent (e.g. suggesting an anxiety management technique adequate for a public place). In this regard, work is ongoing regarding the integration of the emotional state and context of the user.

Acknowledgements. This work is partially funded by IEETA Research Unit funding (UID/CEC/00127/2019), by Portugal 2020 under the Competitiveness and Internationalization Operational Program, and the European Regional Development Fund through project SOCA – Smart Open Campus (CENTRO-01-0145-FEDER-000010).

References

1. Aderka, I.M., Nickerson, A., Bøe, H.J., Hofmann, S.G.: Sudden gains during psychological treatments of anxiety and depression: a meta-analysis. J. Consult. Clin. Psychol. **80**(1), 93 (2012)
2. Bakker, D., Kazantzis, N., Rickwood, D., Rickard, N.: Mental health smartphoneapps: review and evidence-based recommendations for future developments. JMIR Mental Health **3**(1) (2016)
3. Bandelow, B., Michaelis, S., Wedekind, D.: Treatment of anxiety disorders. Dialogues Clin. Neurosci. **19**(2), 93 (2017)
4. Bangor, A., Kortum, P.T., Miller, J.T.: An empirical evaluation of the system usability scale. Intl. J. Hum.-Comput. Interact. **24**(6), 574–594 (2008)
5. Chisholm, D., et al.: Scaling-up treatment of depression and anxiety: a global return on investment analysis. Lancet Psychiatry **3**(5), 415–424 (2016)
6. Cooper, A., Reimann, R., Cronin, D., Noessel, C.: About Face: The Essentials of Interaction Design. Wiley, Hoboken (2014)
7. Cuijpers, P., Sijbrandij, M., Koole, S., Huibers, M., Berking, M., Andersson, G.: Psychological treatment of generalized anxiety disorder: a meta-analysis. Clin. Psychol. Rev. **34**(2), 130–140 (2014)
8. Fenger, M., et al.: Internet-based self-help therapy with fear fighter[TM] versus no intervention for anxiety disorders in adults: study protocol for a randomised controlled trial. Trials **17**(1), 525 (2016)

9. Fitzpatrick, K.K., Darcy, A., Vierhile, M.: Delivering cognitive behavior therapy to young adults with symptoms of depression and anxiety using a fully automated conversational agent (woebot): a randomized controlled trial. JMIR mental health **4**(2) (2017)
10. Gaynes, B.N., et al.: Feasibility and diagnostic validity of the M-3 checklist: a brief, self-rated screen for depressive, bipolar, anxiety, and post-traumatic stress disorders in primary care. Ann. Family Med. **8**(2), 160–169 (2010)
11. Haller, H., Cramer, H., Lauche, R., Gass, F., Dobos, G.J.: The prevalence and burden of subthreshold generalized anxiety disorder: a systematic review. BMC Psychiatry **14**(1), 128 (2014)
12. Kessler, R.C., et al.: The global burden of mental disorders: an update from the WHO World Mental Health (WMH) surveys. Epidemiol. Psychiatr. Sci. **18**(1), 23–33 (2009)
13. Lewis, J.R.: Psychometric evaluation of the pssuq using data from five years of usability studies. Int. J. Hum.-Comput. Interact. **14**(3–4), 463–488 (2002)
14. Mack, S., et al.: Self-reported utilization of mental health services in the adult German population-evidence for unmet needs? Results of the DEGS1-Mental Health Module (DEGS1-MH). Int. J. Methods Psychiatr. Res. **23**(3), 289–303 (2014)
15. Martins, A.I., Rosa, A.F., Queirós, A., Silva, A., Rocha, N.P.: European portuguese validation of the System Usability Scale (SUS). Procedia Comput. Sci. **67**, 293–300 (2015)
16. Michael, T., Zetsche, U., Margraf, J.: Epidemiology of anxiety disorders. Psychiatry **6**(4), 136–142 (2007)
17. Morgan, C., et al.: The effectiveness of unguided internet cognitive behavioural therapy for mixed anxiety and depression. Internet Interventions **10**, 47–53 (2017)
18. Neary, M., Schueller, S.M.: State of the field of mental health apps. Cogn. Behav. Pract. **25**, 531–537 (2018)
19. Nielsen, J.: Heuristic evaluation. In: Nielsen, J., Mack, R.L. (eds.) Usability Inspection Methods. Wiley, New York (1994)
20. Rosa, A.F., Martins, A.I., Costa, V., Queirós, A., Silva, A., Rocha, N.P.: European Portuguese validation of the post-study system usability questionnaire (PSSUQ). In: 2015 10th Iberian Conference on Information Systems and Technologies (CISTI), pp. 1–5. IEEE (2015)
21. Sarkar, U., et al.: Usability of commercially available mobile applications for diverse patients. J. Gen. Intern. Med. **31**(12), 1417–1426 (2016). https://doi.org/10.1007/s11606-016-3771-6
22. Silva, S., Teixeira, A.: Design and development for individuals with ASD: fostering multidisciplinary approaches through personas. J. Autism Dev. Disord. **49**(5), 2156–2172 (2019)
23. Torous, J., et al.: The emerging imperative for a consensus approach toward the rating and clinical recommendation of mental health apps. J. Nerv. Ment. Dis. **206**(8), 662–666 (2018)
24. Wittchen, H.U., Jacobi, F.: Size and burden of mental disorders in Europe–a critical review and appraisal of 27 studies. Eur. Neuropsychopharmacol. **15**(4), 357–376 (2005)

Using Data Distribution Service for IEEE 11073-10207 Medical Device Communication

Merle Baake[1], Josef Ingenerf[2] (ID), and Björn Andersen[2](✉) (ID)

[1] Cardioscan GmbH, Hamburg, Germany
merle.baake@cardioscan.de
[2] Institute of Medical Informatics, Universität zu Lübeck, Lübeck, Germany
{ingenerf,andersen}@imi.uni-luebeck.de

Abstract. The concept of an Integrated Clinical Environment can be implemented by a fully connected operation room containing devices from different manufacturers. An exchange architecture and protocol for this kind of environment is defined by the IEEE 11073 Service-oriented Device Connectivity family of standards. Therein, a Domain Information and Service Model is bound to the Medical Devices Communication Profile for Web Services, which is the specification for the information exchange technology. It is employed as the communication layer in the software library SDCLib/J that implements an Integrated Clinical Environment. In order to demonstrate that the functionality of SDCLib/J is independent of the underlying transport technology, its communication layer was replaced with an implementation of the Data Distribution Service. Therefore, its publish-subscribe pattern needed to be redesigned and transformed so that it matches the library's request-response principle.

Keywords: IEEE 11073 SDC · SOMDA · DDS · ICE · Publish-subscribe · Request-response

1 Introduction

Interconnecting point-of-care medical devices from various manufacturers has been shown to enable technological and economic benefits [8]. Apart from data exchange, remote control is of great importance when connecting medical devices [12]. By monitoring parameters like heart rate or blood pressure and using remote control, functions depending on their current values can be controlled, e.g. pausing the injection of a drug when the patient's vital signs drop out of a previously defined safe range.

Unfortunately, in most cases, a device can only be connected efficiently to another device if it is from the same vendor [5]. In case devices from mixed manufacturers are introduced, additional interfaces are required. Therefore, users have a high dependency on the availability of devices from the same manufacturer.

© ICST Institute for Computer Sciences, Social Informatics and Telecommunications Engineering 2020
Published by Springer Nature Switzerland AG 2020. All Rights Reserved
G. M. P. O'Hare et al. (Eds.): MobiHealth 2019, LNICST 320, pp. 127–139, 2020.
https://doi.org/10.1007/978-3-030-49289-2_10

The *Integrated Clinical Environment (ICE)* describes a clinical workplace such as an operation room, where devices can communicate even if they are from different manufacturers [9]. However, the concept needs to be implemented with specific software technologies. In the IEEE 11073 *Service-oriented Device Connectivity (SDC)* series, a communication protocol is described that aims to fulfil the requirements of an ICE and can be implemented as a software library [12]. Such a library acts as a communication layer under the application layer and provides components for the data exchange in distributed systems of medical devices.

SDC uses the *Medical Devices Communication Profile for Web Services (MDPWS)* as its underlying transport technology. It is thus implemented as the communication layer in the SDC implementation SDCLib/J. Other ICE implementations, like OpenICE, use the communication protocol *Data Distribution Service (DDS)* and demonstrated it to be generally appropriate in a medical context [1].

As the design of the SDCLib/J reflects the loose coupling of the IEEE 11073 SDC standards, the transport technology is exchangeable. The interconnection of medical devices based on the IEEE 11073 data model is therefore not bound to MDPWS. In this work, SDCLib's communication layer is extended so that devices can communicate over DDS, broadening the variety of devices being able to exchange information through the library. To integrate the new communication protocol, DDS' publish-subscribe pattern needed to be mapped to SDCLib's request-response principle.

2   IEEE 11073 SDC

The IEEE 11073 series of standards aims for the interoperability of medical devices and information systems [3]. Three recent additions to it are known as the SDC sub-series [6]:

20701 Service-Oriented Medical Device Exchange Architecture and Protocol Binding (SDC)
10207 Domain Information and Service Model for Service-Oriented Point-of-Care Medical Device Communication (BICEPS)
20702 Medical Devices Communication Profile for Web Services (MDPWS)

2.1   20701: Architecture and Protocol

SDC specifies the technical interface for interconnected medical devices at a clinical workplace, e.g. an operation room, as described in the ICE concept [11]. The specification adheres to the *Service Oriented Medical Device Architecture* (SOMDA) pattern, which assumes that medical devices represent their capabilities in the network as *services*. The focus lies on reducing the complexity and costs that come with the integration of devices into distributed enterprise systems. Dealing with medical data, the exchange is highly safety-critical and underlies strict requirements.

2.2   10207: Information and Service Model

Furthermore, IEEE 11073 defines the *Basic Integrated Clinical Environment Protocol Specification* (BICEPS). In the *Medical Device Information Base* (MDIB), the core of the data model, metrics describe the capabilities of a medical device, like vital parameters, settings, states, and contextual information [3].

The following service operations are defined in BICEPS to exchange information in a medical context [3,16]:

GET   reading access (request-response pattern),
SET   writing access to change values → remote control,
EVENT REPORT reading access (publish-subscribe pattern),
ACTIVATE   execute a predefined job on a remote device → remote control.

To access the metrics, *GET* and *SET* methods allow for reading and possibly writing access as per the request-response pattern: Values can be actively fetched or modified by a client with read/write access. *EVENT REPORTS* are based on reading access as well, but employ the publish-subscribe paradigm – notifications can be sent periodically or when a change of value occurs. The use of an *ACTIVATE* operation triggers an action and thereby allows for external control of a medical device.

2.3   20702: Communication Technology

The communication protocol MDPWS is needed to technically realise the SOMDA [8]. It is implemented as a set of web services, which support interoperability across a network using the *Web Service Definition Language (WSDL)* and SOAP messages. MDPWS fulfils the special requirements of communication between medical point-of-care devices, enabling i.a. remote control and data streaming.

2.4   SDCLib: Communication Library

The Java library SDCLib/J implements IEEE 11073 SDC, thereby putting the ICE concept into effect [18]. Figure 1 shows the setup of devices implementing the library. The application itself serves as the entry and exit point for medical device data into and out of the network. The library establishes the consumer and the provider and processes the exchanged information used by the application. The SDC protocol specification works as a binding between the data model BICEPS and the transport layer MDPWS, which passes on the data and handles the technical details on the information exchange.

Due to the separation of service model and implementation, it does not matter which communication protocol is used to exchange the data as long as the data structure of the BICEPS layer is preserved in the lower layers.

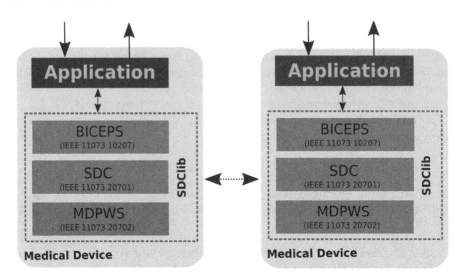

Fig. 1. Based on MDPWS and BICEPS, the library enables the exchange of information between multiple devices. The application using the library serves as the entry and exit point of the data into and out of the network.

3 Data Distribution Service

3.1 A Data-Centric Protocol

The main focus of *Data Distribution Service (DDS)* lies on the data-centrality and timely availability of information [15]. In a global data space, a unit of information – a *Topic* – is transmitted between publishers and subscribers [7]. DDS is designed following the publish-subscribe principle. Instead of the client specifically asking for new information, as in the request-response pattern, clients subscribe to specific types of information and receive the respective data as soon as the server sends it. With a single subscription, nodes can subscribe to many similar data streams to receive data.

Figure 2 shows the interaction between the basic components needed for the communication process. The scenario assumes that all entities are part of the same data space (domain). Each of the two Topics is associated with a DataReader/ DataWriter pair, which is used by the application(s) to exchange information on the specific Topic. The DataWriter for Topic A writes samples, which can only be read by the respective DataReader. The DataReader associated with Topic B has no access to the samples of Topic A and vice versa.

User-specific types for the Topics can be defined comprehensively. Rather than sending general messages, the communication layer understands the types syntactically, creating a type-safe environment.

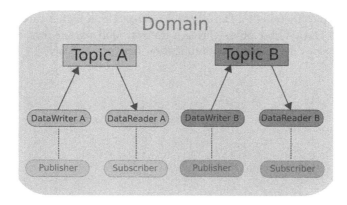

Fig. 2. DataReaders and DataWriters can only communicate through their associated Topic. Although they exist in the same domain and know of each other's existence, DataReader B will not receive any samples written by DataWriter A.

3.2   Exchanging Data Within a Domain

Communication takes place in the *Domain*, which represents a global data space and enables multiple applications to communicate within this data space [7]. It is important to note that the data is not physically located on a central domain storage; it is rather kept decentrally in the caches of its DataWriters and DataReaders.

Creating a DomainParticipant with a specific 'domainId' is the ticket for the application to enter the domain. Based on the DomainParticipant, all other entities which enable communication are created by the software implementation of DDS. Multiple applications can exchange data when initiating their DomainParticipants with the same 'domainId'.

3.3   Quality of Service Parameters

The setting of Quality of Service (QoS) parameters determines how the components of the application behave before, during, and after sending and receiving data [4]. With these parameters, memory preallocation for the samples, the size of the caches, and details of the transport process can be defined comprehensively. The main goal is to maximise the likelihood of readers and writers to match while controlling the entities' behaviour. By default, the QoS parameters are set to fit general use cases.

As visualised in Fig. 3, a DataReader and a DataWriter are in the same Domain and bound to the same Topic. Because their QoS parameters are compliant, they are able to communicate (A). In case of a discrepancy between their defined QoS parameters, the two entities are declared as incompatible by DDS and can not exchange any information (B).

If the QoS parameters of a DataReader request e.g. a higher rate of receiving data than the DataWriter offers through its own QoS parameters, the communication layer does not enable communication between the two.

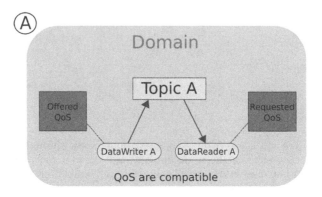

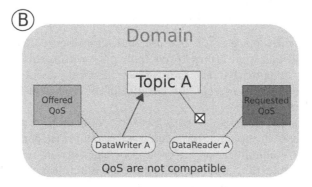

Fig. 3. DataWriter and DataReader must be in the same Domain, bound to the same Topic and have agreeing QoS parameters. If the DataWriter can not fulfil the DataReader's requested QoS parameters, or vice versa, the pair is declared as incompatible.

4   Concept

To recreate the functionality of SDCLib/J with DDS, the communication layer is replaced by the new protocol. For that, the request-response pattern is recreated with the use of DDS' Topics.

The initial implementation of SDCLib/J based on MDPWS is designed so that all information is mapped to messages containing XML before being sent trough the network. After receiving the data, it is transformed to its original form so it can be processed by the upper layers.

With DDS, information types are handled individually. For every *GET* and *SET* operation, as well as the *EVENT REPORTS*, individual Topics need to be created containing the necessary data. Along with the created Topics, the consumer side needs to implement DataWriters for the requests and DataReaders for the responses and the reports. Respectively, the provider's side implements DataReaders for the requests as well as DataWriters for the responses and the reports. Figure 4 exemplifies this based on the entities that are needed to exchange information on the MDIB.

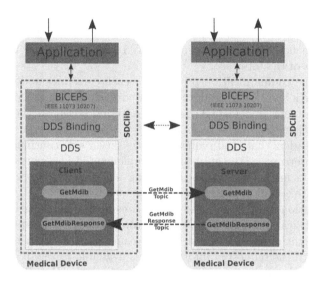

Fig. 4. In the new setup, the library exchanges data through DDS. The consumer requests the MDIB of the provider by sending a sample of a GetMdib Topic, which is received by the provider and answered with a sample of the GetMdibResponse Topic.

ICE emphasises the need for reliable one-to-one communication. Three steps guarantee that the client finds the intended server and exchanges the information needed:

1. When a device enters the domain in order to communicate with other devices, a new DomainParticipant is initiated for the role of the client and another one for the server. All participants are based on the same domainId so that communication takes place in the same data space. Automatic discovery is enabled so that the client is notified when new DomainParticipants enter the domain and can extract information, e.g. the server's endpoint reference. Thereby, the client can directly address the server to request information or to initiate remote control.
2. The endpoint reference of the server is added to the request sample. On the server side, a filter is used to only read requests that hold the server's endpoint reference.
3. The DataReader for the response waits for samples of the response Topic. Only the sample containing the identifier of the previously sent request is processed.

5   Implementation

In SDCLib/J, the concept of the information exchange is basically the same for every use case: the consumer sends a *GET* or *SET* request, which is received by the provider. The provider creates the response and sends it back. Upon receiving a subscribe request, *EVENT REPORTS* are triggered that are sent directly to the subscriber.

SDCLib/J is designed so that the transport layer is connected to the upper layers via a binding interface. Through the extension described in this work, the library user can now switch between MDPWS and DDS to use the respective implementation of the interface.

To enable the communication process, for each consumer and each provider one DomainParticipant is created and initiated with the same 'domainId'. The Topics, DataReaders, and DataWriters are initiated based on the DomainParticipants on both sides.

The DataReaders that read requests on the server side continuously wait for data without interrupting the application. Implemented Listeners allow them to wait for requests in the background, allowing all other processes to run while being ready to take and process new requests at all times.

The information that is requested by the consumer is implicitly asked for and used by the application. Therefore, the DataReaders for the responses start to wait for data right after the request is sent, causing the current thread to stop temporarily until the requested information is available to them.

Furthermore, Listeners are also implemented on the DataReader's side to listen for *EVENT REPORTS*.

6   Evaluation

The implementation process was closely tied to tests, which were initially designed to test the basic functionalities of the library based on MDPWS. Now, the binding interface implemented with DDS is passed as the transportation layer. It was thereby guaranteed that the new transportation layer enables the same functionalities as MDPWS.

6.1   Qualitative Distributed Analysis

As SDCLib's purpose is to enable communication in distributed systems, the implementation was tested on virtual machines representing medical devices. A consumer and a provider with basic information are initialised on one virtual machine each. Communication is possible due to the machines entering the same Domain. Therefore, the consumer's DataWriter for the *request* Topics can exchange data with the respective DataReader on the provider side.

Several tests assure that information is exchanged correctly. This includes basic information being requested and sent, parameters being set remotely, and alerts being triggered correctly.

Indeed, the machines were able to exchange the information accordingly. The *GET* and *SET* methods could be executed as intended and *EVENT REPORTS* were triggered correctly. To enable two or more devices to exchange information, the setting of the QoS parameters was crucial. With the default parameters, information could only be exchanged between instances running on a single machine. Therefore, specific adjustments were necessary as described in Sect. 6.2 to enable communication between multiple devices.

6.2 QoS Parameters for Distributed Systems

Running the application on multiple machines for the purpose of evaluation required adjusting the QoS parameters as the defaults were not feasible. To assure that all requests and the related replies are received, reliable communication was enabled. If a DataReader does not receive a sample, it is repaired and re-sent, making sure it will receive the sample eventually. To further increase safety in the process, acknowledgements are sent automatically after a DataReader has read a sample and returned it to the cache. The number of instances of each sample is limited so that very old instances that are most likely obsolete are deleted and do not occupy memory.

It may occur that a client requests an MDIB of a device that is not on the network (yet). Still, it should be possible for the device to receive the request. The durability parameter is set so that late joiners receive all sent requests.

With limited memory, it proved to be better to reduce the number of samples that are stored after they were sent or received. Only a specific number of samples can be resent if they were not received by the intended DataReader, either because it did not join the network yet or because the sample got lost.

To make sure all participants/applications can be found on the network, discovery through *UDPv4* is enabled. That assures the discovery of applications on different machines.

7   Results

By replacing SDCLib/J's built-in communication protocol MDPWS with the alternative DDS, it has been proven that communication between medical devices based on this library is not limited to one transport technology. This meets the requirement for data exchange between medical devices having to be independent of the underlying communication protocol as described in the ICE concept.

8   Discussion

8.1   Challenges

Whereas MDPWS is able to implement both the request-response pattern (*GET* and *SET* operations) and the publish-subscribe principle (*EVENT REPORTS*),

DDS is specifically designed to support only the latter. Therefore, it was challenging to map the other services to DDS and to support the request-response pattern as DDS does not intend the client to start the communication process by addressing the server directly. Rather, the provider starts the communication process, sending out data to all participants. This had to be considered when integrating the new protocol.

Therefore, our implementation does not think of the consumer/client as one DataReader, which receives information, and the provider/server as a DataWriter, which publishes data. Both sides uphold multiple DataWriters and DataReaders. Different from DDS' initial approach, where a DataWriter starts the information exchange by broadcasting data whenever it is available (except for *EVENT REPORTS*), the DataWriters are triggered by certain events, usually by receiving a request.

8.2   Advantages of Using DDS

The main focus of this work lies on the substitution of the communication layer, enabling information exchange in a distributed system with a different protocol than MDPWS while keeping the functionality and the data model of SDCLib/J.

Similiar to Mastouri and Hasnaoui in [13], it shall be further investigated to which extent the number of created entities (publisher, subscribers, etc.) influences the performance of the implementation. The suitability of the library shall also be evaluated and compared to other implementations, as done by Kasparick et al. in [10]. To decide whether MDPWS or DDS are more appropriate to exchange data with SDCLib/J, the performance and reliability of both communication protocols need to be examined and compared. Implementations of further communication protocols are currently under evaluation and are expected to be available for comparison in the near future as well.

As evaluated by Serrano-Torres et al. in [17], variances in the performance of different implementations of DDS occur as well and need to be considered.

8.3   Security

Although it is not within the scope of this work, it should be noted that there are data security issues when using this implementation of DDS. The basic concept of DDS, the publish-subscribe principle, is designed in a way that every DataReader of a certain Topic receives all samples from every respective DataWriter.

In terms of medical data, patient information may only be sent to certain participants. The way DDS is integrated into SDCLib/J at this point, all samples are sent to every participant. The discovery process only guarantees that the client uses the server's device reference when writing requests. The listeners on the server side filter all samples that are intended for the respective device. Still, the request can technically be read by any DataWriter (of the specific Topic) of all DomainParticipants in the Domain. Furthermore, new DataWriters may be created bound to any Topic, causing false alarms or unwanted operations.

Adjusting the QoS parameters to send authentication details as the participant's metadata or creating a stricter matching process is not sufficient in a real-world medical context. Depending on which DDS implementation is used, plugins can be added to increase the security level. These include *RTI Connext DDS Secure*, based on *RTI Connext DDS*, which offers comprehensive mechanisms to improve security in critical environments, such as autonomous vehicles, medical and defence industries [14].

8.4   QoS Parameters

A big advantage of DDS lies in the QoS parameters [2]. They allow the developer to determine how much memory is preallocated, making the most of the available resources, and how exactly data is transferred. In a medical context, the parameters that control reliability are especially useful, making sure no important data is lost. It is guaranteed that all data is received as intended. Lost or broken samples are being repaired and resent. Running the application on multiple devices with limited memory, adjusting the resource limits is inevitable. Developers can not only specify the structure of the types by creating Topics, but the QoS parameters also allow for them to determine how the data moves around in the distributed system [4].

When using SDCLib/J with DDS in a practical environment, optimal QoS parameters should be determined beforehand. They must be sufficiently restrictive, especially in a distributed system of medical devices. With the knowledge of available memory capacity, the QoS parameters for memory allocation can be adjusted to process sufficiently large amounts of data.

9   Conclusion

The variety of medical devices from different manufacturers in an operation room demands libraries that allow communication between different medical devices independent of the underlying communication protocol [1]. This principle is specified as part of the ICE concept, which describes a fully connected clinical environment. Within the scope of this work, the communication protocol of the library SDCLib/J is exchanged, proving independence in the choice of communication protocol. It has been shown that the library SDCLib/J is not limited to exchanging data over MDPWS. Replacing MDPWS with DDS as its communication layer shows that the upper layers are agnostic to which communication protocol is used below.

To integrate DDS into the library, the publish-subscribe pattern of the protocol needed to be mapped to the request-response pattern of SDCLib/J. Though being profoundly different, it was possible to recreate this communication pattern with DDS to integrate it into SDCLib/J as its transportation layer. Thereby, the functionalities of the library and the data model remained unaffected.

The data-centric principle of DDS provides certain advantages for the library. With DDS, user-specific data types can be modelled comprehensively, allowing for a type-safe communication process. Furthermore, the QoS parameters are of great advantage, especially for enabling and optimising communication in distributed systems. This is especially important when using DDS in a real-world medical scenario, which imposes stringent safety requirements.

In the future, other communication protocols could be integrated as well, broadening the variety of devices being able to communicate using SDCLib's comprehensive data model.

References

1. Kavya, K.A., Annapurna, V.K.: Integration of medical devices into MIOT using OPENICE. Int. J. Eng. Sci. Comput. **6**, 7323–7324 (2016)
2. Basem, A.M., Ali, H.: Data Distribution Service (DDS) based implementation of Smart grid devices using ANSI C12. 19 standard. Procedia Comput. Sci. **110**, 394–401 (2017). https://doi.org/10.1016/j.procs.2017.06.082
3. Andersen, B., et al.: Interoperabilität von Geräten und Systemen in OP und Klinik. Technical report, Frankfurt, Germany (2015)
4. Arney, D., Plourde, J., Goldman, J.M.: OpenICE medical device interoperability platform overview and requirement analysis. Biomed. Eng. Biomed. Tech. **63**(1), 39–47 (2018). https://doi.org/10.1515/bmt-2017-0040
5. Beger, F., Janß, A., Kasparick, M., Besting, A.: Der Operationssaal OP 40 - Für mehr Sicherheit und Effizienz durch offene Vernetzung in Operationssälen und Kliniken der Zukunft. meditronic-journal - Fachzeitschrift für Medizin-Technik, **4**, 20–24 (2017)
6. Besting, A., Stegemann, D., Bürger, S., Kasparick, M., Strathen, B., Portheine, F.: Concepts for developing interoperable software frameworks implementing the new IEEE 11073 SDC standard family, vol. 1, pp. 258–263. CAOS, 13 June 2017
7. Corsaro, A., Schmidt, D.C.: The data distribution service-The communication middleware fabric for scalable and extensible systems-of-systems. Syst. Syst. **2**, 19 (2012). https://doi.org/10.5772/30322
8. Gregorczyk, D., Fischer, S., Busshaus, T., Schlichting, S., Pöhlsen, S.: An approach to integrate distributed systems of medical devices in high acuity environments. In: 5th Workshop on Medical Cyber-Physical Systems 2014. Schloss Dagstuhl-Leibniz-Zentrum fuer Informatik (2014)
9. Hatcliff, J., King, A., Lee, I., Macdonald, A., Fernando, A., Robkin, M., Vasserman, E., Weininger, S., Goldman, J.M.: Rationale and architecture principles for medical application platforms. In: 2012 IEEE/ACM Third International Conference on Cyber-Physical Systems, 17 April 2012, pp. 3–12. IEEE (2012). https://doi.org/10.1109/ICCPS.2012.9
10. Kasparick, M., Beichler, B., Konieczek, B., Besting, A., Rethfeldt, M., Golatowski, F., Timmermann, D.: Measuring latencies of IEEE 11073 compliant service-oriented medical device stacks. In: IECON 2017-43rd Annual Conference of the IEEE Industrial Electronics Society, October 2017, pp. 8640–8647. IEEE (2017). https://doi.org/10.1109/IECON.2017.8217518
11. Kasparick, M., Schlichting, S., Golatowski, F., Timmermann, D.: Medical DPWS: new IEEE 11073 standard for safe and interoperable medical device communication. In: 2015 IEEE Conference on Standards for Communications and Networking (CSCN), 28 October 2015, pp. 212–217. IEEE (2015). https://doi.org/10.1109/CSCN.2015.7390446

12. Kasparick, M., Schmitz, M., Golatowski, F., Timmermann, D.: Dynamic remote control through service orchestration of point-of-care and surgical devices based on IEEE 11073 SDC. In: 2016 IEEE Healthcare Innovation Point-Of-Care Technologies Conference (HI-POCT), 9 November 2016, pp. 121–125. IEEE (2016). https://doi.org/10.1109/IC.2016.7797712
13. Mastouri, M.A., Hasnaoui, S.: Performance of a publish/subscribe middleware for the real-time distributed control systems. Comput. Sci. Netw. Secur. **7**(1), 313–319 (2007)
14. Real-Time Innovations, I.: RTI Connext DDS Secure. https://www.rti.com/products/secure (2018). Accessed 09 July 2018
15. Rowstron, A., Druschel, P.: Pastry: scalable, decentralized object location, and routing for large-scale peer-to-peer systems. In: Guerraoui, R. (ed.) Middleware 2001. LNCS, vol. 2218, pp. 329–350. Springer, Heidelberg (2001). https://doi.org/10.1007/3-540-45518-3_18
16. Schlichting, S., Pöhlsen, S.: An Architecture for distributed systems of medical devices in high acuity environments - a technical whitepaper (2014)
17. Serrano-Torres, R., García-Valls, M., Basanta-Val, P.: Performance evaluation of virtualized DDS Middleware. In: Simposio de tiempo real, Madrid, pp. 18–19 (2014)
18. SurgiTAIX: SDCLib Bitbucket Repository. https://bitbucket.org/surgitaix/sdclib. Accessed 09 July 2018

Enabling Multimodal Emotionally-Aware Ecosystems Through a W3C-Aligned Generic Interaction Modality

David Ferreira[1], Nuno Almeida[1,2], Susana Brás[1,2], Sandra C. Soares[3,4], António Teixeira[1,2], and Samuel Silva[1,2(✉)]

[1] DETI - University of Aveiro, Aveiro, Portugal
sss@ua.pt
[2] IEETA – University of Aveiro, Aveiro, Portugal
[3] DEP – University of Aveiro, Aveiro, Portugal
[4] William James Center for Research, University of Aveiro, Aveiro, Portugal

Abstract. Emotions play a key role in our life experiences. In interactive systems, the user's emotional state can be relevant to provide increased levels of adaptation to the user, but can also be paramount in scenarios where such information might enable us to help users manage and express their emotions (e.g., anxiety), with a positive impact on their daily life and on how they interact with others. However, although there is a clear potential for emotionally-aware applications, they still have a long road to travel to reach the desired potential and availability. This is mostly due to the still low translational nature of the research in affective computing, and to the lack of straightforward, off-the-shelf methods for easy integration of emotion in applications without the need for developers to master the different concepts and technologies involved. In light of these challenges, we advance our previous work and propose an extended conceptual vision for supporting emotionally-aware interactive ecosystems and a fast track to ensure the desired translational nature of the research in affective computing. This vision then leads to the proposal of an improved iteration of a generic affective modality, a key resource to the accomplishment of the proposed vision, enabling off-the-shelf support for emotionally-aware applications in multimodal interactive contexts.

Keywords: Affective interaction · Generic modality · Multimodal interfaces · W3C

1 Introduction

Emotions govern our daily life experiences and much of our motivated behaviour [17,19]. The stimuli and events that capture our attention, the information we learn and recall, and the decisions we make, widely depend on the emotions we experience (e.g., happiness, sadness, fear and anxiety).

© ICST Institute for Computer Sciences, Social Informatics and Telecommunications Engineering 2020
Published by Springer Nature Switzerland AG 2020. All Rights Reserved
G. M. P. O'Hare et al. (Eds.): MobiHealth 2019, LNICST 320, pp. 140–152, 2020.
https://doi.org/10.1007/978-3-030-49289-2_11

The assessment of implicit measures of emotion (e.g., elevated heart rate, angry facial expression) can, nowadays, be easily performed continuously, with minimally invasive equipment and less dependent on compliance, hence offering an excellent opportunity to monitor emotional states in the context of interactive systems [5]. Gathering an insight on the user's emotional state can improve our ability to understand how the user is experiencing the environment (e.g., discomfort [1]) or task (e.g., complexity), but can also be of particular interest in aiding users understand [9], manage and communicate their emotional state, which may then result in significant improvements in their quality of life [12]. A paradigmatic example in which implicit measures of emotions may offer an added value is the case of individuals who lack their ability to communicate emotions, such as in Autism Spectrum Disorders [16]. In this line of thought, bringing the emotional state into interactive systems as an implicit interaction [14] can be a valuable resource to foster more natural and adapted forms of interaction [18]. For instance, the word "No", as an answer to a system query, is always recognised as the command "No", but, if uttered in a neutral or angry emotional state, it might be regarded differently, by the system.

Affective Computing [13] is the scientific area responsible for the study and development of systems and devices that can recognize, interpret, process, or simulate human affects. Even though the field has strongly evolved, in the past few years, and several contributions have been made in making the proposed methods available, to developers, e.g., through the proposal of affective libraries, much is yet to be done in bringing this work to its full potential in a broad set of interactive scenarios. First, developers should be able to deploy emotionally-aware interactive systems without having to master the different available technologies, or having to develop custom application logic, every time a new affective computing method needs to be integrated or a different application scenario is addressed. Second, affective computing researchers should be able to more rapidly deploy their methods into interactive scenarios, to favor the translational nature of affective computing research. This should enable a 'fast track' for the assessment of novel methods in more ecological scenarios. In this context, a solution that could be used off-the-shelf, by developers and researchers, to transparently support the design and development of emotionally-aware interactive systems would be a useful resource. To this end, and evolving a first proof-of-concept for a generic affective modality proposed in [10], this article presents the work carried out aiming at: (a) a broader vision on how affective inputs can be provided on a variety of scenarios, considering a common approach; (b) an improved conceptualisation of the modality's architecture and how it can encompass, for instance, affective fusion; (c) an enhanced compliance with the W3C recommendations for multimodal interactive systems, particularly when considering mobile scenarios; (d) an explicit consideration regarding how to deal with multiple users; and (e) a redesign of how the data required to determine the emotional state of the user reaches the modality and is subsequently processed.

The remainder of this document is organised as follows: Sect. 2 briefly presents an overview of relevant background and related work; then, Sect. 3

presents the adopted vision for the role and utility of an affective modality in the context of multimodal interactive systems and defines the main requirements to take in consideration to evolve previous work; these requirements then lead to the proposal of the enhanced modality's overall architecture presented, in Sect. 4, along with a summary of the main aspects of its development; in Sect. 5 a proof-of-concept application is presented to illustrate the integration of the modality in a simple use scenario; finally, Sect. 6 presents some conclusions and ideas for future work.

2 Background and Related Work

This section briefly provides a background on the main aspects and work deemed relevant to contextualise the presented work: affective computing, previous work, by the authors, on affective interaction deployment in multimodal ecosystems, and the support to the development of such systems.

2.1 Affective Computing

The field of affective computing studies different input variables in order to determine and understand human emotions. The extracted user's emotional state can, for instance, enable interactive systems to provide more adapted environments or react to how the user is experiencing it. Given the potential of these technologies, there is a growing interest in affective computing in the industry of video games, marketing, and mental health applications [6].

Humans communicate their emotions in many ways, and these can be inferred from a wide range of physiological and behavioural data, such as physiological signals (e.g., electrodermal activity (EDA), heart rate (HR)), speech data, text, facial expression analysis, behaviour, amongst others. With advances in the field, different technologies are now available to extract information from those humans' expressions. Although the current technologies are not yet totally confident in the results, merging information from different inputs would increase that confidence.

Different libraries are available that allow the extraction of affective information from different kinds of data. For instance Microsoft Face API[1] can extract emotion from facial images, SightCorp[2] from images or video, Tone Analyzer[3] from text, and Empath from audio. However, the libraries that are available with their pre-trained models require some effort, from developers, to include each of them in their applications, having to acquire new knowledge about each library as well.

The proposal of novel affective computing methods is a very active field of research [13] and, with the proliferation of novel sensing technologies, new methods are continuously being proposed. However, the path from the research

---

[1] Face API: https://azure.microsoft.com/en-us/services/cognitive-services/face/.

[2] SightCorp: https://sightcorp.com/.

[3] Tone Analyzer: https://tone-analyzer-demo.ng.bluemix.net/.

lab (e.g., with controlled data collection environments, or considering a wide range of software technologies), to real scenarios is sometimes hard to achieve. In this context, our team is not only interested in improving how developers can deploy emotionally-aware systems, but also in how translational multidisciplinary approaches to tackle complex problems, for instance regarding Mental Health, can be supported. This requires that not only affective computing researchers need to have a fast track to the interactive applications, but also that the research in sensing devices needs to be brought into the picture in a way that it can rapidly reach end-applications. How this might be articulated will be one of the key points of our conceptual vision, presented ahead.

2.2 Previous Work on an Affective Modality

In Henriques et al. [10], the authors have identified a set of challenges that need to be tackled to more effectively and profusely bring affective computing to interactive ecosystems. First, it is important to support developers in adding this feature to their applications without requiring them to master the different technologies involved; and, secondly, the research in new and improved methods for affective computing should have an easier and faster way to reach interactive systems, also with advantages on how it can be validated. This latter aspect is often hindered by a mismatch between the technologies used for developing interactive systems and those used for prototyping novel affective computing methods (e.g., Matlab). Therefore, an approach should be devised that completely decouples these two aspects and makes changing or updating the methods completely transparent to both the interactive system developers and the users.

In light of these challenges, we proposed a first affective modality, i.e., a module that could be connected to applications to provide affective inputs, and showed [10] that it was feasible to integrate the management of any available methods to extract affective information in a way that it became transparent to the developers. Nevertheless, this first effort, while extracting requirements from a broad conceptual vision of how affective interaction could be made available in complex interactive ecosystems, some requirements that would enable its easier adoption were left behind, for instance, in mobile scenarios, or the support for multiple users. Additionally, while the possibility of multiple sources of data for computing affective parameters was considered, the proposed vision did not make any consideration regarding how, conceptually, multiple affective information could be simultaneously tackled.

2.3 Developing Multimodal Interactive Systems

The development of multimodal interactive systems is a complex task, and a major effort has been done, by the W3C consortium, in proposing an architecture and a set of standards to support multimodal interaction (MMI) [7].

A few frameworks have been proposed to support the development of MMI systems, such as HephaisTK [8], OpenInterface [15], MUDRA [11], and AM4I [4]. One distinguishing characteristic of the latter is that it is based on the open standard for MMI, which was proposed by the W3C. A simplified model of the architecture is presented in Fig. 1. The most notable aspect of the implemented architecture is that the different modules are fully decoupled: a set of modalities (i.e., ways of interacting with the system) communicate, using a standard markup, with a central Interaction Manager. The application logic receives and sends messages to and from the modalities also by communicating with the Interaction Manager [4].

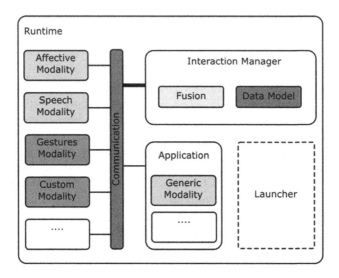

Fig. 1. Multimodal interactive architecture.

The framework reduces much of the work required to deploy interactive systems and allows the fast creation of new applications. One of its key aspects is the decoupled and modular approach: by configuring a new application with the requirements that are needed to communicate with the framework, it can immediately take advantage of its capabilities. For instance, the framework already provides an off-the-shelf modality to support speech interaction, and the developer only has to configure a few parameters with no need to master the development of speech synthesis and recognition logic. Also, the framework includes multiplatform and multi-device interaction capabilities, enabling the use of different devices, simultaneously, to interact with one application [3].

One of the interesting aspects of AM4I is that it explicitly embraces the concept of generic modalities. A generic modality, like other modalities, enables interaction with the system. Additionally, these modalities are an integral part of the framework, i.e., they come off-the-shelf when the framework is adopted and allows developers to easily deploy them with little to no effort to configure the modality. One notable example of a generic modality, which is already part of the AM4I framework, is the speech modality [2].

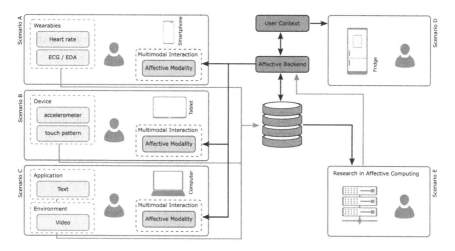

Fig. 2. Overview of the deployment of emotionally-aware applications in diverse scenarios. The sensing data and the affective computing logic are decoupled from the interactive systems, being an affective generic modality providing affective inputs to the various interactive contexts.

In this regard, any effort that results in a generic Affective Modality, which can be integrated within the framework and, thus, made available to all systems that adopt it, is an important step to bring affective interaction to a broad range of applications, for instance, in a smart-home environment.

3 Generic Affective Modality

In a first stage, we aim to have a conceptual vision on how affective computing would be deployed (and useful) in the diversity of scenarios where interaction is, nowadays, a possibility and a necessity, extending, as well, the ideas that were previously presented in [10].

3.1 Conceptual Vision on Affective Computing in a Diverse Multimodal Interactive Ecosystem

In line with what was said, Fig. 2 depicts a set of illustrative scenarios where affective interaction and affective contexts are important features.

One of the distinguishing marks of this illustrated vision is the fact that the data that is used for affective state extraction can be obtained from a wide range of sensors, which may eventually be completely decoupled from the applications. Scenarios A, B and C depict this mentioned diversity, with the sensing being performed at different levels and not only using wearables or the sensors in the user's device. For instance, a sensor in the environment, e.g., a surveillance camera, can capture facial expressions that might be used to compute the user's affective state. If the user is, for example, moving around a building, taking, at each time, different devices with him (e.g., smartphone, tablet), the interactive ecosystem should be able to make the most out of the available sensing data to adapt itself to the obtained affective information.

Another important aspect to retain is that the interactive systems do not need to have direct access to the sensing data, but only to the extracted affective information, enabling a higher degree of data privacy. For instance, if the data used to compute the affective state comes from ECG data, no application will ever have access to it, but to the extracted affective information; or an application that is indirectly obtaining affective states, derived from locally acquired accelerometer data, will never have access to it or know where it came from.

Scenario D represents the cases where the system does not explicitly receive an affective input (i.e., from an affective modality). Instead, it can access the available affective information in the user's context, which can be populated through the features that are available in the affective backend. The main difference is that the affective information on the user's context is not necessarily instantaneous, e.g.,, it can result from a full day representative history that will enable adaptation anyway, e.g., of a smart fridge to the user's mood in that day.

Additionally, Scenario E depicts the Affective Computing research environment. Naturally, it does not entail any interaction. Instead, it provides the means for the researchers to rapidly access relevant data and deploy (improvements of) their methods into interactive ecosystems. This entails that the Affective Backend should be able to integrate novel methods in a way that is transparent for the remaining modules.

3.2   Requirements

Considering a first exploratory work [10], presenting a first proof-of-concept affective modality, and the extended context and vision presented in the previous section, we established a set of requirements that, adding to the features already considered for the first version of the modality, should be central in this novel iteration of the modality, namely:

– **Cleaner integration with mobile platforms** — The first version of the Affective Modality did not fully respect the W3C standards for Multimodal Interaction, particularly, in how the communication between the modality and the remaining modules of the architecture was performed, with some of the communication logic being tightly coupled with the application's core. Thus, to fully abide to the W3C standard, the new modality should only communicate with the Interaction Manager by resorting to MMI Lifecycle Events. Such consideration would allow the modality to be fully decoupled from the mobile systems, facilitating its integration in a wider range of scenarios;
– **Multiuser support** — To bring the Affective Modality closer to real-world scenarios, one needs to consider that multiple users may be using systems in a simultaneously way, being necessary to ensure that the modality and its backend can properly manage their different requests. This implies user identification to be possible, for cases when data is selected to identify the affective

state of a specific user and the result is made available to be consumed by its corresponding application.

- **Storage and Processing of Sensing Data** — Previously, a Firebase data storage was considered for collecting the sensing data to be subject to affective information extraction. While being a reasonable approach, for demonstration purposes, it raises several scalability and versatility concerns, considering the actual envisaged extended scenario. Therefore, a novel method should be devised to properly deal with the stream and transient natures of the arriving data and its subsequent processing;

- **Affective fusion** — Considering that multiple streams of sensing data can be simultaneously available for each user (e.g., ECG, video, text typed in an email), that means an equal number of possibilities to extract affective states. Therefore, at a particular time, multiple affective states may be available, and it is important to determine how they are considered to provide a final decision. As such, the novel iteration of the Affective Modality should be able to support affective fusion, that is, know how multiple affective states, if available, can be used together;

4   Generic Affective Modality

In light of the presented conceptual vision, we designed and implemented a generic affective modality, improving our earlier work, and adopting the features and standards of the AM4I framework [4].

4.1   Architecture

Regarding the development of the Affective Modality, three main modules (stream data processor, hub fusion, modality controller) were deemed relevant for it to properly serve its purpose, being an overview depicted in Fig. 3. Their main characteristics and roles are as follows:

- The **modality controller** is responsible for creating a session of data stream consumption whenever a client connects to it. It is responsible for beginning the stream consumption session and for managing the communication with the Interaction Manager, for instance, to convey changes of the user's affective state.

- The **stream data processor** is a module that runs in the backend and which is bound to a specific client's session, waiting for incoming streams of data that are relevant for that specific user. After a data stream is successfully consumed, it is analysed to determine its data type, e.g., GPS, video, audio, or image. With both the data type and the content in its possession, the module looks for services that can process that type of data (whether local or external) to successfully identify the user's emotional state and further relay it to the **hub fusion** module.

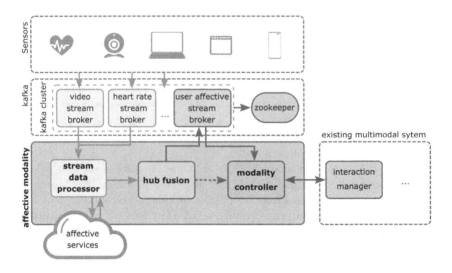

Fig. 3. Affective Modality's Architecture and supporting modules.

– The **hub fusion** module's purpose is to fuse all the events and emotions that arrive from the **stream data processor**. It tries to combine multiple affective state inputs, which result from the possibility of multiple streams of data being available for the same user, within specific time-windows, resulting in an emotion that characterises the current emotional state of the user that the inputs belong to.

4.2 Implementation

Although the mechanism to communicate the data streams from the sensors/devices is not part of the Affective Modality, it is important to note how it was implemented. For that, a distributed streaming platform, Apache Kafka[4], was considered to handle all the data streams derived from the available sensors.

These streams are subscribed by the Affective Modality, in the **stream data process**, which then identifies their types by using some supported **affective service**, such as Affectiva[5] or Kairos[6], to extract affective information. The **affective services** are a collection of computational methods, which either run locally or remotely, to support the extraction of affective information. The output of this module is delivered to the **hub fusion**, which then merges the information from different sources, and, at this stage, adopts an unsophisticated approach to choose the affective information with the highest confidence level.

After merging the available data and determining the affective state with the highest confidence level, the **hub fusion** then publishes it in a new stream, so

---

[4] Apache Kafka: https://kafka.apache.org/.
[5] https://www.affectiva.com/.
[6] https://www.kairos.com/.

that it can be available for consumption in other places, such as in the **modality controller** which it effectively does. This module then interprets the stream's semantics, and, if a new affective state is detected for that specific user, an MMI life cycle event, containing that data, is generated and sent to the Interaction Manager. After sending the event, all the applications that are part of the multimodal ecosystem, and which are interested in obtaining the affective state of the user to which it belongs, can consume the message so that they can adapt themselves to the detected emotional state.

4.3   Integration in the Application's Context

The versatility and decoupled nature of the used multimodal architecture enabled the Affective Modality to be easily integrated with the multimodal framework. Whenever the Affective Modality detects a change in the user's affective state, it sends a new event, containing that information, to the Interaction Manager. After the event is sent, it is the responsibility of the Interaction Manager to deliver it to any interested application, that is currently running, and in which the user that the event belongs to is currently logged.

The applications that are present in the multimodal ecosystem will continuously receive the new events that are generated by the Affective Modality, which contain the affective states of their users to allow them to adapt themselves accordingly. It is important to mention that, for the applications to be able to deploy the Affective Modality and subsequently receive their users' emotional updates, they need to implement and be able to communicate with the Interaction Manager.

5   Proof-of-Concept Results

With the integration process of the modality already described, it is now presented an illustrative proof-of-concept depicting the modality in action (Fig. 4). To this end, a simple proof-of-concept Android application has been developed, adopting the AM4I framework [4], and integrating the proposed Affective Modality. The main purpose of such integration was to enable the developed application to react to whichever user's emotional state updates received.

For the sake of simplicity, the webcam of the user's laptop is active and forwarding the video feed to his corresponding Kafka topic. The application, as soon as the user logs in, informs the modality that it has an interest in being updated regarding possible changes in its user's emotional state. When the video data reaches the user's topic, the Affective Modality backend processes it using one of the available affective services. As soon as the user's emotional state is identified, it is then redirected to the developed application so that it can react accordingly, as depicted in Fig. 4.

As seen in this practical example, by integrating the developed modality, the app developers simply need to declare that they want to know the users' affective states and deal with the semantic contents of the events that reach

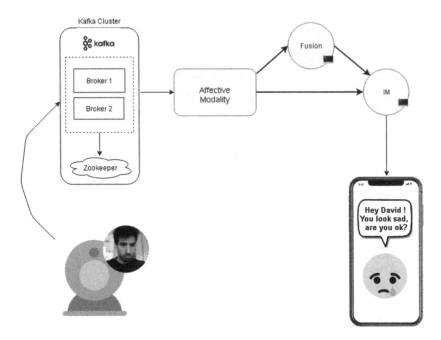

Fig. 4. Practical example of the Modality's Integration. An ambient camera captures the user's face, and that video data serves as a source for the Affective Modality to compute the associated affective state, subsequently notifying an application, on the user's smartphone, about that emotional update.

their system. This way, most of the complexity that is inherent to emotional extraction is transparently handled by remote services or toolkits, thus allowing them to focus on their system's development.

6   Conclusions

This article evolves early work, by the authors, in proposing a conceptual vision for the deployment of multimodal emotionally-aware ecosystems and showcases an improved version of a key component in this vision, a generic Affective Modality. This modality is proposed in the scope of a multimodal interactive framework, the AM4I, enabling any system that adopts it to have off-the-shelf support for affective inputs. In this regard, the full adoption of the standards proposed by the W3C also enabled a fully decoupled communication between mobile applications and the proposed modality, which was not possible in our previous proposal [10]. Additionally, the proposed vision advances how the research in affective computing can more rapidly integrate with real scenarios, and the proposal of a sensing repository based on Kafka should enable the consideration of technologies, such as Kafka Streams, to support the development of affective methods, thus facilitating their faster integration with the Affective Modality. This, should be the goal of our future efforts.

Acknowledgement. This work is partially funded by IEETA Research Unit funding (UID/CEC/00127/2019), by Portugal 2020 under the Competitiveness and Internationalisation Operational Program, the European Regional Development Fund through project SOCA – Smart Open Campus (CENTRO-01-0145-FEDER-000010), and project Smart Green Homes (POCI-01-0247-FEDER-007678), a co-promotion between Bosch Termotecnologia S.A. and the University of Aveiro.

References

1. Alavi, H.S., Verma, H., Papinutto, M., Lalanne, D.: Comfort: a coordinate of user experience in interactive built environments. In: Bernhaupt, R., Dalvi, G., Joshi, A., Balkrishan, D.K., ONeill, J., Winckler, M. (eds.) INTERACT 2017. LNCS, vol. 10515, pp. 247–257. Springer, Cham (2017). https://doi.org/10.1007/978-3-319-67687-6_16

2. Almeida, N., Silva, S., Teixeira, A.: Design and development of speech interaction: a methodology. In: Kurosu, M. (ed.) HCI 2014. LNCS, vol. 8511, pp. 370–381. Springer, Cham (2014). https://doi.org/10.1007/978-3-319-07230-2_36

3. Almeida, N., Silva, S., Teixeira, A., Vieira, D.: Multi-device applications using the multimodal architecture. In: Dahl, D.A. (ed.) Multimodal Interaction with W3C Standards, pp. 367–383. Springer, Cham (2017). https://doi.org/10.1007/978-3-319-42816-1_17

4. Almeida, N., Teixeira, A., Silva, S., Ketsmur, M.: The am4i architecture and framework for multimodal interaction and its application to smart environments. Sensors **19**(11), 2587 (2019)

5. Barrett, L.F.: How Emotions are Made: The Secret Life of the Brain. Houghton Mifflin Harcourt, Boston (2017)

6. Brigham, T.J.: Merging technology and emotions: introduction to affective computing. Med. Reference Serv. Q. **36**(4), 399–407 (2017)

7. Dahl, D.A. (ed.): Multimodal Interaction with W3C Standards. Springer, Cham (2017). https://doi.org/10.1007/978-3-319-42816-1

8. Dumas, B., Lalanne, D., Oviatt, S.: Multimodal interfaces: a survey of principles, models and frameworks. In: Lalanne, D., Kohlas, J. (eds.) Human Machine Interaction. LNCS, vol. 5440, pp. 3–26. Springer, Heidelberg (2009). https://doi.org/10.1007/978-3-642-00437-7_1

9. Gay, V., Leijdekkers, P., Agcanas, J., Wong, F., Wu, Q.: CaptureMyEmotion: helping autistic children understand their emotions using facial expression recognition and mobile technologies. Stud. Health Technol. Inform. **189**, 71–76 (2013)

10. Henriques, T., Soares, S.C., Silva, S., Almeida, N., Brás, S., Teixeira, A.: Emotionally-aware multimodal interfaces: preliminary work on a generic affective modality. DSAI 2018, 20–22 June 2018, Thessaloniki, Greece (2018)

11. Hoste, L., Dumas, B., Signer, B.: Mudra: a unified multimodal interaction framework. In: Proceedings of the 13th International Conference on Multimodal Interfaces, pp. 97–104. ICMI 2011, ACM, New York (2011). https://doi.org/10.1145/2070481.2070500

12. Picard, R.W.: Emotion research by the people, for the people. Emotion Rev. **2**(3), 250–254 (2010)

13. Poria, S., Cambria, E., Bajpai, R., Hussain, A.: A review of affective computing: from unimodal analysis to multimodal fusion. Inf. Fus. **37**, 98–125 (2017)

14. Schmidt, A.: Implicit human computer interaction through context. Personal Technol. **4**(2–3), 191–199 (2000)

15. Serrano, M., Nigay, L., Lawson, J.Y.L., Ramsay, A., Murray-Smith, R., Denef, S.: The openinterface framework: a tool for multimodal interaction. In: Proceeding of the Twenty-Sixth Annual CHI Conference Extended Abstracts on Human Factors in Computing Systems - CHI 2008, p. 3501. ACM Press, New York, April 2008. https://doi.org/10.1145/1358628.1358881
16. Sucala, M., et al.: Anxiety: there is an app for that. a systematic review of anxiety apps. Depression and Anxiety 34, 518–525 (2017)
17. Solovey, E.T., Afergan, D., Peck, E.M., Hincks, S.W., Jacob, R.J.K.: Designing implicit interfaces for physiological computing (2015)
18. Teixeira, A., et al.: Design and development of Medication Assistant: older adults centred design to go beyond simple medication reminders. Univ. Access Inf. Soc. **16**(3), 545–560 (2016). https://doi.org/10.1007/s10209-016-0487-7
19. Tyng, C.M., Amin, H.U., Saad, M., Malik, A.S.: The influences of emotion on learning and memory. Front. Psychol. **8**, 1454 (2017)

A SmartBed for Non-obtrusive Physiological Monitoring During Sleep: The LAID Project

Marco Laurino[1]([✉]) [ID], Nicola Carbonaro[2,3] [ID], Danilo Menicucci[4] [ID], Gaspare Alfì[4], Angelo Gemignani[1,4], and Alessandro Tognetti[2,3] [ID]

[1] Institute of Clinical Physiology, National Research Council, Pisa, Italy
laurino@ifc.cnr.it
[2] Department of Information Engineering, University of Pisa, Pisa, Italy
[3] Research Centre "E. Piaggio", University of Pisa, Pisa, Italy
[4] Department of Surgical, Medical and Molecular Pathology and Critical Care Medicine, University of Pisa, Pisa, Italy

Abstract. The individual experience of inadequate or insufficient sleep is one of the most common health issues in the industrialized world. The 65% of Italian population reports disturbed sleep experiences, while chronic sleep disorders affect about 10% of the population. The people with inadequate and unsatisfactory sleep often suffers drowsiness during the day associated with both somatic and mental disorders. For these reasons, the systematic and continuative monitoring of sleep is one of the main objectives in preventive, personalized and participatory sleep medicine. The purpose of this paper is to describe the architecture of a "smart mattress" (SmartBed) that is the main outcome of the Italian R&D project called LAID. SmartBed will be able to non-obtrusively collect physiological and environmental parameters and signals, to processing them and to provide information about the quality of sleep, the levels of stress, and more generally the well-being of an individual. Specifically, SmartBed will be able to estimate data relating to cardiorespiratory activity, movements, body position, snoring and environmental parameters. SmartBed aims to obtain a continuative and ecological assessment of sleep and well-being of a person, in order to improve his quality of life. SmartBed will be a fundamental tool for carrying out both longitudinal and epidemiological studies on the quality of sleep and life on general population.

Keywords: Sleep · Sensorized mattress · Non-obtrusive sensors

1 Introduction

The inadequate sleep and insomnia are the most common human health issues in the industrialized societies. As the experiences during the day deeply influences sleep quality, sleep also influences the efficiency of activities during wakefulness. In fact, insomnia correlates with high rates of absenteeism from work, with the reduction of performance capabilities, and with accidents at work or on the road. Sleepless people have more frequent medical issues, indeed they use healthcare facilities and drugs much more

G. M. P. O'Hare et al. (Eds.): MobiHealth 2019, LNICST 320, pp. 153–162, 2020.
https://doi.org/10.1007/978-3-030-49289-2_12

than non-sleepless. Among the health problems related to insomnia the best known are metabolic diseases (diabetes and dyslipidemia), some cardiovascular diseases (myocardial infarction and hypertension), as well as cognitive impairment [1]. In addition, chronic insomnia increases the probability of death due to myocardial infarction as well as the vulnerability to affective psychopathology (Depression and Anxiety Disorders) [2]. In order to obtain a new tool to identify sleep disorders in the general population, we conceived an R&D project called **LAID** "Linking Automation to artificial Intelligence for revealing sleep Dysfunctions". LAID project aims to develop an innovative smart mattress (**SmartBed**) able to identify insomnia or preclinical sleep disorders early, with the final goals of reducing the socio-economic cost due to sleep disorders and increasing individual well-being condition. More specifically, LAID project is concern about the research and development of: i) a sensorized smart mattress for non-obtrusive physiological data collecting, ii) an innovative algorithms for physiological data processing and iii) a software for extraction of sleep quality index. With respect to previous developed smart mattress (e.g. [3]), LAID project aimed to obtain a low-cost product, with multi-sensors integration and innovative algorithm for sleep quality estimation.

2   Materials and Methods

2.1   Overall Architecture

In order to estimate the global quality of sleep, it is important to evaluate not only the physiological state of the subject but also the environmental conditions. Besides, it will also possible to associate sleep issues with both physiological alterations and specific features of environment where the subject sleeps.

The overall architecture of SmartBed is composed by the following functional blocks (see Fig. 1):

- Physiological data collector (PDC)
- Environmental data collector (EDC)
- Docking station (DS)

Both PDC and EDC are wired to DS via serial communication interface. The DS of the first prototype is windows 10 based system with a tailored software for managing PDS and EDC, processing the signals and parameters from PDS/EDC, storing the collected data, and finally extracting the sleep quality and well-being indices. The future version of DS will be managed also by a user-friendly interface by mobile device and the data will be sent and stored on specific cloud database.

The most innovative aspects of SmartBed is the PDC and the integration between PDC/EDC data. PDC is made of a custom designed acquisition unit and it has two kind of sensors: three-axial accelerometers and a pressure matrix. The mattress of SmartBed is made by Materassificio Montalese S.P.A. (Pistoia, Italy), the PDC is design and develop by EB Neuro S.P.A (Firenze, Italy), EDC and DS by BP Engineering S.P.A. (Carrara, Italy).

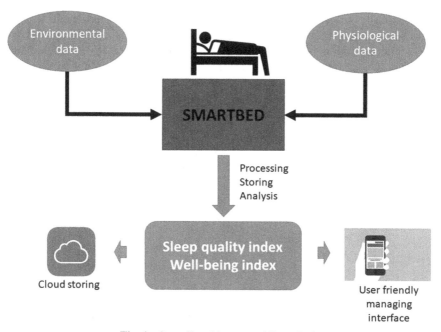

Fig. 1. Overall architecture of SmartBed.

2.2 Accelerometers

The accelerometric signals collected by SmartBed will be used to evaluate the cardiac and respiratory activities and movements of the subject during the night in a non-obtrusive way. The used accelerometers are the PNADXL362 (Analog Device), their specifications are reported in Table 1.

Table 1. Accelerometer specifications

Number of axes	3
Range	± 2 g
Supply voltage	3.3 V
Sensitivity	1 mg/LSB
Raw data noise level	175 μg/$\sqrt{}$Hz (ultralow noise mode)
Bit resolution	12 bits
Sampling frequency	128 Hz
Shape and dimension	Circular, diameter 2.2 cm

We used three accelerometers simultaneously but in different positions of the mattress. One was placed in a central area of the mattress, and the other two in lateral and contro-lateral sites (as shown in Fig. 2). In this way, by mediating the signals from different accelerometers we can reduce the noise. Furthermore, if the subject places itself on non-centered positions our idea is to select or set a higher weight to the accelerometer closer to the subject. Indeed, we can obtain the exact body position of the subject on the mattress by using the pressure matrix.

The accelerations collected from PDC are used to estimate the movements, the cardiac and respiratory activities of the subjects on SmartBed during the night.

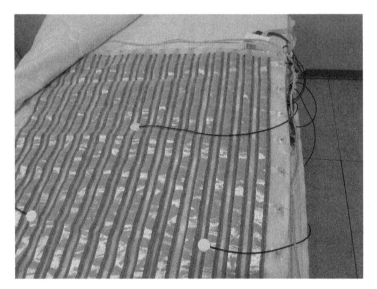

Fig. 2. Position of accelerometers (white dots) over the pressure matrix.

2.3 Pressure Matrix

Starting from the analysis of the literature and considering the lower complexity, the lower cost and the greater tolerance to external disturbances, we have considered the resistive sensor matrix solution, similar to the one reported in [4]. Considering the project specifications (spatial resolution <10 cm, single mattress measuring 190 × 90 cm), we have built a mattress cover based on a resistive matrix of 15 × 13 uniformly spaced sensing areas that cover a surface of 125 × 75 cm (i.e. head and feet will not be considered in this first version of the prototype). Figure 3 shows a schematic description of the proposed solution: the central layer is a pressure sensing semi-conductive fabric while the additional two layers are fabrics with integrated row and column conductors (note that row and column conductors are perpendicular).

Two analog multiplexers are used to scan rows (row mux) and columns (column mux) in order to select all the sensing areas of the resistive matrix. The row mux sequentially connects each row conductor to Vcc (3.3 V) through a pull-up resistor R1 (2 KΩ). When a row is selected (i.e. powered), the col mux sequentially connects each col conductor

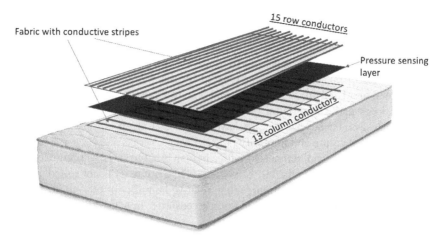

Fig. 3. Proposed solution: mattress cover based on a resistive matrix with 13 column conductors and 15 row conductors for a total of 195 sensing areas.

to a voltage divider stage (pull down resistor R2, 10 KΩ). In this way, each crossing between a row and a column represents a sensing area whose electrical resistance will decrease as the applied pressure increases.

For the pressure-sensing layer, we have used the semi-conductive fabric CARBOTEX 03-82 by SEFAR AG. The top and bottom layers are made of a PET fabric (from SEFAR AG) with integrated evenly spaced metallic stripes. According to our indications, the metallic stripes have 2 cm width and are separated 3 cm in the top layer and 8 cm in the bottom layer. As described in [5], this sensing architecture has parasitic resistivity on the transversal directions due to the conductivity of the pressure-sensing layer. To reduce the cross-talk due to the parasitic resistivity we have built our prototype by additionally cutting the sensing layer in stripes parallel to the column direction (around 3.5 cm width). The stripes were then sewn to the top layer to be centered with respect to the row conductors. Figure 4 reports the details of the pressure sensing matrix prototype.

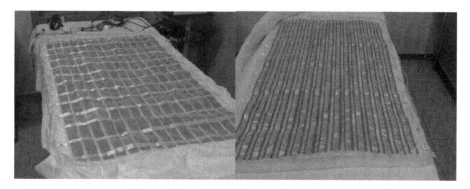

Fig. 4. Pressure sensing matrix: on the left the top layer, on the right the bottom layer.

2.4 Environmental Data

As expected, environmental acoustic noise also influences sleep [6–9]. Ohrstrom [7] has shown that intermittent acoustic noise causes a worsening of sleep with respect to constant levels of noise. In a report prepared for the World Health Organization in 1995, Berglund and Lindvall [11] recommend a continuous noise level no higher than 30/35 dB indoors and a maximum of 45 dB for intermittent noise exposure caused by single noisy events. Several studies have shown that sleep is influenced by both environmental temperature and humidity [9, 12, 13].

The comfortable range of temperature for a human is between 22.8 °C and 26.1 °C in summer and between 20 °C and 23.9 °C in winter. High humidity is not suited to higher temperatures than to lower temperatures (e.g. relative humidity of 60% at 26.1 °C and 85% at 20 °C are both optimal) [10]. In addition, exposure to light can alter sleep, through the inhibition of melatonin secretion in humans.

Therefore, all these studies have shown that is extremely important to monitor and evaluate environmental conditions in order to assess the quality of sleep and overall well-being.

The EDC module is based on Seeeduino V4.2 board. It is composed by several sensors to collect the following environmental variables: i) sound intensity, ii) temperature, iii) relative humidity, iv) luminosity and v) atmospheric pressure. All the variables, except for the sound intensity, is collected with a sampling frequency of 1 Hz. Since the environmental sound intensity is the only parameter that has a potentially fast dynamic and it is also be used to evaluate the respiratory activity and snoring, its sampling frequency is set to 20 Hz. All the signals and parameters are collected synchronized with respect to the data from PDC.

2.5 Processing Algorithm

In the first prototype of SmartBed, the DS module is a windows 10 based system with a tailored software able to collect simultaneously all the signals from PDC and EDC. The software on DS on the next prototype of SmartBed will also contain the processing algorithm to estimate the sleep quality index that is now in a preliminary version. The sleep quality index will be mainly obtained from the integration of two kind of information: macrostructure of sleep (sleep stages, sleep duration and sleep apnea episodes) and environmental condition. The macrostructure of sleep will be estimates from the following parameters: the cardiac activity, the respiratory activity, the movements and the body position during the night. The cardiac activity (heart rate and heart rate variability) will be estimated from the ballistocardiogram obtained from the accelerometer signals and by using validated algorithms available in literature [14–16]. The respiratory activity (breathing rate) will be obtained from signals of accelerometers, pressure matrix and sound sensor [17–19]. The movements of the subject will be evaluated from the accelerometers and the pressure matrix. Finally, the body position will be assessed with pressure matrix (Fig. 5).

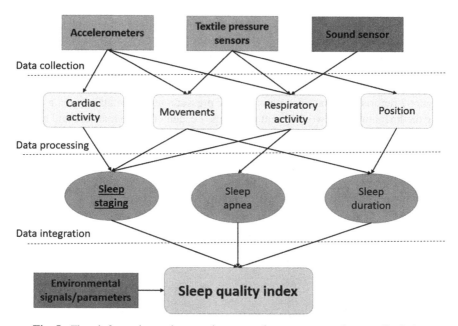

Fig. 5. Flow information and processing stages from sensors to sleep quality index.

3 Results

The actual prototype of SmartBed can acquire and store the data from both PDC and EDC. In Fig. 6 the signals (60 s) of each axis of the three accelerometers are reported during a recording of a subject laying on SmartBed.

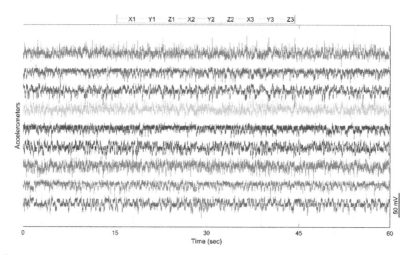

Fig. 6. Signals from the three 3-axial accelerometers of 60 s with a subject standing on SmartBed.

The accelerometers respond consistently to the accelerations to which they are subjected by the person on the mattress, it is possible to clearly detect the macroscopic movements by the subject on the mattress. The next step of the project will be dedicated to the evaluation of the quality of the signals for the estimation of indexes of the cardiac and respiratory activity.

Figure 7 reports the processed output of the pressure-sensing matrix when a subject is lying on the mattress in two different positions (i.e. center of the mattress and towards his right). The chest, the upper arms and the legs can be easily recognizable. The image reported in the figure is obtained by a linear interpolation of the raw output values in each sensing area. In addition, a threshold algorithm is applied to compensate for the sensor bias.

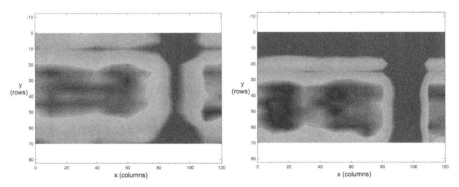

Fig. 7. Pressure maps with same subject in two different positions on the mattress (on the left the subject is centered on the mattress, while on the right the subject has moved to his right).

4   Conclusion

Years of scientific evidence have reported the importance of the sleep that is strictly related to our psychophysical wellbeing, the stability of our mood, our memories and cognitive abilities, and to the quality of our health. It is also well known that sleep alterations can completely modulate homeostatic condition and adaptive functions of subjects during the day.

The main aim of LAID project will be the design and development of a "smart mattress" (SmartBed) able to record vital and environmental signals/parameters in a non-obtrusive way, to analyze them and to provide information about the quality of sleep and more generally about the well-being and on quality of life of an individual.

The first stage of the LAID project is concluded and now the first hardware and software prototype of SmartBed is available and well-working.

In conclusion, the first prototype of SmartBed has good performances regarding the acquisition of measures related to the physiology of the subject on the sensorized mattress and the environmental parameters. At now, the signals and parameters collected that can be collected are: i) 3-axial accelerations, ii) pressure matrix, iii) environmental parameters (noise, temperature, relative humidity, atmospheric pressure and luminosity). Future activities will be aimed at integrating the signals and testing the system with an adequate number of subjects.

Acknowledgment. LAID project is co-funded by Tuscany POR FESR 2014−2020 (DD 3389/2014 call 1). We would to thank all our industrial partners: Materassificio Montalese S.P.A, EB Neuro S.P.A and BP Engineering S.P.A.

References

1. Terzano, M.G., et al.: Studio Morfeo: insomnia in primary care, a survey conducted on the Italian population. Sleep Med. **5**(1), 67–75 (2004)
2. Leger, D., Guilleminault, C., Bader, G., Levy, E., Paillard, M.: Medical and socio-professional impact of insomnia. Sleep **25**(6), 625–629 (2002)
3. Hao, J., Jayachandran, M., Kng, P.L., Foo, S.F., Aung, P.W.A., Cai, Z.: FBG-based smart bed system for healthcare applications. Front. Optoelectron. China **3**(1), 78–83 (2010). https://doi.org/10.1007/s12200-009-0066-0
4. Cheng, J., Sundholm, M., Zhou, B., Hirsch, M., Lukowicz, P.: Smart-surface: large scale textile pressure sensors arrays for activity recognition. Pervasive Mob. Comput. **30**, 97–112 (2016)
5. Zhou, B., Lukowicz, P.: Textile pressure force mapping. In: Schneegass, S., Amft, O. (eds.) Smart Textiles, pp. 31–47. Springer, Cham (2017). https://doi.org/10.1007/978-3-319-50124-6_3
6. Marquis-Favre, C., Premat, E., Aubree, D.: Noise and its effects - a review on qualitative aspects of sound. Part II: noise and annoyance. Acta Acustica United Acustica **91**(4), 626–642 (2005)
7. Ohrstrom, E., Skanberg, A.: Sleep disturbances from road traffic and ventilation noise - laboratory and field experiments. J. Sound Vib. **271**(1–2), 279–296 (2004)
8. Bonnet, M.H., Arand, D.L.: The impact of music upon sleep tendency as measured by the multiple sleep latency test and maintenance of wakefulness test. Physiol. Behav. **71**(5), 485–492 (2000)
9. Okamoto-Mizuno, K., Tsuzuki, K., Mizuno, K., Iwaki, T.: Effects of partial humid heat exposure during different segments of sleep on human sleep stages and body temperature. Physiol. Behav. **83**(5), 759–765 (2005)
10. Wickens, K., et al.: The determinants of dust mite allergen and its relationship to the prevalence of symptoms of asthma in the Asia-Pacific region. Pediatr. Allergy Immunol. **15**(1), 55–61 (2004)
11. Berglund, B., Lindvall, T.: Community noise: Center for Sensory Research. Stockholm University and Karolinska Institute (1995)
12. Libert, J.P., Dinisi, J., Fukuda, H., Muzet, A., Ehrhart, J., Amoros, C.: Effect of continuous heat exposure on sleep stages in humans. Sleep **11**(2), 195–209 (1988)
13. Dewasmes, G., Telliez, F., Muzet, A.: Effects of a nocturnal environment perceived as warm on subsequent daytime sleep in humans. Sleep **23**(3), 409–413 (2000)
14. Vehkaoja, A., Rajala, S., Kumpulainen, P., Lekkala, J.: Correlation approach for the detection of the heartbeat intervals using force sensors placed under the bed posts. J. Med. Eng. Technol. **37**(5), 327–333 (2013)
15. Brueser, C., Winter, S., Leonhardt, S.: Robust inter-beat interval estimation in cardiac vibration signals. Physiol. Meas. **34**(2), 123–138 (2013)

16. Choe, S.-T., Cho, W.-D.: Simplified real-time heartbeat detection in ballistocardiography using a dispersion-maximum method. Biomed. Res. India **28**(9), 3974–3985 (2017)
17. Sanchez Morillo, D., Rojas Ojeda, J.L., Crespo Foix, L.F., Leon Jimenez, A.: An accelerometer-based device for sleep apnea screening. IEEE Trans. Inf. Technol. Biomed. **14**(2), 491–499 (2010)
18. Nam, Y., Kim, Y., Lee, J.: Sleep monitoring based on a tri-axial accelerometer and a pressure Sensor. Sensors. **16**(5), 750 (2016)
19. Ren, Y., Wang, C., Yang, J., Chen, Y.: IEEE fine-grained sleep monitoring: hearing your breathing with smartphones. In: 2015 IEEE Conference on Computer Communications (Infocom) (2015)

A Prototype System of Acute Stroke Type Discrimination and Monitoring Based on a Annulus Antenna Array: A Pilot Study

Mingsheng Chen, Jia Xu, Jingbo Chen, Haisheng Zhang, and Mingxin Qin[✉]

Department of Biomedical Engineering and Medical Imaging, Army Medical University,
Chongqing 400038, China
qmingxin@tmmu.edu.cn

Abstract. Objective: Timely and effective discrimination of hemorrhagic stroke and ischemic stroke can significantly improve the prognosis. Current discrimination is expensive and has the disadvantage of having to be in contact with the patient. Based on animal experiments, in this paper, microwave measurement technique is used to study the discrimination of two stroke types. Method: In the experiments, 10 rabbits (5 cerebral hemorrhage and 5 cerebral ischemia) are selected. Cerebral hemorrhage is induced by injecting autologous blood (1 to 4 mL) into the brain of rabbits, and the cerebral ischemia is induced by bilateral common carotid artery ligation and femoral artery blood extraction. The two groups are monitored by a 16-channel microwave detection system to obtain the reflection parameter caused by pathological changes in the brain. After redundancy removed from original data, support vector machine (SVM) is used to identify the type and severity of two types of stroke. Findings: The study shows that the microwave-based stroke identification system can effectively distinguish the cerebral hemorrhage model and the cerebral ischemia model. The experimental system is very promising in pre-hospital stroke type identification because of low cost, non-invasive, simple operation and rapid measurement.

Keywords: Stroke type discrimination · Cerebral hemorrhage · Cerebral ischemia · Microwave detection · Support Vector Machine

1 Introduction

The treatments of hemorrhagic stroke and ischemic stroke are significantly different, which make the stroke type diagnosis imperative before treatment (Lancet 2015). According to European clinical guideline (Committee 2008; Appelros 2015), within 4.5 h after ischemic stroke, it is the golden period of receiving thrombolytic therapy. Therefore, it is of great significance to develop an instrument for pre-hospital stroke type diagnosis which is portable, fast, and easy to operate.

Recently, mobile CT (Computed Tomography) equipment has been used for pre-hospital stroke diagnosis (Gierhake 2013; John et al. 2016). It significantly shortens the

© ICST Institute for Computer Sciences, Social Informatics and Telecommunications Engineering 2020
Published by Springer Nature Switzerland AG 2020. All Rights Reserved
G. M. P. O'Hare et al. (Eds.): MobiHealth 2019, LNICST 320, pp. 163–168, 2020.
https://doi.org/10.1007/978-3-030-49289-2_13

intervening time between ischemic stroke attack and thrombolytic therapy (Fassbender et al. 2013), but its application is limited by the medical vehicles it installed, the required professional medical staff, the stable environment and good communication. Also, it can't be used to continuously monitor rapid pathologic lesions in the acute phase of stroke. Transcranial doppler ultrasound (TCD), Near infrared spectroscopy (NIR) can be used for continuously monitoring in neurocritical intensive care unit (N-ICU) to detect large-scale vascular occlusion of stroke (Schlachetzki et al. 2012; Nakae 2012; Erdoes et al. 2018). But these methods are difficult to detect accurately when the vascular is small or the position is deep, and also cannot be used to identify bleeding caused by ischemic. Electrical impedance tomography (EIT) has been reported to detect cerebral hemorrhagic in animal experiments (Xu 2010), and to detect intracranial tissue displacement caused by stroke (Bonmassar et al. 2010). However, the measurement accuracy is easily affected by the contact resistance and the high resistivity of the skull. Microwave imaging technology has been gradually applied to brain function monitoring after several decades of development (Crocco 2018). Unlike its research applications in breast cancer detection (Byrne et al. 2017; Chen et al. 2016), the complex structure of the brain limits the imaging quality of its disease diagnosis. Therefore, using microwave scattering parameters to discriminate stroke type without imaging deserves studying.

This study combines microwave detection and pattern recognition method to rapidly diagnose and monitor stroke type without imaging of brain. This study has the following innovations, (1) A new parameter Euclidean distance is proposed here mapping the original scattering parameters, which improves the discrimination between hemorrhagic stroke and ischemic stroke. (2) Before the SVM classification, we firstly carry out the dimensionality reduction to improve the diagnostic accuracy and the efficiency of the classifier. (3) The in vivo animal experiment under controlled conditions is validated by the microwave-based stroke detection system, which not only diagnoses the type of stroke but also monitors the development of stroke.

Based on the multi-channel detection system in this study, it realizes the classification of different types and different degrees of stroke in rabbit model with discrimination accuracy of 90%. Experiments have shown that different degrees of cerebral hemorrhage and ischemia will lead to differences in microwave reflection signals, which demonstrate the feasibility of non-contact discrimination of stroke types and stroke severity based on electromagnetic properties of brain tissue.

2   Methodology

2.1   Detection Principle

The theoretical basis for the microwave reflection detection is to detect dielectric properties of different tissues in brain (Peyman et al. 2007; Schmid et al. 2003). Under pathological conditions, these changes in dielectric properties cause changes in reflection parameters.

2.2   Detection System

To detect the spatial electromagnetic properties of the whole brain, a multi-channel microwave measurement system is built here. The system is mainly composed of an antenna array sensor, a microwave monitoring device and a multiplexing switch controlled by a computer, connection as Fig. 1 shown.

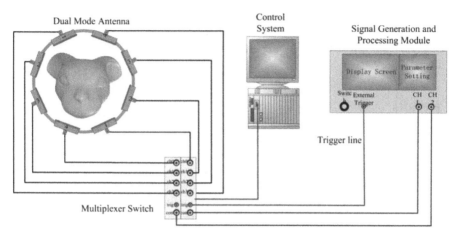

Fig. 1. System schematic

The antenna array is composed of 8 microwave patch antennas (4 Receiver and 4 Transmitter) which fixed on an acrylic loop, as shown in Fig. 1. The multiplexer switch controls 16 channels (4 Receiver × 4 Transmitter) in turn to launch the microwave measurement system. The measurement frequency ranges from 300 kHz to 3 GHz. The rabbit head is placed in the center of the sensor array during experiment, and the active antenna emits microwave through it. By detecting the reflected microwave, the parameters of the measured object are calculated, which reflect the dielectric properties of the object.

2.3 Experimental Process

Detection of cerebral hemorrhage model
The cerebral hemorrhage rabbit (inner capsule cerebral hemorrhage model) is placed on the measuring platform, and the data is measured before the blood injection as the origin experimental data (0 ml). Blood injected with the pump, and 1 ml blood is injected within 1 min. When each injection is completed (1 ml), the data is recorded and stored. The steps are repeated to complete the data acquisition at 2, 3, and 4 ml.

Detection of cerebral ischemia model
After ischemic model of bilateral carotid artery ligation, rabbits are placed on the measurement platform. The initial (0 min) ischemic data is recorded and saved at this time. Then set the multiplexer switch to automatically measure 1 time every 6 min. The measurement is repeated 6 times and the total recording time is 42 min.

2.4   Classification Algorithm

The number of samples in this experiment is small. The statistical learning theory is suitable for small sample cases according to machine learning theory. Therefore, we choose the SVM classification algorithm based on statistical learning. This paper mainly uses the LIBSVM toolkit provided by Chih-Chung Chang and Chih-Jen Lin (Fan et al. 2005; Chang and Lin 2011), and compares different parameters affecting classification accuracy.

3   Results

Since the cerebral hemorrhage model and cerebral ischemia model are different, and the pathological mechanisms are different, the data of hemorrhage (maximum 4 ml, minimum 1 ml) and ischemia (maximum 42 min, minimum 6 min) are discriminated here, preliminarily. The classification results are shown in Fig. 2. It can be seen that for the classification of hemorrhage and ischemia, the classification accuracy is above 85%, and a higher classification accuracy is achieved under linear kernel function.

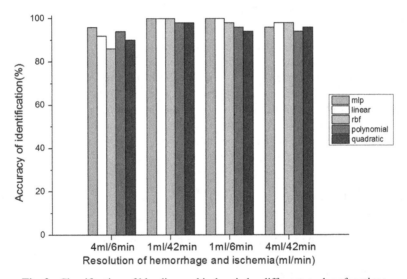

Fig. 2. Classification of bleeding and ischemia by different nuclear functions

4   Conclusions

Based on the multi-channel detection system described in this study, this paper realizes the classification of different types and different degrees of stroke on rabbit models with 90% identification accuracy. Experiments have shown that different degrees of cerebral hemorrhage and ischemia will lead to differences in microwave reflection signals, which confirm the feasibility of non-contact discrimination of stroke types based on electromagnetic properties of brain tissue. It is indicated that the electromagnetic-based method for detecting stroke is a very promising method. There will be more stroke patients benefit from its portability and low cost. And it is hopeful that more cerebral ischemia patients will be received timely thrombolytic therapy. At the same time, it indicates that the data preprocessing, the selection of classification features and the classifier are the critical factors to determine the final detection accuracy in the research.

References

Appelros, P.T.A.: Thrombolysis in acute stroke. The Lancet **9976**, 1394 (2015)

Bonmassar, G., Iwaki, S., Goldmakher, G., Angelone, L.M., Belliveau, J.W., Lev, M.H.: On the measurement of electrical impedance spectroscopy (EIS) of the human head. Int. J. Bioelectromagn. **12**, 32–46 (2010)

Byrne, D., Sarafianou, M., Craddock, I.J.: Compound radar approach for breast imaging. IEEE Trans. Biomed. Eng. **64**, 40–51 (2017)

Chang, C., Lin, C.: LIBSVM: a library for support vector machines. ACM Trans. Intell. Syst. Technol. **2**, 27:1–27:27 (2011)

Chen, B., Zhang, Y., Wang, L., Wang, F.: Microwave tomography for early breast cancer detection based on the alternating direction implicit finite-difference time-domain method. Acta Physica Sinca, 65 (2016)

Committee, E.S.O.E.: Guidelines for management of ischaemic stroke and transient ischaemic attack 2008. Cerebrovascular Diseases **25**, 457–507 (2008)

Crocco, L, Karanasiou, I., James, M.: Emerging Electromagnetic Technologies for Brain Diseases Diagnostics, Monitoring and Therapy‖Microwave Technology for Brain Imaging and Monitoring: Physical Foundations, Potential and Limitations. (Chapter 2), 7–35 (2018)

Erdoes, G., et al.: Limitations of current near-infrared spectroscopy configuration in detecting focal cerebral ischemia during cardiac surgery: an observational case-series study. Artif. Organs **42**, 1001–1009 (2018)

Fan, R.E., Chen, P.H., Lin, C.J.: Working set selection using second order information for training SVM. J. Mach. Learn. Res. **6**, 1889–1918 (2005)

Fassbender, K., Balucani, C., Walter, S., Levine, S.R., Haass, A., Grotta, J.: Streamlining of prehospital stroke management: the golden hour. Lancet Neurol. **12**, 585–596 (2013)

Gierhake, D, et al.: Mobile CT: technical aspects of prehospital stroke imaging before intravenous thrombolysis. Rofo, 1, 55–59 (2013)

John, S., et al.: Brain imaging using mobile ct: current status and future prospects. J. Neuroimag. **26**, 5–15 (2016)

Lancet, T.: Achieving respectful care for women and babies. Lancet **385**, 1366 (2015)

Nakae, R.Y.H.Y.: Transcranial doppler ultrasounography for diagnosis of cerebral vasospasm after aneurysmal subarachnoid hemorrhage: mean blood flow velocity ratio of the ipsilateral and contralateral middle cerebral arteries. J. Vascular Surgery **4**, 1220 (2012)

Peyman, A., Holden, S.J., Watts, S., Perrott, R., Gabriel, C.: Dielectric properties of porcine cerebrospinal tissues at microwave frequencies: in vivo, in vitro and systematic variation with age. Phys. Med. **52**, 2229–2245 (2007)

Schlachetzki, F., et al.: Transcranial ultrasound from diagnosis to early stroke treatment – part 2: prehospital neurosonography in patients with acute stroke – the regensburg stroke mobile project. Cerebrovascular Dis. **33**, 262–271 (2012)

Schmid, G., Neubauer, G., Mazal, P.R.: Dielectric properties of human brain tissue measured less than 10 h postmortem at frequencies from 800 to 2450 MHz. Bioelectromagnetics **24**, 423–430 (2003)

Xu, C.H., et al.: Real-Time imaging and detection of intracranial haemorrhage by electrical impedance tomography in a piglet model. J. Int. Med. Res. **5**, 1596–1604 (2010)

Patient Monitoring and Robotics

Smart System for Supporting the Elderly in Home Environment

Eleni Boumpa[✉][iD] and Athanasios Kakarountas[iD]

Intelligent Systems Laboratory, University of Thessaly, Lamia, Greece
{eboumpa,kakarountas}@uth.gr

Abstract. This work presents the development of an assistive system for the elderly in their home environment. The purpose of this system is to provide them support and extend their autonomy in order to extend life expectancy and improve quality of life when living at home. This work explores various technological innovations and technology building blocks, such as open software and open hardware. In this work, a low-cost and small-scale ubiquitous system was developed that does not disrupt the prevailing conditions in the elderly's home. Also, a part of this work has been developed, keeping in mind elderly people suffering from dementia, offering a sufferer-centered solution.

Keywords: Smart home · Assisted living · Internet of Things · Dementia

1 Introduction

Global demographic trends show that the population aging is very fast. According to the report [1], the population of the European Union in 2017 amounted to 511.5 million, of which 19.4% consisted of people over 65 years of age. The percentage of the population aged over 65 increased in all EU Member States as it rose by 0.2% compared to the corresponding 2016 and by 2.4% compared to 10 years ago.

Furthermore, dementia is a collective name for progressive brain syndromes that affect memory, thought, behavior and emotions of the elderly. Dementia is a major cause of disability and dependability for the elderly. Dementia affects about 50 million people worldwide, with a new case of dementia happening every 3 s worldwide. Until today, there is no cure for most types of dementia, but there are treatment and support [2].

Also, the desire of the elderly is to extend the time they live in their preferred environment, i.e. their home, increasing their autonomy, self-confidence, and mobility. These reasons have led the world scientific community to develop solutions for the assistive living of the elderly, as living independently in their own homes is an important goal for an increasing part of the world population.

Thus, with the help of constantly evolving technology, there have been developed solutions which mainly offer an environment that provides facilitation, like

© ICST Institute for Computer Sciences, Social Informatics and Telecommunications Engineering 2020
Published by Springer Nature Switzerland AG 2020. All Rights Reserved
G. M. P. O'Hare et al. (Eds.): MobiHealth 2019, LNICST 320, pp. 171–185, 2020.
https://doi.org/10.1007/978-3-030-49289-2_14

safety, well-being, etc., in the daily lives of the elderly. This work proposes an open software/hardware system to assist the elderly in their home environment. Its aim is the support, protection, well-being, and maintenance of their health and functional abilities, without discriminating between a sufferer of dementia or someone aging healthy. This system will consist of individual subsystems that will operate independently but will also be able to communicate with each other. The subsystems concern the safety of the elderly within the limits of their residence, prosperity, and support.

2   Exploration of Smart Homes

In recent years, a variety of home assistive systems for elderly people have been proposed. Already there are various assistive living systems, either in the experimental or research phase, which in the near future will be able to meet all the needs and requirements of the elderly for their controlled and autonomous life. For categorization reasons, we have divided the projects into two groups, those that refer to support the elderly, and those that refer to support dementia elderly people. Some of these works are presented below.

2.1   Supporting Systems for the Elderly

In [3] the proposed system oversees and helps the elderly maintain their level of physical activity balanced as well as perform their rehabilitation exercises after a serious illness in their home. A platform with various services aiming to enable older people to participate in social networks to prevent isolation and loneliness and improve their well-being is presented in [4]. An open hardware and software home-based system has been proposed in [5], which provides an integrated and easy-to-use residential system through which the elderly will have the means and technologies to have control of their lives for a longer period of time. In [6] a Personal Virtual Assistant allows the elderly to live independently for a longer period of time, with the use of assistive technology. The system at [7] aims to maintain the independence of older people by monitoring their physical state with mobile devices, assessing their neurological status using mobile phones and promoting self-care. The project in [8] provides to the elderly a set of services to organize their daily routine and monitor their health through an easy-to-use online platform. In [9] a virtual assistant is proposed to facilitate communication and cooperation between the elderly and their carers. A system that has smart internet applications to provide the elderly with personalized and environmentally-friendly help in their homes, to improve their quality of life, to be assisted whenever needed, to monitor their medication and rehabilitation physiotherapy and to reduce the cost of their health care is proposed in [10]. A proposed integrated, mobile and adaptive solution for remote sensing to support both patients, relatives, and friends with abnormal heart failure, as well as cardiologists and health professionals, in general, is presented in [11]. In [12] the development of mental health tools for the elderly and their families are presented, as well as for specialists, to measure and visualize the mental changes of the elderly.

2.2 Supporting Systems for the Elderly Focusing on Dementia

In [13], a system has been proposed to monitor the activities of dementia people, using sensors, to maintain their autonomy and quality of life, to provide them with a sense of security at home and to delay, as much as possible, their hospitalization in a care center for dementia people. A platform that allows remote monitoring and personalized intervention and care of the dementia people in order to support and maintain their health and functional and cognitive abilities is presented in [14]. In [15], various devices have been developed to support sufferers and their carers, such as memory support devices (e.g. medication reminders, etc.), devices that provide entertainment, and devices to facilitate communication (e.g. pre-programmed telephone). A service that supports the increase of the independence and well-being of dementia sufferers in their home environment, and reduces their social isolation, increases their participation in their daily activities, stimulate their cognitive skills and access to Internet services, is presented in [16]. Another innovative tool for supporting people with mild dementia for the provision of remote care, which exploits the transmission of data via television and the interplay of video between health professionals, sufferers, carers and sufferers' families using the Internet is presented in [17]. In [18] is presented a complete solution for the care, treatment, and diagnosis for dementia sufferers, which motivates them to perform personalized, emotionally oriented exercises, to stimulate cognitive processes, to cope with physical activities and promoting their social inclusion. The system in [19] helps dementia people in their daily routine, creating a room atmosphere that supports their feelings, activity, and mood. It consists of light, sounds and smells so that the atmosphere of the room is shaped to improve the mood and behavior of both the sufferers and the caregivers. The room's atmosphere creation is achieved by checking the calculated data of the people involved in their daily routine. A platform to monitor the movements of dementia people indoors and outdoors to identify them, to satisfy the desire of their relatives to monitor the location of the sufferers in order to avoid situations of danger, and to provide information when they leave a particular area, such as their home, hospital, etc. has been proposed in [20]. A platform capable of monitoring the behavior of users (movements, speech, interactions) and supporting individualized control of lights and devices in their environment, is presented in [21]. This project aims to help people with mild dementia to stay oriented at what they are supposed to do, by providing intelligent support capable of controlling devices in such a way as to flexibly drive their attention and behavior towards their goals.

2.3 Commercial Smart Home Solutions

There exist nowadays commercial smart home solutions covering partially the needs of elderly people. They mainly focus on safety and security services, however, some of the systems intervene in the elders home, disrupting their day-to-day life, or require extensive training, while others cost a few hundred dollars for installation and operation. Selected promising and well established smart home solutions are presented below.

The smart home system in [22] provides safety and security services like smart locks that sends alerts to the cell phone when a door opens, indoor cameras for two-way communication, doorbell cameras that permit the home's residents to check and respond to a person at the door either they are at home or not, and thermostats that adjust automatically home temperature to the preferences of the home's residents. The control of smart devices via voice and an application for smartphones and tablets for remote control is offered in [23]. In this way, the system can provide monitoring, warnings, safety, and security to the elders. The commercial solution in [24] provides elderly people remote control on heating, remote monitoring of their home, measurement of the indoor and outdoor conditions of the home environment. In parallel, the system allows optimization of their comfort and well-being at home, via smart devices in their house like smart thermostats, smart door and window sensors, a smart video doorbell, etc. In [25] smart home services via different kinds of sensors and actuators that set up at home are provided. These services are the focus on safety, security, and improvement of the elderly's well-being. Different kinds of services, via actuators and embedded systems, provide to older people the remote control of the home's lighting, blinds, switches, heating, and cameras in [26].

The main characteristic of the previously mentioned systems is the high cost, which is a significant issue for the elderly people. Furthermore, although the systems are based on high technology, it is not open and available to others. This affects not only the cost but also the availability worldwide.

3 Proposed System

This work aims at proposing an elderly care system for use in their home environment to support, protect, prosper and maintain their health and functional abilities, based on open technologies. According to [27] the main needs of elderly people are safety and well-being at their homes and their support of their daily life routine. The contribution of the proposed system is to assist the needs of either the older people in general or specifically the older people suffering from dementia, with the use of low-cost and small-scale Information and Communication Technologies (ICT) solutions. Thus, this system will consist of autonomous subsystems that will operate independently but will also be able to communicate with each other. The subsystems that make up the main system are three: *the safety subsystem, the subsystem of well-being*, and *the support subsystem*.

3.1   The Safety Subsystem

The purpose of the safety subsystem is to detect the movements of the elderly within their home space. In order to achieve this, sensors can be placed in specific locations within the house to detect any activity - movement of the elderly. Thus, in the absence of movement sense of the person for a certain period, the subsystem undertakes to communicate with the elderly.

The communication between the subsystem and the elderly will be achieved using smart speakers within the house. Thus, communication is performed via physical language and doesn't require extra training. Through smart speakers, the subsystem will ask the elderly specific and predetermined questions about his/her state of health. If the elderly respond, with a predefined response for the subsystem, that he/she is well, then the subsystem does not perform any action. If the elderly respond, with a predefined response for the system that he/she is not well in his/her health, or does not respond at all, then the subsystem will undertake to inform his/her relatives that something has happened to him/her.

Furthermore, in order to avoid false alarms from the subsystem, during installation, a categorization of the house rooms will be performed in terms of a safe place and potentially dangerous room. For example, motion sensors may not record some movement for a long time in a room classified as 'low risk', such as a bedroom. A fact that will lead the subsystem not to alert the elderly's relatives, as it is most likely to, he/she was lying down. On the other hand, if motion sensors did not record any movement in a home area characterized as 'high risk', such as the bathroom, then the subsystem will immediately update his/her relatives.

In addition, sensors will be placed at the entrances of the house in order to inform the relatives that the elderly person has gone out of the 'limits' of the house (geofencing) so that it can be traced promptly and directly by his relatives (geolocation). While the elderly will carry on a wearable device that will act as a panic button, to call his/her family immediately in case of an emergency.

In the context of the present work, only the typical infrastructure and basic functions of the subsystem were implemented, such as the infrastructure of geofencing and geolocation for the elderly. Details of their implementation are offered at the next Section.

3.2   The Well-Being Subsystem

The purpose of the well-being subsystem is to provide confidence and instill a sense of safety to the elderly, but also their relatives. This is accomplished with the placement of specific sensors at critical points into the home, as well as the use of wearable devices that the elderly will bear on them.

The wearable devices for the elderly will provide information about their location (geographic location). These devices will help to make easy and accurate the localization of the elderly if they are away from their home and are searched for by their relatives.

The location of the sensors was selected to be the kitchen and the bathroom, based on high risk categorization, for easy management of the electrical appliances and the faucets. In particular, sensors will be placed to detect whether a cooker has been left switched on, without having a pot on it or even having a superheated utensil that has been forgotten on it. In this case, the subsystem will either be able to alert the home's owners that a device remains unnecessarily switched on or even shut down the cooker. A similar case will also happen with home faucets. If a faucet is left switched on for no reason, the subsystem will either alert the occupants of the house or switch off the faucet itself.

3.3   The Support Subsystem

The objectives of the support subsystem are two; the first is to remind the elderly to receive their medication, and the second is the recognition of their familiars, in case of the elderly suffer from dementia.

The reminder of receiving the medication of the elderly will be achieved by using a device that will be adjusted according to the needs of the older people and will reproduce a distinctive sound at the time of day that medications should be taken.

The recognition of familiar people from the elderly who suffer from dementia is achieved through a specially designed infrastructure that focuses on the sufferer and uses the sound stimuli, that we have proposed in [28]. In particular, its function is to reproduce characteristic sounds for each of the familiar faces of the elderly sufferer, so that the sounds help him/her recognize more easily who is the favorite person that has entered his/her home. The reproduction of the characteristic sound for each of the familiar faces of the elderly is done by using smart speakers, that located in the elderly's home, and an identifying wearable device that will bring upon it every familiar face of the elderly. The identifying wearable device acts as the unique identifier for each familiar. Thus, whenever one of the familiar faces of older person enters his/her home, the identification device will be recognized by the smart speaker. In effect, this will reproduce the corresponding characteristic sound for that person, which will act as stimuli for the elderly who suffers from dementia, to recognize his/her beloved people.

4   Implementation

In the implementation of the proposed system, we initially implemented the basic infrastructure of each subsystem, as we wanted to keep the cost and complexity of the entire system at low levels. The basic infrastructure of each subsystem is detailed below.

4.1   The Safety Subsystem

The safety subsystem consists of two devices. The first device (D1) is the one that is installed at the home of the elderly and checks to detect the old people or not at their home. While the second device (D2) is the wearable device that the elderly bear on, so that it can be located by D1. The device D1 searches for D2 at regular intervals to create communication between them. When D2 is not detected by D1, i.e. it is out of its range, D1 generates a warning.

Both subsystem's devices were implemented with the use of special-purpose hardware, namely Raspberry Pi micro-computers. For the device D1, a Raspberry Pi 3 B+ micro-computer was used because of its programming capabilities, its operating system availability and its built-in communication protocols. While for the device D2 a Raspberry Pi Zero W was used, due to its small size and features, such as programming and operating system availability, wireless LAN connection and Bluetooth.

The communication between the two devices is achieved by using Bluetooth communication protocol, while the recognition of device D2 by D1 is achieved based on the unique MAC address identifier of each device. In the case that D1 pairs with the device D2, then it does not perform any action. Otherwise, it sends a message that the D2 device, and hence the elderly who bears it on, is not in the house.

4.2 The Well-Being Subsystem

The subsystem of well-being also consists of two devices. The device D3 is designed to monitor and control the environmental conditions prevailing in the elderly's home, by using temperature, humidity, and gas leakage sensors in the home. While, the device D4 oversees the cooker hobs if a hob has been forgotten in operation, using a sensor that provides information about the temperature of the object that supervises.

For the implementation of both devices of the well-being subsystem, the Arduino Uno was selected, an open software/hardware board, to which the sensors were connected to collect the measurements/environmental data. The sensors selected for D3 and D4 device, measure, at regular intervals, specific environmental characteristics, that often refer to critical situations that lead to accidents. Humidity and temperature are metrics that affect the quality of living in their home, while gas is associated with various reports of elderly deaths from fumes or gas leakage. Finally, frequent is the case of failure or omission to switch off cooker hobs, leading to a fire. Thus, for the device D3, a sensor is used, which measures the temperature and humidity of the environment, and a sensor for detecting leakage of natural gas and carbon gas in the room, as shown in Fig. 1. While in Fig. 2, the D4 device is using an IR temperature sensor for remotely measuring the surface temperature of a target object, while it also measures the average ambient temperature.

The communication with the central system and the transmission of the collected data was selected to implements via a wireless channel, in order to reduce the complexity of connection and to make the system safe (i.e. allow it to be used for example in the kitchen where no exposed cables are allowed). The Bluetooth HC-05 unit was selected, for the wireless communication and transmission of the device's data to the rest of the system. The transmission of data follows a structured information packet format, exploiting JSON messages. Each device initially transmits its identifier allowing information parsing to be made easily, and then the fields, as well as the values, of the measurable metrics. For example, {*id: 1, temp: 25.0, humidity: 56.5, gas: 0 leak: no leak*}.

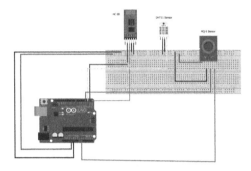

Fig. 1. Schematic representation of the D3 device.

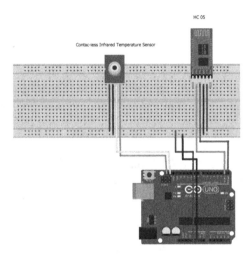

Fig. 2. Schematic representation of the D4 device.

4.3   The Support Subsystem

The support subsystem is an information system at home to support elderly people with dementia and their relatives. The information system consists of two main applications: the client application, and the server application.

The client application runs on the identifying device of the individuals (e.g. smartphone). Communication is achieved via Bluetooth with the server. At the server, the collected ID is matched to a predefined sound. Then, the corresponding sound is reproduced, which will act as a stimulus for the sufferer to recognize his/her beloved person. The identification of each device, that leads to the recognition of the right person and eventually the reproduction of the right sound, is achieved through the unique MAC address that has each device and transmits to the server.

The server application is embedded in a micro-computer Raspberry Pi 3 B+ model, which acts as a smart speaker at the patient's home. The role of the server is to handle communication with identifying devices. In addition, the server has a list of all identifying devices and their corresponding sound, which we can modify whenever necessary. So, the server searches for identifying devices, via the unique MAC address that has each device, at regular intervals to create communication between them, via Bluetooth. When the in-between communication is achieved, the server application is searching in the sounds' list for the associated sound with that device, and reproduce it.

5   Results

In this section, the functionality of the implemented system is tested and evaluated. Specifically, for the evaluation of the proper functionality of the system, experimental tests were carried out for each subsystem separately.

5.1   The Safety Subsystem

The experiments conducted for the safety subsystem concerned the ability of the device D1 to search for and locate the device D2 when the second device was in the range of the first. The tests of the safety subsystem were carried out in various rooms of a building, in order to study all possible distances between the two devices (different rooms, different floors, etc.). The test results are presented in Table 1.

Table 1. Safety subsystem tests results.

Test	Tracking the device D2	Distance of devices
1	Yes	3.7 m
2	Yes	5.2 m
3	No	19.5 m
4	No	13.0 m
5	Yes	1.9 m
6	Yes	3.1 m
7	No	2.1 m
8	Yes	3.0 m
9	No	13.9 m
10	No	16.3 m

The first six tests, as shown in Table 1, were carried out with both devices (D1 and D2) on the same floor of the building, while the remaining 4 tests were conducted with the device D1 being located on the first floor and the device D2 on the ground floor of the building. This also explains the result of test 7 against the tests 1 and 2, in which although the distance is shorter, the device D2 is not detected by D1 due to the difference in the floor. On the other hand, in test 8, although the floor difference continued to exist, the two devices were almost one below the other, so D2 was able to be identified by D1. Note that the device D1 throughout the tests was located at a specific point in the building, while the device D2 was the one that constantly changed its position. Finally, the distance between the two devices in each test was calculated using the GPS, taking in each test the different coordinates of D2, since the coordinates of D1 remained constant.

5.2   The Well-Being Subsystem

The experiments conducted for the well-being subsystem aimed to evaluate the D3 device to monitor the environmental conditions of a room (humidity and temperature). While the device D4 has been evaluated for its ability to detect the different temperatures of a cooker in operation, when there is a pot on it or when it does not, but the cooker is still in operation.

For the experiments of the D3 device, the device was placed in a room to measure the prevailing conditions of temperature, humidity and gas leakage for 1 h. Every 15 min, we affected the room conditions, near the sensor, to evaluate and validate the value fluctuations in the measurements. The measurements, lasting 1 h, took place for 5 days in 2 different rooms of a house. The results of the measurement values of the temperature are depicted in the graph in Fig. 3, the measurement values of the humidity are shown in the graph in Fig. 4, and the measurement values of the gas leakage are offered in the graph in Fig. 5.

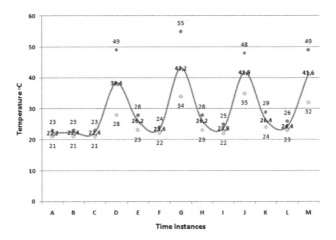

Fig. 3. Results of the measurements of the temperature of the D3 device; the blue line in the graph shows the average value of the temperature of the total measurements of the experiments, the red dots correspond to the maximum values of the temperature and the yellow ones to the minimum. (Color figure online)

Every time instance in the graph $(A–M)$ corresponds to 5 min, with A being the minute 0 and the M the 60th min for each measurement. The blue line in the graph shows the average value of the temperature of the total measurements of the experiments, while the red dots correspond to the maximum values of the temperature and the yellow ones to the minimum.

At the *Time instances D, G, J, and M* we notice an increase in the temperature values, as they correspond to the 15th, 30th, 45th and 60th min, respectively, during which we affected the temperature.

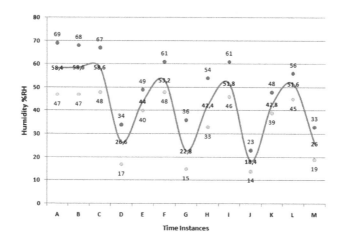

Fig. 4. Results of the measurements of the humidity of the D3 device; the blue line in the graph shows the average value of the humidity of the total measurements of the experiments, the red dots correspond to the maximum values of the humidity and the yellow ones to the minimum. (Color figure online)

As in the temperature graph, thus and in the humidity graph, every time instance in the graph $(A–M)$ corresponds to 5 min. The blue line in the graph shows the average value of the humidity of the total measurements of the experiments, while the red dots correspond to the maximum values of the humidity and the yellow ones to the minimum.

At the *Time instances D, G, J, and M* we notice a decrease in the humidity values, as they correspond to the 15th, 30th, 45th and 60th min, respectively, during which we affected the humidity.

As in the temperature and humidity graphs, thus and in the gas leakage graph, every Time instance in the graph $(A–M)$. The blue line in the graph shows the average value of the gas leakage of the total measurements of the experiments, while the red dots correspond to the maximum values of the gas leakage and the yellow ones to the minimum.

At the *Time instances A, B, C, E, F, H, I, K, and L* the gas value is 0, as there is no gas leakage in the room. While, at the *Time instances D, G, J, and*

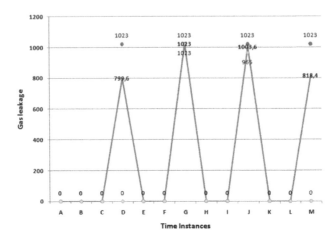

Fig. 5. Results of the measurements of the gas leakage of the D3 device; the blue line in the graph shows the average value of the gas leakage of the total measurements of the experiments, the red dots correspond to the maximum values of the gas leakage and the yellow ones to the minimum. (Color figure online)

M we notice an increase in the gas value, as they correspond to the 15th, 30th, 45th and 60th min, respectively, during which we affected the gas leakage.

The results of the measurements values of the D4 device are shown in the graph in Fig. 6. The blue line in the graph shows the average value of the total measurements of the experiments of the temperature of the object that was monitored (e.g. cooker hob and pot), while the red dots correspond to the maximum values of the temperature and the yellow ones to the minimum.

For the experiments of the D4 device, we placed the device over the cooker hobs at the height of the cooker hood, focusing on a particular hob, supervising it for 21 min, for 5 days. During the 21 min, a number of actions were carried out, such as placing a pot with water in the cooker, removing the pot with the hob remaining in operation, etc. The time duration between each action (*Time instances*) lasted a fixed time for all experiments to facilitate experiments.

Specifically, at the *Time instance A* was put the pot with water in the hob and was turned it on. After 3 min (*Time instance B and C*), we added another cold water to the pot. The value at *Time instance B* is the temperature of the pot with the water just before putting cold water, while the value at *Time instance C* is the temperature of the utensil after the cold water has been placed. At the *Time instance D*, we have measured the temperature of the pot as it continues to stay above the hob. After 3 min (*Time instance E and F*) was removed the pot from the hob, while the cooker remains lit. The value at *Time instance E* is the temperature of the pot just before removing it from the hob, while the value at *Time instance F* is the temperature of the lit hob immediately after the pot has been removed. Three minutes later (*Time instance G and H*) the pot was put back in the hob with the value at the *Time instance G* being the temperature

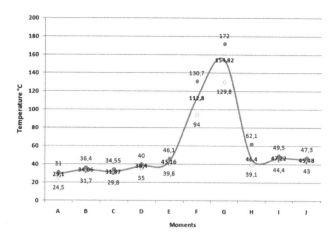

Fig. 6. Results of the measurements of the D4 device; the blue line in the graph shows the average value of the total measurements of the experiments of the temperature of the object that was monitored (e.g. cooker hob and pot), while the red dots correspond to the maximum values of the temperature and the yellow ones to the minimum. (Color figure online)

of the hob shortly before placing the utensil, while the value at *Time instance H* is the temperature of the utensil that was just put again. After 3 min (*Time instance I*), was turned off the hob while the pot stays on it. While 6 min later (*Time instance H*), were measured the temperature of the pot for the last time.

5.3   The Support Subsystem

The experiments conducted for the support subsystem aimed to evaluate-validate the identification of the client from the server, as well as the successful reproduction of the sound by the server.

In total, 20 different tests were performed. In particular, two series of 10 trials were conducted, in which two *Familiars* were examined to assess the Familiar's identity in a room and a patient. The difference between the two test groups was the device that each *Familiar* carried with. In both series, the identifier was a smartphone. While the tests were done within the limits of a room, thus the support subsystem would be located in every room of the elderly home.

The first 10 tests in the Table 2 correspond to *Familiar 1*, while the other 10 in *Familiar 2*. Both *Familiars* had a 100% success rate in their identification from the system, while in the sound reproduction *Familiar 1* had an 80% success rate since in *Test 1* was not reproduced the characteristic sound, while *Familiar 2* had a 100% success rate.

Table 2. Support subsystem tests results.

Test	Identification of the client	Reproduction of the sound
1	Yes	No
2	Yes	Yes
3	Yes	Yes
4	Yes	Yes
5	Yes	Yes
6	Yes	Yes
7	Yes	Yes
8	Yes	Yes
9	Yes	Yes
10	Yes	Yes
11	Yes	Yes
12	Yes	Yes
13	Yes	Yes
14	Yes	Yes
15	Yes	Yes
16	Yes	Yes
17	Yes	Yes
18	Yes	Yes
19	Yes	Yes
20	Yes	Yes

6   Conclusion

In this paper, a smart home supporting system for elderly people is proposed, based on low-cost building blocks, such as open software and open hardware. The aim is the protection of the elderly life, the enhancement of life quality and assistance to day-life activities, which however have a critical character. A collection of smart installments was proposed for achieving three goals, namely safety at home, smart home support and well-being. In this work, a significant part of smart sensors and devices of the proposed system are considered and implemented.

The experimental results showed that this system can offer integrated assistance for the elderly at home. The integrated assistance, in combination with the low-cost and the small-scale of the system, gives it a lead over other similar proposed systems.

As future work, the rest of the proposed system will be implemented. Also, for the safety subsystem, the aim is to include bio-metrics algorithms to take into account behavioral characteristics. While in the support subsystem the aim is the integration of the solution using smart speakers. Furthermore, as future work, the authors wish to evaluate the system's effectiveness in real conditions.

Acknowledgment. The authors would also like to thank Dr. Vasileios Kokkinos, for the fruitful discussion, his comments on dementia and the appropriate guidance.

References

1. Eurostat. https://ec.europa.eu/eurostat/statistics-explained/index.php?title=Population_structure_and_ageing. Accessed 26 Mar 2019
2. Alzheimer's Disease International. https://www.alz.co.uk/research/statistics. Accessed 26 Mar 2019
3. PAMAP. http://www.aal-europe.eu/projects/pamap/. Accessed 4 Mar 2019
4. WE CARE. http://www.aal-europe.eu/projects/we-care/. Accessed 4 Mar 2019
5. Vizier Homepage. https://aalvizier.eu/. Accessed 4 Mar 2019
6. MyLifeMyWay Homepage. http://www.mylifemyway-aal.eu/. Accessed 6 Mar 2019
7. Innovcare Homepage. https://www.innovcare.org/project. Accessed 6 Mar 2019
8. Maestro Homepage. https://www.maestro-aal.eu/en/. Accessed 6 Mar 2019
9. OLA. http://www.aal-europe.eu/projects/ola/. Accessed 6 Mar 2019
10. PersonAAL Homepage. http://www.personaal-project.eu/. Accessed 6 Mar 2019
11. SmartBEAT Homepage. https://www.smartbeatproject.org/. Accessed 6 Mar 2019
12. M3W Homepage. https://m3w-project.eu/. Accessed 6 Mar 2019
13. ROSETTA. http://www.aal-europe.eu/projects/rosetta/. Accessed 8 Mar 2019
14. ALADDIN. http://www.aal-europe.eu/projects/alladin/. Accessed 8 Mar 2019
15. Enable Homepage. http://www.enableproject.org/. Accessed 8 Mar 2019
16. Mylife Homepage. http://www.karde.no/mylife-project.org/. Accessed 8 Mar 2019
17. TV Assist Dem Homepage. http://www.tvassistdem-aal.eu/. Accessed 8 Mar 2019
18. PLAYTIME Homepage. http://aal-playtime.eu/. Accessed 9 Mar 2019
19. GREAT Homepage. http://uct-web.labs.fhv.at/index.php?id=264&L=1. Accessed 9 Mar 2019
20. Follow.Me Homepage. http://www.followmeproject.eu/overview.html. Accessed 9 Mar 2019
21. PETAL. http://www.aal-europe.eu/projects/petal/. Accessed 9 Mar 2019
22. SMARTHOME+. https://www.gosmarthomeplus.com/control/. Accessed 28 May 2019
23. D-Link Smart Home. https://eu.dlink.com/uk/en/for-home/smart-home. Accessed 28 May 2019
24. NETATMO. https://get.netatmo.com/renovation-en/. Accessed 28 May 2019
25. Homematic. https://www.eq-3.com/solutions/smart-home.html. Accessed 28 May 2019
26. iNELS. https://www.inels.com/apartment. Accessed 28 May 2019
27. Alzheimer Hellas. https://www.alzheimer-hellas.gr/index.php/en/. Accessed 28 May 2019
28. Boumpa, E., Charalampou, I., Gkogkidis, A., Ntaliani, A., Kokkinou, E., Kakarountas, A.: Assistive system for elders suffering of Dementia. In: 2018 IEEE 8th International Conference on Consumer Electronics-Berlin (ICCE-Berlin), pp. 1–4, IEEE (2018)

A Wearable Exoskeleton for Hand Kinesthetic Feedback in Virtual Reality

Emanuele Lindo Secco[1](✉) and Andualem Maereg Tadesse[1,2]

[1] Robotic Laboratory, Department of Mathematics and Computer Science,
Liverpool Hope University, Liverpool L16 9JD, UK
{seccoe,maerega}@hope.ac.uk
[2] The Manufacturing Technology Centre, Coventry, UK

Abstract. This paper presents a novel two-fingers exoskeleton kinesthetic inter-action in Virtual Reality (VR): the proposed design of the exoskeleton prioritizes the performance of the device in terms of low weight, good adaptability to differ-ent size of the human hand. This design made also the exoskeleton well wearable and allows strong force feedback which is an important parameter for a realistic kinesthesis of manipulated objects in VR.

Keywords: Haptic device · Wearable device · Kinesthetic feedback · Virtual reality

1 Introduction

Human beings are constantly interacting with objects on their daily life: this interaction is made possible through the manipulation and explorations of objects, devices and things, which are explored, touched and grasped by the hand of the user.

To perform such an interaction, multiple sensors are available on the human hands: the limbs, in fact, are equipped with a set of 'transducers' allowing the perception of posi-tion, temperature, roughness and movement and much more. These sensors are embedded within our limbs, muscles and skin [1]: from an anatomical viewpoint, the perception is induced by different *receptors* and *mechanoreceptors*, which provide kinematic and dynamic sensations, such as the Ruffini and Merkel cells and corpuscles.

Kinesthetic devices are wearable systems, which stimulate such receptors in order to provide a realistic 'kinesthetic' sensations in terms of movement and position. These devices are particularly useful when the end-user is interacting with a medical Virtual Reality (VR) environment allowing, for example, a remote surgical procedure. Typi-cal kinesthetic devices are combining wearable sensors with mechanical components assuming the set of an exoskeleton or a robotic manipulator. They have been used for a variety of applications, including studies on human perception [2], development of training systems for MIS (Minimally Invasive Surgery) [3], rehabilitation devices [4, 5] and remote-control platforms [6].

Despite these progresses, the development of haptic devices for Virtual Reality sys-tems requires a set of performance, which are not easy to be simultaneously achieved:

© ICST Institute for Computer Sciences, Social Informatics and Telecommunications Engineering 2020
Published by Springer Nature Switzerland AG 2020. All Rights Reserved
G. M. P. O'Hare et al. (Eds.): MobiHealth 2019, LNICST 320, pp. 186–200, 2020.
https://doi.org/10.1007/978-3-030-49289-2_15

these systems, in fact, should exhibit high accuracy, low inertia, high range of stiffness, combined with a small size of the equipment which is worn by the hand of the user. On the other side, the VR environment should require a minimum set of parameters to be controlled and interact with the haptic system. In this context, haptic exoskeletons are wearable force feedback devices that allow users to mechanically interact with the VR environment. They are becoming increasingly common and they are usually designed to guide the user's motion and give force feedback by attaching the exoskeleton to the human body, such as the user can control the position and movement of the fingers joints precisely [7, 8].

Exoskeletons for haptics may vary for their mechanical design, actuation system, and type of control. Force can be applied directly or indirectly through a transmission cable drive system. However, existing haptic exoskeletons cannot usually provide high fidelity force feedback in wearable setup. A high-quality haptic interface is typically characterized by low inertia and damping, high structural stiffness and absence of mechanical singularities. Other considerations in the design of wearable haptic exoskeletons are the space and weight limitation and the kinematic constraints induced by the human arm. The size of the overall design and mechatronics counterparts have to be smaller and lightweight to fit on human hand and therefore to increase the portability and flexibility, without affecting the dexterity of the hand.

Unlike other force feedback devices, haptic exoskeletons allow users to feel virtual and physical objects more naturally. This expands their applications in Virtual and Augmented Reality (VR, AR, respectively), medical and surgical training, teleoperation and others. Even though many researchers have developed different kinds of haptic exoskeletons, most exoskeletons with high fidelity force feedback restrain natural hand movement because of their complex mechanism. Moreover, the range and resolution of the force applied by the actuators should also be bigger enough to match with the human hand sensitivity.

Exoskeletons offer an intuitive method of actuating multiple Degress Of Freedom (DOFs) of the hand. These make them more valuable for application where the coupling of the force feedback devices with the fingers is needed. In this context, this paper presents the design and development of an exoskeleton for force feedback. The design of the exoskeleton focuses on the selection of a suitable kinematic, allowing the full reach of the finger's workspace, while combining under actuation with a proper wearable design.

2   Haptic Exoskeletons

The capability to be worn (i.e. the *'wearability'*) of haptic devices broadened the application of haptic devices in a variety of new areas such as social interaction, health care, virtual reality, remote assistance, and robotics. However, smaller form factor and wearability bring a challenge in the design requirement of kinesthetic haptic devices. There are various types of hand exoskeletons developed for commercial and research purposes. For example, the *CyberGrasp* is a commercial haptic exoskeleton developed by CyberGlove Systems LLC, USA [9]. It uses electrical actuators placed on the dorsal side of the hand as drive system; low friction tendons are used to transmit forces from the actuators to the fingertips with a joint position resolution of 0.5° and a peak force of 12 N on the fingertip. CyberGrasp has relatively large weight, 350 g, which can cause fatigue if it is used for long hours. The mechanical bandwidth is also limited at 40 Hz due to the friction and backlash effect of the tendons. The *Rutgers Master II-ND* (RMII-ND) glove is another type of force feedback devices [10], which uses a direct drive actuation system with actuators placed on the palm. Compared to Cybergrasp, this exoskeleton weights less and is able to control four independent fingers thorough four pneumatic actuators, providing force feedback up to 16 N. Pneumatic actuators have also used in other exoskeletons presented [11–13]. Unlike other devices, the RMII-ND provide forces on the intermediate phalanx, leaving fingertips free to interact. Arata et al. [14] presented an exoskeleton mechanism, which is driven through large deformation of a compliant mechanism. The system is an underactuated mechanism which converts 1 DOF of linear motion into rotation of three finger joints causing extension and flexion. Similar mechanism with remote actuation system has been developed by Nycz et al. [15]. The remote actuation system used pull-push Bowden cable that transmits force from the back of the hand to the fingertip. This cable transmission system reduces the overall weight of the exoskeleton without affecting the functionality of the system.

Choi et al. [16] introduce the *Wolverine*, a mobile, wearable haptic device designed for virtual simulation of the interaction with rigid objects. This device renders a force directly between the thumb and the three fingers to simulate the grasp. The device can simulate grasping rigid bodies by leveraging low-power brake based locking sliders which can withstand up to 100 N force between each finger and the thumb. Time-of-flight sensors are used to track the position of each finger and an Inertial Measurement Unit (IMU) is used for orientational tracking.

Chiri et al. developed *Handexos*, a hand exoskeleton featuring a kinematic coupling with users joints [17, 18]. The self-aligning structure is made of revolute joint aligned with the user PIP and DIP joint, whereas the MCP joint uses a parallel chain made of two rotational and one linear DOFs. The mechanism uses a cable actuation system with an idle pulley to drive the joints of the exoskeleton. Iqbal et al. [19] developed a wearable mechanism which can provide forces up to 45 N at the proximal phalanx of the thumb and the index fingers. The design uses three revolute mechanisms (RRR). The same design has been revised considering multi-finger mechanism and overall wearability and performance [20, 21]. Othe authors presented a four-link serial mechanism which provides kinesthetic force feedback to the fingertip of the user [22]. Allotta and Conti et al. [23, 24] developed a 330 g *four-fingers parallel kinematic chain mechanism*. The device is grounded on the palm, and it can provide feedback in 1 DOF on the intermediate phalanx.

Achibet et al. [25] presented *Flexifingers*, a passive wearable exoskeleton with independent finger modules using bendable metal strips. The device provides kinesthetic feedback to four fingers up to 2.5 N. Each strip allows a 7.3 cm range of movement to the fingertip. Agrawal et al. [26] presented a wearable hand exoskeleton capable of bidirectional and independent joint torque control. The very light (80 g) mechanism uses *Series Elastic Actuation* (SEA) cables. The stiffness elements can be replaced to adjust for different users. Yang et al. [27] presented a jointless tendon-driven hand exoskeleton, which enables to couple the PIP and DIP movements as well as the MCP and PIP during flexion to replicate the natural finger motion during grasping.

3 Design

3.1 Optimization Criteria

In order to design a proper exoskeleton, different requirements and specifications that affect the performance and the ergonomics of the hand exoskeleton should be considered. Some primary design characteristics are:

- *Transparency* - A wearable exoskeleton haptic device should be a transparent interface to the remote and virtual environment, namely the user should be able to feel the interaction with the virtual objects as if this interaction occurs with the real ones.
- *Stiffness* - The maximum stiffness that can be achieved by the exoskeleton depend on the mechanical rigidity of the system and the achievable stability of the controller [28, 29]. Moreover, the device performance has a significant impact on the overall performance of the haptic display, irrespective of the used control algorithm.
- *Actuation* - The type of actuation and transmission systems are crucial factors in determining the performance. There are a variety of actuation technologies ranging from electric motors, hydraulic, pneumatic, magneto-rheological, electro-rheological, electroactive polymers, shape memory alloys, etc. This factor can compromise the portability of the system.
- *Force Feedback* - The maximum range or limits of force, velocity, and acceleration the haptic device can render should be enough for high force fidelity. The performance of an active force feedback control could suffer from actuator saturation to apply high forces or fast deceleration to display impulsive forces during interaction with hard contacts [30].
- *Wearability* - The kinematic design should accommodate different hand sizes without significant adjustment. The actuation system should allow a light-weight, portable and compact system. The device should be comfortable to wear. The way of attaching the device to the fingers should not obstruct the hand motions. There are basically two typical ways, namely (1) single location attachment and (2) multi-phalangeal attachment (see also Fig. 1).
- *Single point attachment* is simpler and provides haptic transparency by reducing unwanted internal forces between the mechanical structures and the finger phalanges.
- *Multiple attachments* to the phalanges provide an easier way of articulation of the finger and provide direct feedback forces to the attached phalanges. Such kind of design considers the number of DOF achievable by the hand and the size of the workspace reachable by the human hand.

Proper alignment of the exoskeleton joint and hand joint must be preserved during the use of these devices. There are various reasons which caused improper alignment of the exoskeleton joints from the finger joints: the first one is the inherently compliant mounting of the exoskeleton onto the hand, which leads to inaccurate positioning of the exoskeleton joints during movements. The other one is that the inter-subject variability of

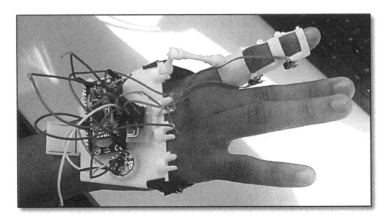

Fig. 1. A 3D printed index exoskeleton developed at the Robotic Laboratory of Liverpool Hope University.

the anatomical structure, size and shape of the hands requires an adjustable mechanism to align the joints.

3.2 Hand Kinematics

Understanding the kinematics of the human hand is essential to design a proper exoskeleton. For multi-phalangeal design, the joint degrees of freedom, joint ranges, and phalanx length should match the average human hand kinematic parameters.

Human hand grasping capability is amazing (Fig. 2). Its kinematics can be considered using a skeletal structure. The first link is the meta carpal joint, which is located in the palm. The base of each finger is connected to Metacarpus Phalangeal joints (MCP). Three phalanges, called the Distal Phalanx (DIP), the Middle Phalanx, and the Proximal Phalanx (PIP) are connected through the Inter-Phalangeal (IP) joints. The MCP joint connects the metacarpal and proximal phalanx. The PIP joint connects the proximal and middle phalanx, and the DIP joint connects the middle and distal phalanx. The thumb has only one IP joint. The motion of each finger includes flexion and extension as well as abduction and adduction.

The Index finger can be considered as three link mechanism with 4-DOF motion. However, human anatomy studies show that the motion of the DIP is naturally coupled with the PIP motion. Levangie et al. [32] shows that the maximum range of the index finger joints is 90° for the MCP, 100°–110° for the PIP, 80° for the DIP in flexion and extension movements, 40° for the adduction and abduction movements. This motion ranges vary for different fingers and different users according to the bone geometry and tendon and muscle structure of the hand. The thumb's kinematic is different from the other fingers. Unlike the index finger, the thumb has only three joints: the first two joints, MCP and DIP have revolute joints whereas the MC joint of the thumb can execute 3 DOF motion.

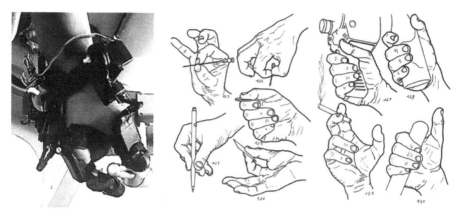

Fig. 2. Human hand grasping capability - from [31] - vs the proposed exoskeleton grasping performance.

3.3 Exoskeleton Design

According to the aforementioned optimization criteria and the human hand kinematics, the design and manufacturing of an underactuated, cable-driven hand exoskeleton is implemented. This process has required different steps as it is shown in Fig. 3. The Exoskeleton is designed to fit on two fingers of the human hand, i.e. on the index and thumb fingers which are the most used limbs to perform pinching and grasping. The design embeds lightweight links with low inertia. The overall system weighs around 120 g including the 3D printed mechanical system, the control electronics, and the actuators. Such a lightweight system will enable the user to use the exoskeleton without feeling fatigue.

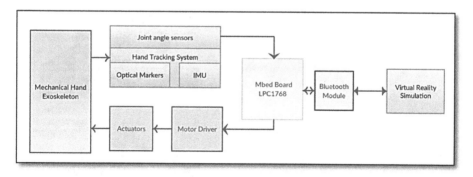

Fig. 3. Block diagram of the integration of the exoskeleton control and communication units.

a. Mechanical Design

In this section, the mechanical design of two fingers haptic hand exoskeleton that allows exerting forces on the index and thumb fingertip of the user is developed. The exoskeleton structure consists of a wrist and palm bracket, the palm mounting box, and the finger assemblies (Fig. 4). The wrist bracket and palm bracket are used to fix the exoskeleton on the hand, functioning as a ground for the finger assemblies. The palm is used to mount actuators and control electronics system. All finger lengths, joint positions, and widths of each finger were taken from measurements of an average size human hand. Velcro strap connected to each finger phalanx allows accommodating the different size of human fingers. A passive and adjustable MC joint mechanism is also used to fit the exoskeleton over hands of different size.

The complexity of the human hand structure makes it difficult to design an utterly similar hand exoskeleton, which controls the movement of the joints in all DOFs. Therefore, some consideration must be taken based on the physical assessment of the hand function. Based on some studies the finger adduction and abduction motion is not essential for achieving the critical hand functions including grasping and pinching [33]. Therefore, we do not include the abduction and adduction of the fingers on the design of the index finger exoskeleton. In addition, the index and the thumb finger joints have a limited range of motion (Table 2): therefore, the mechanism is designed to restrict unnecessary motions, apart from the natural movement of the finger joints. This is very important for the safety of the user, to reduce damage, which might be caused by a faulty and unstable control system.

The Exoskeleton fingers consist of three links corresponding to the DIP, MCP and PIP links. Rather than implementing a direct mechanical bar transmission (Fig. 1), a cable transmission is used to obtain a compact and lightweight assembly. Two cables are routed through the mechanical links, from the exoskeleton fingertip to the actuators on the hand, via a passive pulleys and bearings.

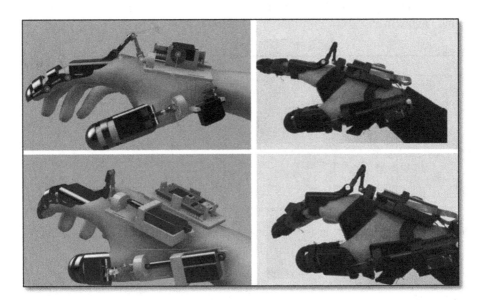

Fig. 4. 3D model and 3D printed haptic exoskeleton (left and right panels, respectively).

A first version of the hand exoskeleton was integrated where rotary servo motors (EMAX ES08MA-II) were used (Fig. 4). However, during some preliminary tests, tests revealed that these actuators do not have enough torque to resist vs the reactive force.

As a consequence, the actuation unit of a second version of the exoskeleton consists of two linear actuators (PQ12-P), one for index finger and another one for the thumb; each actuator is coupled with a cable driven system. The PQ12-P linear actuators weigh about 15 g and feature a stroke length of 20 mm with speed of 28 mm/s. The actuators can apply a maximum force of about 50 N (at 12 V). These forces exceed the maximum force which are needed to match a human hand maximum output force, which is around a value of 35 N. The commercial CyberGrasp haptic glove can output only up-to 12 N force. These actuators work as a linear servo, therefore, no external encoders are needed. The exoskeleton design is implemented with 3D printed parts which have been manufactured in PolyLactic Acid (PLA) material.

Table 1. Length of the exoskeleton *linkages*.

Linkages	Index [mm]	Thumb [mm]
L_1	52	0
L_2	58	45
L_3	21	25

b. Modelling

b.1. *Kinematic Model*

A simplified kinematic model of the finger is used to study the kinematic properties and trajectories of the hand. The index finger mechanism provides three rotary joints that allow extension and flexion of the finger. Accordingly, a planar model with three Revolute or Rotational joints (RRR) have been used as the kinematic model of the index finger. The Thumb also considers a planar model with two R joints. All the joints in the design use revolute pin connections. Extension and flexion are possible for both the index and the thumb mechanisms, whereas abduction and adduction movements are locked.

A schematic representation of the exoskeleton kinematic model is shown in Fig. 5. The revolute joint R_1 and R_2 mimic the PIP and DIP joints, respectively, while the third joint R_3 refers to the MCP joints. All three joints have parallel rotation axes forming a planar mechanism. The model follows the precise articulation of the index finger. The position of the exoskeleton's joint carefully matches the joint position of the human hand on the lateral side. The last MC joint uses two links to allow both rotation and translation of the finger assemblies with respect to the palm. Each joint is coupled with passive pulleys, which corresponds to the R joints. In addition, the exoskeleton is designed to keep the fingertip and the palm area free from additional tactile feedback. This also helps to reduce the weight of the overall system.

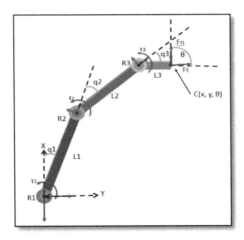

Fig. 5. The Kinematic model of the exoskeleton.

The human thumb kinematics is complicated because of the six degrees of freedom motion of the MC joint. In addition to the flexion, extension and adduction, abduction, the thumb performs a strategic opposition. Therefore, the thumb kinematics is simplified to allow the extension and flexion of the IP and MP joints. The abduction and adduction of the MC joint and the opposition movements are accommodated by the free passive motions of the elastic textile connector between the palm and thumb motor mounts.

Each finger of the exoskeleton can be modeled as planar and serial three link mechanism (Fig. 5), where the mount on the dorsum of the hand (i.e. the MC link) is considered as the ground link. The planar method ignores lateral movements of the finger, namely the adduction and abduction. Therefore, the overall exoskeleton device can be considered as an independent three-link (i.e. the index) and two-link (i.e. the thumb) mechanism, respectively. A separate thumb kinematic analysis is not necessary as the two links kinematic model of the thumb can be easily calculated by setting the first link length and the joint value of the index kinematic model to zero. Therefore, only the index finger kinematics is discussed.

The link parameters of both fingers are given in Table 1 and the joint constraints of the mechanism are reported within Table 2. These angular ranges are chosen to match the effective anthropomorphic articular ranges of the human hand.

The position and orientation of each fingertip are calculated using the forward kinematics equation. The position and orientation of the fingertip with respect to the MC link (ground) can be expressed using the 3×3 2D homogeneous transformation matrix, which consists of the rotation of each link with respect to the previous link, and the translation of each joint from the previous joint. It holds:

$$C = R(q_1)\, T(L_1)\, R(q_2)\, T(L_2)\, R(q_3)\, T(L_3) \tag{1}$$

Table 2. Anthropomorphic angular excursions of the rotational exoskeleton *joints*.

Joints	Index [°]	Thumb [°]
R_1	−30, +90	0
R_2	0, +110	0, +180
R_3	−5, +90	−5, +90

where

$$C = \begin{pmatrix} \cos(q_1 + q_2 + q_3) & -\sin(q_1 + q_2 + q_3) & x \\ \sin(q_1 + q_2 + q_3) & \cos(q_1 + q_2 + q_3) & y \\ 0 & 0 & 1 \end{pmatrix} \tag{2}$$

The 2D position and orientation of the fingertip can be extracted from the above transformation matrix. Precisely, the fingertip contact point $C\,(x, y, \vartheta)$ can be expressed by transforming the joint coordinates:

$$\begin{aligned} x &= L_1 \cdot \cos(q_1) + L_2 \cdot \cos(q_1 + q_2) + L_3 \cdot \cos(q_1 + q_2 + q_3) \\ y &= L_1 \cdot \sin(q_1) + L_2 \cdot \sin(q_1 + q_2) + L_3 \cdot \sin(q_1 + q_2 + q_3) \end{aligned} \tag{3}$$

and the rotational part is expressed as:

$$R = \begin{pmatrix} \cos(q_1 + q_2 + q_3) & -\sin(q_1 + q_2 + q_3) \\ \sin(q_1 + q_2 + q_3) & \cos(q_1 + q_2 + q_3) \end{pmatrix} \tag{4}$$

This component is similar to the rotation matrix occurring when a rotation of an angle of ϑ is performed around the z-axis. Therefore, the fingertip orientation can be expressed as:

$$\vartheta = q_1 + q_2 + q_3 \tag{5}$$

The forward kinematic equation can be generalized as $x = f(q)$ where x is position and orientation of the fingertip and q is the Lagrange joint variables. The derivative of this equation returns the Jacobian matrix, $J(q)$:

$$\dot{x} = J(q) \cdot \dot{q} \tag{6}$$

Accordingly, the linear velocity is expressed as a function of the Jacobian and of the joint velocities:

$$\begin{pmatrix} \dot{x} \\ \dot{y} \end{pmatrix} = \begin{pmatrix} m_{11} & m_{12} & m_{13} \\ m_{21} & m_{22} & m_{23} \end{pmatrix} \cdot \begin{pmatrix} \dot{q}_1 \\ \dot{q}_2 \\ \dot{q}_3 \end{pmatrix} \tag{7}$$

where it holds:

$$\begin{aligned} m_{11} &= -L_1 \cdot \sin(q_1) - L_2 \cdot \sin(q_1 + q_2) - L_3 \cdot \sin(q_1 + q_2 + q_3) \\ m_{12} &= -L_2 \cdot \sin(q_1 + q_2) - L_3 \cdot \sin(q_1 + q_2 + q_3) \\ m_{21} &= L_1 \cdot \cos(q_1) + L_2 \cdot \cos(q_1 + q_2) + L_3 \cdot \cos(q_1 + q_2 + q_3) \\ m_{22} &= L_2 \cdot \cos(q_1 + q_2) + L_3 \cdot \cos(q_1 + q_2 + q_3) \\ m_{32} &= -L_3 \cdot \sin(q_1 + q_2 + q_3) \\ m_{23} &= L_3 \cdot \cos(q_1 + q_2 + q_3) \end{aligned}$$

And, finally, then the rotational velocity can be expressed in function of the fingertip velocities, namely:

$$\begin{pmatrix} \dot{q}_1 \\ \dot{q}_2 \\ \dot{q}_3 \end{pmatrix} = \begin{pmatrix} m_{11} & m_{12} & m_{13} \\ m_{21} & m_{22} & m_{23} \\ 1 & 1 & 1 \end{pmatrix} \cdot \begin{pmatrix} \dot{x} \\ \dot{y} \\ \dot{\vartheta} \end{pmatrix} \tag{8}$$

b.2. *Workspace*

When exploring a free space in a remote or VR environment, the haptic device should not restrict the human users' motion (see also Sect. 3). Thus, the DOFs of the haptic device should match the natural ones of the human hand. According to Gruebler's formula, the mobility of the overall mechanism can be calculated as:

$$F = 3(n - l) - 2l - h \tag{9}$$

Where F is the total DOFs of the mechanism, n is the number of links (including the frame), l is the number of lower pairs (i.e. one DOF), h is the number of higher pairs (i.e. two DOF). According to the used kinematics, the results of Eq. (9) provide a 3-DOF mechanism for the index and a 2-DOF for the thumb, respectively. Enough workspace of the haptic device is also needed to achieve the desired motion which is achievable with the natural hand movement. The multi-link mechanism considered in this design is suitable for a multi-finger interaction and also it enables larger workspace for the haptic device. Accordingly, the 2D workspace for the index finger, as well as the joint trajectories, are shown in the Figs. 6 and 7.

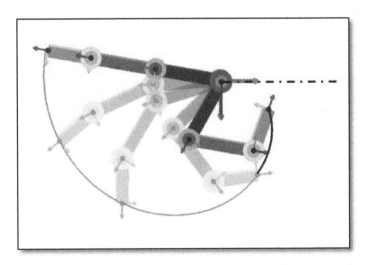

Fig. 6. Reachable workspace of the mechanism of the index finger.

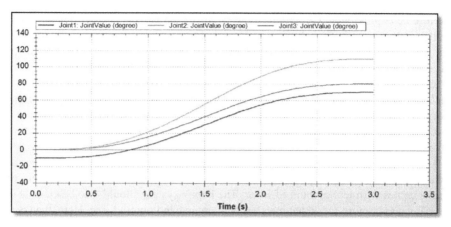

Fig. 7. Angular joint trajectories of the index finger mechanism - from the fully open configuration to the fully closed one.

b.3. *Actuation and Force Transmission*

An underactuated mechanism has been chosen to match the requirements such as a compact size, low weight, and low power system. The underactuated system allows having a number of actuators which is lower than the number of DOFs as performed with the hand. They also enable the exoskeleton mechanism to passively adapt to the finger structure.

Both the exoskeleton fingers are actuated via a cable transmission system, which is routed from the actuators on the palm to each joint of the finger up to the fingertip (Fig. 8). The cable transmission systems provide adequate power in order to also reduce the weight and inertia of the moving parts, and it allows remote actuation from the palm.

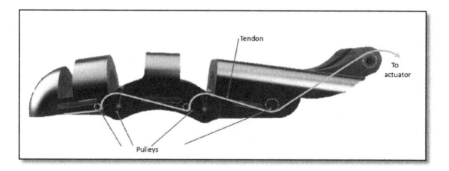

Fig. 8. The tendon and pulley mechanism of the index finger exoskeleton.

All revolute joints are driven by applying a tension force F to the cable which is wrapped around the finger joints of radius r. Assuming that the friction force is negligible, and that the cables are ideally rigid, the applied torque on each joint can therefore be expressed as a function of the radius of the pulleys and the tension force. Finally, an underactuated mechanism, with cable force transmission system, couples the joint torques with the cable tension F through the equation $\tau_i = F \cdot r_i$. The tension forces are also assumed to be constant for the same cable. This happens considering that the tension torque on the pulleys is negligible and the torque due to the pulley inertia is small. Unlike rehabilitation exoskeleton - which requires two cables for the extension and flexion movements - haptic exoskeleton requires a single cable to restrict the extension movement. The flexion can be passively performed not to restrict the natural movement of the finger (Fig. 8).

A DC motor actuation system pulls the cable. The haptic system needs either an active control of the cable position or should be back derivable so that the user can pull the cables with less amount of force. The haptic system should also be capable of delivering a maximum force that matches the human hand output force. Here, thanks to the adopted motors, the maximum thumb and finger force output is in the order of 35 N. The CyberGrasp, commercial force feedback device, can apply 12 N maximum output force, which is enough to provide a realistic force feedback sensation. As a consequence, in our design, a 10-12 N maximum force is considered.

4   Conclusions

In this paper, the design, and implementation of a wearable haptic exoskeleton is presented. A two-fingered (index-thumb) exoskeleton haptic device with force feedback function is developed. The exoskeleton consists of links corresponding to each phalange of the two finger which are connected with rotary joints. The determination of the position and orientation of each link relative to the previous one is solved by using a multi-body kinematics. The kinematic model also provides the necessary velocity and acceleration of the fingertip.

A VR system has been also developed around the exoskeleton: this VR component consists of a human hand physical model. The device can be used as a motion capture system, and as an input to a teleoperated control system, as a master device.

Even though the literature has presented different exoskeletons for haptics and rehabilitation purposes, there are still several problems which prevent those devices to be used in daily life [34]. Some of these constraints and limitations regard the fact that the exoskeletons are very large mainly because they use a direct drive system combined with mechanical links. Such a solution limits the natural movement of the end-user fingers, the joint angle positions, and the fingertip positions which may not properly measured. In this context the proposed haptic exoskeleton device should improve and by-pass some of these limitations thanks to its design.

We believe that the proposed device may have interesting application on rehabilitation and, in particular, in all medical application where the patient or the medical operator will benefit of haptic feedback.

Acknowledgment. We thank all staff of the Department of Mathematics and Computer Science for their valuable support.

This work was presented in thesis form in fulfilment of the requirements for the PhD in Robotics of the student A.M. Tadesse from the Robotics Laboratory, Department of Mathematics & Computer Science, Liverpool Hope University.

References

1. Jones, L.A.: Peripheral mechanisms of touch and proprioception. Canadian J. Physiol. Pharmacol. **72**(5), 484–487 (1994)
2. Fritschi, M., Ernst, M.O., Buss, M.: Integration of kinesthetic and tactile display-a modular design concept. In: Proceedings of the EuroHaptics, pp. 607–612 (2006)
3. Ueberle, M., Mock, N., Peer, A., Michas, C., Buss, M.: Design and control concepts of a hyper redundant haptic interface for interaction with virtual environments. In: Proceedings of the IEEE/RSJ International Conference on Intelligent Robots and Systems IROS, Workshop on Touch and Haptics (2004)
4. Bergamasco, M., et al.: An arm exoskeleton system for teleoperation and virtual environments applications. In: 1994 IEEE International Conference on Robotics and Automation, 1994, Proceedings, IEEE, pp. 1449–1454 (1994)
5. Gupta, A., O'Malley, M.K.: Design of a haptic arm exoskeleton for training and rehabilitation. IEEE/ASME Trans. Mechatron. **11**(3), 280–289 (2006)
6. Carignan, C.R., Cleary, K.R.: Closed-loop force control for haptic simulation of virtual environments (2000)
7. Bouzit, M., Popescu, G., Burdea, G., Boian, R.: The rutgers master II-nd force feedback glove. In: Haptics, p. 145. IEEE (2002)
8. Turner, M., Gomez, D., Tremblay, M., Cutkosky, M.: Preliminary tests of an arm-grounded haptic feedback device in telemanipulation. In: Proceedings of the ASME Dynamic Systems and Control Division, vol. 64, pp. 145–149 (1998)
9. CyberGlove Systems LLC (2019). CyberGlove Systems LLC. http://www.cyberglovesystems. com/. Accessed 8 Mar 2019
10. Kerber, F., Löchtefeld, M., Krüger, A., McIntosh, J., McNeill, C., Fraser, M.: Understanding same-side interactions with wrist-worn devices. In: Proceedings of the 9th Nordic Conference on Human-Computer Interaction. p. 28. ACM (2016)
11. Pabon, S., et al.: A data-glove with vibrotactile stimulators for virtual social interaction and rehabilitation. In: 10th Annual Intl Workshop on Presence (2007)
12. Pacchierotti, C., Chinello, F., Malvezzi, M., Meli, L., Prattichizzo, D.: Two finger grasping simulation with cutaneous and kinesthetic force feedback. In: Isokoski, P., Springare, J. (eds.) Euro-Haptics 2012. LNCS, vol. 7282, pp. 373–382. Springer, Heidelberg (2012). https://doi.org/10. 1007/978-3-642-31401-8_34
13. Paggetti, G., Cizmeci, B., Dillioglugil, C., Steinbach, E.: On the discrimination of stiffness during pressing and pinching of virtual springs. In: 2014 IEEE International Symposium on Haptic, Audio and Visual Environments and Games (HAVE), pp. 94–99. IEEE (2014)
14. Pai, D.K., Reissell, L.-M.: Haptic interaction with multiresolution image curves. Comput. Graph. **21**(4), 405–411 (1997)
15. Pang, X.D., Tan, H.Z., Durlach, N.I.: Manual discrimination of force using active finger motion. Perception & Psychophys. **49**(6), 531–540 (1991)
16. Papetti, S., Järveläinen, H., Giordano, B.L., Schiesser, S., Fröhlich, M.: Vibrotactile sensitivity in active touch: effect of pressing force. IEEE Trans. Haptics **10**(1), 113–122 (2017)
17. Chiri, A., et al.: HANDEXOS: towards an exoskeleton device for the rehabilitation of the hand. In: IEEE/RSJ International Conference on Intelligent Robots and Systems, 2009, IROS 2009, pp. 1106–1111. IEEE (2009)

18. Chiri, A., et al.: On the design of ergonomic wearable robotic devices for motion assistance and rehabilitation. In: 2012 Annual International Conference of the IEEE Engineering in Medicine and Biology Society (EMBC), pp. 6124–6127. IEEE (2012)
19. Iqbal, J., Tsagarakis, N.G., Caldwell, D.G.: Design of a wearable direct-driven optimized hand exoskeleton device. In: 4th International Conference on Advances in Computer-Human Interactions (ACHI), pp. 142–146. Citeseer (2011)
20. Iqbal, J., Tsagarakis, N.G., Fiorilla, A.E., Caldwell, D.G.: A portable rehabilitation device for the hand. In: 2010 Annual International Conference of the IEEE Engineering in Medicine and Biology Society (EMBC), pp. 3694–3697. IEEE (2010)
21. Iqbal, J., Tsagarakis, N.G., Caldwell, D.G.: A multi-DOF robotic exoskeleton interface for hand motion assistance. In: 2011 Annual International Conference of the IEEE Engineering in Medicine and Biology Society, EMBC, pp. 1575–1578. IEEE (2011)
22. Scott, L., Ferrier, N.J.: Design and control of a force-reflecting haptic interface for teleoperational grasping. J. Mech. Des. **124**(2), 277–283 (2002)
23. Allotta, B., Conti, R., Governi, L., Meli, E., Ridolfi, A., Volpe, Y.: Development and experimental testing of a portable hand exoskeleton. In: 2015 IEEE/RSJ International Conference on Intelligent Robots and Systems (IROS), pp. 5339–5344. IEEE (2015)
24. Meli, C.E., Ridolfi, A.: A novel kinematic architecture for portable hand exoskeletons. Mechatronics **35**, 192–207 (2016)
25. Achibet, M., et al.: FlexiFingers: multi-finger interaction in VR combining passive haptics and pseudo-haptics. In: 2017 IEEE Symposium on 3D User Interfaces (3DUI), pp. 103–106. IEEE (2017)
26. Agarwal, P., Fox, J., Yun, Y., O'Malley, M.K., Deshpande, A.D.: An index finger exoskeleton with series elastic actuation for rehabilitation: design, control and performance characterization. Int. J. Robot. Res. **34**(14), 1747–1772 (2015)
27. Yang, J., Xie, H., Shi, J.: A novel motioncoupling design for a jointless tendon-driven finger exoskeleton for rehabilitation. Mech. Mach. Theory **99**, 83–102 (2016)
28. MacLean, K.E.: The 'haptic camera': a technique for characterizing and playing back haptic properties of real environments. In: Proceedings of Haptic Interfaces for Virtual Environments and Teleoperator Systems (HAPTICS), pp. 459–467 (1996)
29. Lin, M., Gottschalk, S.: Collision detection between geometric models: a survey. In: Proceedings of IMA Conference on Mathematics of Surfaces, vol. 1, pp. 602–608 (1998)
30. Howe, R.T.: Applications of silicon micromachining to resonator fabrication. In: 48th Proceedings of the 1994 IEEE International Frequency Control Symposium, 1994, pp. 2–7. IEEE (1994)
31. Kapandji, I.A.: The Physiology of the Joints, E & S Livingstone, Edinburgh and London, 2nd edition, vol. 1 (1970)
32. Levangie, P.K., Norkin, C.C.: Joint structure and function: a comprehensive analysis, FA Davis (2011)
33. Freeman, W.T., Weissman, C.D.: Hand gesture machine control system. US Patent 5,594,469 (1997)
34. Leon, B., et al.: Grasps recognition and evaluation of stroke patients for supporting rehabilitation therapy. Biomed. Res. Int. **2014**, 1 (2014)

Development of an Intuitive EMG Interface for Multi-dexterous Robotic Hand

Emanuele Lindo Secco[✉], Daniel McHugh, David Reid, and Atulya Kumar Nagar

Robotic Laboratory, Department of Mathematics and Computer Science, Liverpool Hope University, Liverpool L16 9JD, UK
{seccoe,13005235,reidd,nagara}@hope.ac.uk

Abstract. This paper presents an integrated EMG-based system for controlling a 5-fingers robotic hand: the system combines two commercial products, namely an Open-Bionics Hand and a wearable MYO controller in a new fashion where the end-user can control different postural grasping through an intuitive menu, cycling among different pre-set grasping configurations. According to preliminary tests, such a solution may represent an interesting novelty for a user-centered experience of patients with an upper limb prosthetic device.

Keywords: Smart prosthetics · Human-centered healthcare · Electromyography

1 Introduction

Nowadays there is a huge demand for dexterous and user-friendly devices for robotic and prosthetic manipulation. Human subjects, who has suffered from the loss of a limb, need to recover their daily life ability to manipulate and interact with objects and the other human beings. On the other side, current humanoid robots have increased the capability to interact with us and, therefore, to perform actions which belong to our nature [1–3, 14].

Unfortunately, even if many devices have been developed with high movement capability and dexterity, a lack of simplicity on the usage of the interface between such devices and the end-user is still occurring.

Here we are trying to show a simple and low-cost architecture where some of these drawbacks are overcome. This paper looks at the relationship between a prosthetic hand and an *ElectroMyoGraphy* (EMG) sensor to simulate different grasp types. These ones allow the user to interact with different objects in the real world through a robotic hand [4–6]. The approach is based on the integration of an Arduino Mega and an OpenBionics hand [7, 8]. The aim is to propose a novel and improved robotic and prosthetic system that can closely simulate a real limb via EMG which is used to control the robotic hand [9].

G. M. P. O'Hare et al. (Eds.): MobiHealth 2019, LNICST 320, pp. 201–211, 2020.
https://doi.org/10.1007/978-3-030-49289-2_16

2 Materials and Methods

2.1 Hardware

In this section of the paper details of the hardware are reported. The main reasons of specific hardware selection are also mentioned.

The Open Bionics Robotic Hand
The robotic hand which has been used in this project is a 3D printed hand from Open Bionics (Fig. 1): each part of the hand is printed and assembled together to integrate the motion capability; the 4 fingers and the thumb in the hand can reach different positions allowing the manipulator to perform different types of grasping. This is performed through linear actuators, which are installed in the palm of the hand. Each finger and thumb are connected to a single actuator via a fishing wire.

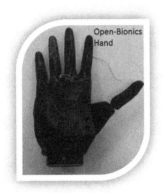

Fig. 1. The 5-finger Open-Bionics robotic hand.

The hand's task is to replicate different grasping configurations when a human input is given. The reason why such a device was chosen is because of how easy it is to interface and control the device itself: all you need to provide is the power supply and then to plug in the hand's controller into a computer through its USB cable: then the user may upload code to an Arduino-compatible controller which is embedded within the hand.

The MYO Band
MyoBand is a wearable device from Thalamic Labs which allows the end-user to collect electrical muscle activity or ElectroMyoGraphic signals (EMG) – Fig. 2. EMG are used in gesture control and many other applications, such as, for example, to develop a MyoWare muscle sensor. This device allows receiving 8 amplified and rectified EMG signals from the human forearm muscles: the larger is the amount of EMG signals, the higher is the information about the human gesture that may be collected by the sensor [10, 11].

When the device is worn on the arm, it will start to read the muscle electrical activity; data are then sent over a wireless Bluetooth protocol to a dongle that will be inserted

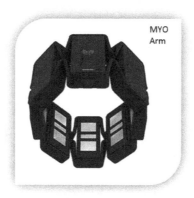

Fig. 2. The 5-finger Open-Bionics robotic hand.

into a PC. The PC reads the transmitted data and perform the action that relates to what the users are intended to do with their arm. The reason why this device was selected is because it is a wearable well integrated system, it is easy to be interfaced given the availability of software libraries and, moreover, it can get accurate readings.

In this project the Myoband will read the electrical activity of the user, transmit that data to a PC; this latter one will communicate to the robotic hand what to do, namely a proper type of grasping configuration, depending on which action and gesture the user has performed.

2.2 Software

In this section the software that has been used in the project is detailed.

The MyoConnect
MyoConnect is the Thalmic Labs software interface which allow the user to perform gesture control vs. a PC operative system: it basically allows to use your PC without having to manipulate the mouse or keyboard. The interface also allows to perform a calibration procedure in order to use the MyoBand irrespective of the orientation of the device when you wear it. Among all the available features of the software, the typical MyoConnect mask is reported in Fig. 3.

MyoConnect can be conceived as the hub to the MyoBand, since all the preliminary information can be accessed from this software. Basic commands can be sent to the wearable device; a "ping" will vibrate the band if it is wirelessly connected to the software; this also allows the user to perform basic tasks and have a direct understanding of how the band and the software work together.

The Myo system inherently embeds a human gesture classifier. 6 gesture can be recognised such as (see also Fig. 3):

- *Fist*
- *Rest*

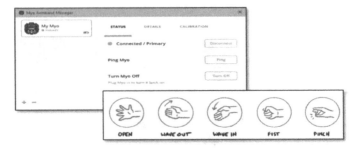

Fig. 3. The MYO Arm bracelet

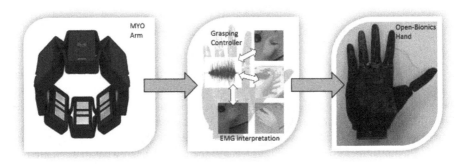

Fig. 4. The hardware architecture with the MyoBand and the open bionics robotic hand

- *Wave in*
- *Wave out*
- *Double tap*
- *Finger spread (i.e. Open Hand)*

Clearly custom gestures may be designed by using the SDK of the device, however – at this stage – this project is going to make use of these 6 available classes.

MyoConnect is also used as a bridge to talk to another software, called MyoDuino, that is used to send data to the robotic hand. Meanwhile the MyoConnect is also used in order for the band to send data to the PC and then be able to understand what is happening on the human-user side. An overall overview of the system is also shown in Fig. 4.

The Arduino IDE

Arduino Software is an open-source Integrated Development Environment (IDE), which uses C/C++ programming language. It provides the user with the ability to write code known as a sketch and in turn the ability to upload the sketch within an Arduino board.

An Arduino sketch is split into four different sections, where Sect. 1 is where the necessary libraries are included: in this project a *FingerLib* library has been embedded within the software. This library is used by the robotic hand in order to move the actuators

```
#include <MyoController.h>
#include <FingerLib.h>

Finger Pinky;
Finger Ring;
Finger Middle;
Finger Index;
Finger Thumb;
```

Fig. 5. The mapping of the 5-fingers robotic hand

and then the fingers. A *MyoController* is also used to allow the MyoBand and the Open Bionics hand to work in synergy. Section 2 is the setup section where the initial values of the variables are set, such as the starting positions of the servos. Also, in the set up all the pin modes are declared. The 3rd section is the loop section, which houses the main body of the code. The 4th and final section are where the functions of the program are declared.

The MyoDuino Software

MyoDuino is a third-party software that can be downloaded on GitHub: this element interfaces the two devices, namely the Myoband - i.e. its Bluetooth I/O - with the Arduino board – i.e. its Serial I/O. MyoDuino allows the user to see what is happening on the Myoband side as a visual display can be seen once the wearable system has been detected.

3   Design of the Interface

An Arduino IDE is used to develop the interface, due to the fact that the robotic hand embeds an Arduino-compatible controller board. The main code also needs to incorporate the *FingerLib* library, which allows each finger and thumb to be assigned a label name and to be actuated. This element makes the design of the grasping configuration easier: all that is needed is (a) to call the finger that you want to move and (b) then to write the position the finger has to reach. The finger labelling as it was performed in the project is reported within Fig. 5.

After setting the labelling, the further step is to make the Myoband able to set some actions into the hand device: this task is performed by using another library in Arduino IDE called *Myocontroller* which allowed the Myoband and the Arduino to dialogue each other: this is done by assigning the library to a variable such as *myo* and then using the functions inside the library to extract the classification output of the human movement from the Myoband itself. In particular, one of the attribute or function that was used in the project is the *myo.getcurrentposistion*. The function returns the current output of the Myoband allowing the Arduino board (i) to recognise a certain configuration of the end-user hand, such as, for example, the *fist* or *rest* configuration and therefore (ii) to trigger the robotic hand. An overview of this process is shown in Fig. 6.

In order to connect the Myoband and the Arduino a third party software called *MyoDuino* is used. MyoDuino acts as the bridge that allows communication between the two devices and it runs alongside the Arduino IDE: it connects the Myoband to the

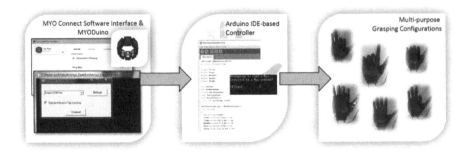

Fig. 6. Software architecture and functional diagram of the MYO-OpenBionics interface

MyoDuino via the Bluetooth dongle that comes with the Myoband and the MyoDuino to the hand via a COM port. Given such an interaction between the parts, a code to map the signals vs the hand movements can be designed. Figure 7 displays some of these movements that were implemented. Such a code should allow the hand to follow the human movements such that the robotic device will mirror the movements of the user. This process inherently requires a continuous stream of data from the Myoband to the hand which collides with the limited amount of memory of the Arduino board, unless the data that was being sent would be delayed (which would cause the unacceptable behaviour of having the hand performing the movement with a delay).

```
void Rock() {
  Pinky.open();
  Ring.close();
  Middle.close();
  Index.open();
  Thumb.open();
}
void graspCylindrical(){
  Pinky.writePos(600);
  Ring.writePos(600);
  Middle.writePos(600);
  Index.writePos(600);
  Thumb.close();
}
```

```
void Fist() {
  Pinky.close();
  Ring.close();
  Middle.close();
  Index.close();
  Thumb.close();
}
void graspSpherical() {
  Pinky.writePos(800);
  Ring.writePos(800);
  Middle.writePos(800);
  Index.writePos(800);
  Thumb.writePos(900);
}
```

Fig. 7. A set of available grasping configuration that were coded into the Arduino board

To bypass this issue a *SavedStatus* was designed within the Arduino IDE, which would allow the user to perform more movement using the same gestures (Fig. 8): namely, all the band gestures are recognised in every state, then each label will call its own function giving the robotic hand an unlimited set of movements.

The action will change based on what *savedstatus* the user is in: for example, a *fist* status will move the hand into the homologous fist configuration, whereas other savedstatus will perform different action allowing for more movements of the robotic device. Similarly, to switch to a next status, the user have to perform a *waveIn*; to go

```
SavedStatus=1;
PreviousTime=millis();
LastPosition=myo.getCurrentPose();
switch ( myo.getCurrentPose() ) {
case rest:
  ResetPosition();
  break;
case fist:
  Fist();
  Serial.print("Correct");
  break;
case waveIn:
  Status=2;
  delay(500);
  break;
```

```
case waveOut:
  Status=4;
  delay(500);
  break;
case fingersSpread:
  Rock();
  break;
case doubleTap:
  Status=10;
  SavedStatus=1;
  ResetPosition();
  delay(500);
  break;
```

Fig. 8. An example of *SavedStatus* setting

back to the last savedstatus the user has to perform a *waveOut*; finally, to reset the device into the home position the user needs to perform a *double tap*.

An overall view of this architecture is reported within the Fig. 9. The complete system is here shown: the MyoBand sends the information to the MyoDuino which in turn sends a command to the hand. This latter one will perform the action and loop back to the Myoband to get the new end-user command.

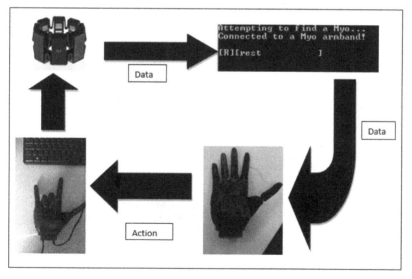

Fig. 9. Overview of the MyoBand and Open Bionics hand controller

4   Results

In this section of the paper, the results of some preliminary laboratory trials are reported. These results are shown in block diagrams to make clear which *savedstatus* were associated with which movements. Only few status are reported as representative of the overall set of the available status.

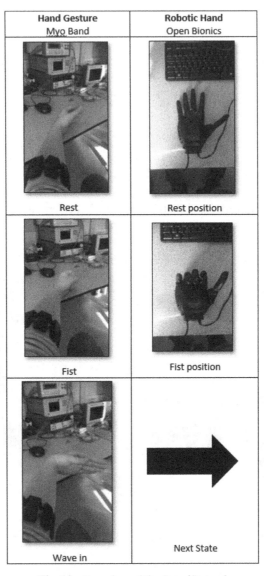

Fig. 10. Overview of the *SavedStatus 1*

Figure 10 shows the movement in *SavedStatus 1*: (i) waving in will change to the next savedstatus and (ii) waving out will go back to the last savedstatus, whereas (iii) double tap is used in case of any errors that happen while the hand is working.

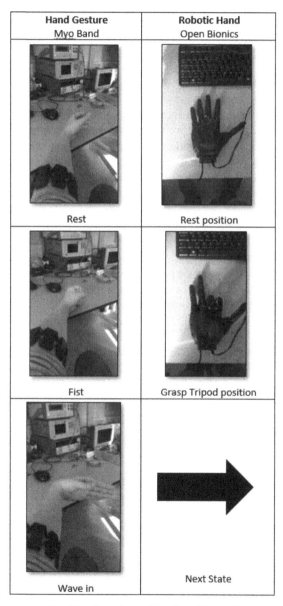

Fig. 11. Overview of the *SavedStatus 2*

This latter command will just set the hand in its reset or home position but the user will still be in the same savedstatus. A similar approach is followed for the *SavedStatus 2*, which is illustrated within the Fig. 11.

A set of 4 different status has been designed: fopr each one of these four stata, different configurations are available, according to the chosen one.

Thanks to this set of status, a menu with different movements allows the hand to switch and move in relation to the gesture that the user has done.

5 Conclusions and Future Works

A low-cost system combining EMG signal detection and classification with a 5 fingers robotic hand has been presented. The proposed system allows controlling the robotic hand in a set of various grasping configuration. Thanks to the choice of the design and experimental set-up, a variety of configuration is also available and easily adaptable [12–14]. Even if the validation has been only performed with some preliminary experiments, results are quite encouraging in view of developing such a system on a real prosthetic application where the patient may benefit of a low-cost system for daily life activity.

The proposed system embeds open-source software, namely the Arduino IDE software interface, and therefore it represents the possibility of developing integrated and human-centered prosthetic system with small budgets.

This approach could go beyond the present scope as the used hardware could be modified to look at many different uses. For example, the robotic hand may be combined with a Brain Computer Interface such as - when the user wears the device interface – brain activity could condition the hand, which would finally result in some movement [15].

Acknowledgements. This work was presented in project & coursework form in fulfilment of the requirements for the MSc in Robotics Engineering for the student Daniel McHugh under the supervision of E.L. Secco from the Robotics Laboratory, Department of Mathematics & Computer Science, Liverpool Hope University.

References

1. Secco, E.L., Moutschen, C.: A soft anthropomorphic & tactile fingertip for low-cost prosthetic & robotic applications. Liverpool: EAI Endorsed Trans. Pervasive Health Technol. **1**, 10 (2018)
2. Secco, E.L., Magenes, G.: Bio-mimetic finger - human like morphology, control & motion planning for intelligent robot & prosthesis. In: Mobile Robotics, Moving Intelligence, pp. 325–348 (2006)
3. Matrone, C., Cipriani, C., Secco, E.L., et al.: A biomimetic approach based on principal components analysis for multi-D.O.F. prosthetic hand control. In: Corner Workshop (2009)
4. Hand Gesture Controlled Robot Using Arduino: Int. J. Recent Trends Eng. Res. **4**(4), 336–342 (2018)
5. Llop-Harillo, I., Pérez-González, A.: System for the experimental evaluation of anthropomorphic hands. Application to a new 3D-printed prosthetic hand prototype. Int. Biomech. **4**(2), 50–59 (2017)

6. Explore & Learn. MyoBand (2019). https://learn.adafruit.com/myo-armband-teardown/inside-myo. Accessed 1 Mar 2019

7. Mounika, M., Phanisankar, B., Manoj, M.: Design & analysis of prosthetic hand with EMG technology in 3-D printing machine. Int. J. Curr. Eng. Technol. 7(1), 115, 119 (2019)

8. Pizzolato, S., Tagliapietra, L., Cognolato, M., Reggiani, M., Müller, H., Atzori, M.: Comparison of six electromyography acquisition setups on hand movement classification tasks. PLOS ONE 12(10), e0186132 (2017). https://journals.plos.org/plosone/article?id=10.1371/journal.pone.0186132

9. Shibata, T.: A study on our new prosthetic hand control method using a low-cost sEMG device. In: The Proceedings of JSME Annual Conference on Robotics and Mechatronics (Robomec), pp. 2A2–E01 (2018)

10. Welcome to Myo Support. Getting starting with Myo on Windows (2019). https://support.getmyo.com/hc/en-us/articles/202657596-Getting-starting-with-Myo-on-Windows. Accessed 4 Mar 2019

11. GitHub. CurrentlyAWey/Arnold-Palm-er (2019). https://github.com/CurrentlyAWey/Arnold-Palm-er. Accessed 4 Mar 2019

12. Secco, E.L., Magenes, G.A.: Feedforward neural network controlling a 3 D.O.F. finger. 5th International Conference on Cognitive & Neural Systems, 2001

13. Secco, E.L., Magenes, G.: Control of a 3 DOF artificial finger by a multi-layer perceptron. In: International Federation of Medical and Biological Engineering (IFMBE) Proceedings Medicon, pp. 927–930 (2001)

14. Magenes, G., Secco, E.: Teaching a robot with human natural movements. In: Pascolo, P.B. (ed.) Biomechanics and Sports. CCL, vol. 473, pp. 135–145. Springer, Vienna (2004). https://doi.org/10.1007/978-3-7091-2760-5_15

15. Elstob, D., Secco, E.L.: A low cost EEG based BCI prosthetic using motor imagery. Int. J. Inf. Technol. Converg. Serv. 6(1), 23–36 (2016)

Kinesthetic Feedback for Robot-Assisted Minimally Invasive Surgery (Da Vinci) with Two Fingers Exoskeleton

Emanuele Lindo Secco[1(✉)] and Andualem Maereg Tadesse[1,2]

[1] Robotic Laboratory, Department of Mathematics and Computer Science,
Liverpool Hope University, Liverpool L16 9JD, UK
{seccoe,maerega}@hope.ac.uk
[2] The Manufacturing Technology Centre, Coventry, UK

Abstract. Minimally Invasive Surgery and, in particular, Robotic Minimally Invasive Surgery may benefit from the integration of Haptic device: here we propose a preliminary study on a two-finger exoskeleton for kinesthetic feedback of surgeon thumb and index finger while controlling a Da Vinci Robotic Device through its Master Tool Manipulator (MTM). Simulation of contact between rigid and soft objects with the Patient Side Manipulator (PSM) are integrated with Force Feedback on the MTM coupled with the exoskeleton.

Keywords: Haptic device · Kinesthetic feedback · Da Vinci

1 Introduction

Minimal Invasive Surgery (MIS) is a surgical technique started during the mid 20th century. MIS uses specially designed surgical tools with multiple Degrees Of Freedom (DOF) wrist. The tools are long but very small, which enables their use inside small incisions of a patient skin. Such system benefits in the reduction of surgical trauma to the tissue decreased pain during surgery and the time to heal the wound. It also creates smaller visible scars compared to conventional surgical procedures. However, the loss of direct touch and contact with the operation site creates some disadvantages for the surgeon [1]. During MIS, in fact, the surgeon will not be able to assess the tissue properties by direct touch or palpation.

Even though multiple DOF endo-wrist (Fig. 1) helps to access the operation site in many directions, the tools need to move at the fixed point of the incision; therefore the DOF motion by the tool is lost, decreasing dexterity inside the operation site. Direct hand-eye coordination is also lost in such scenarios, which makes complex tasks such as knot tying very time consuming and require intensive training.

Robot-assisted Minimally Invasive Surgery (RMIS) was introduced to help reduce some of the disadvantages of MIS. RMIS can improve the accuracy and dexterity of the surgeon. It also minimizes trauma and pain to the patient. Current RMIS system enables hand-eye coordination through motion scaling and tremor filtering. However,

G. M. P. O'Hare et al. (Eds.): MobiHealth 2019, LNICST 320, pp. 212–225, 2020.
https://doi.org/10.1007/978-3-030-49289-2_17

when the surgeon operates the gripper, there is no feedback about the amount of forces exerted other than tissue deformation and other visual cues. Thus, the lack of direct haptic feedback is still a limitation in most of the RMIS systems.

Haptic Feedback - i.e. force and tactile feedback - can be provided from tool-tissue interaction forces and torques during grasping, palpation and tissue manipulation. Such kind of feedback may significantly improve patient safety and reduce operation time in RMOS. Excess grip force, in fact, could result in tissue damage for the patient [3] and also hand fatigue for the surgeon [4]. On the other hand, insufficient grip force may cause slipping of the tissue and increases the task difficulty.

Previous studies have explored different tactile and force feedback methods to provide Haptic Feedback for the surgeon. Many studies have shown that force feedback is essential in telesurgery [5–7] and it is favourable by the operator compared to other types of feedback, mainly visual and auditory [8–10]. Macfiled et al. [11, 12] demonstrated that the mechanoreceptors in the fingertip are essential for grip force control. The importance of tactile feedback for grip force control has been also largely explored [8, 13–15].

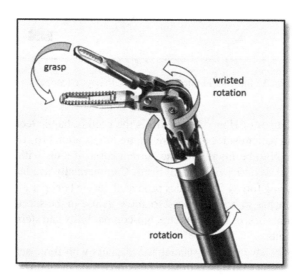

Fig. 1. A typical multi-DOF Endowrist for RMIS (modified from [2]).

In this paper we present a new design of a 2-fingers exoskeleton for haptic feedback combined with one of the most worldwide used robotic device: the application of this haptic Exoskeleton to display gripping force feedback for operation using the Da Vinci Surgical Research Kit (DVRK) is studied. Such kind of force feedback can reduce unintentional tissue injuries, and benefits the surgical procedure since it has been shown that force feedback reduces the grasping force in robot-assisted surgery.

2 Haptics in RMIS

Haptics generally describes touch feedback, which consists of Kinaesthetic (force) and Cutaneous (tactile) feedback. Currently, most RMIS systems do not include haptic feedback system however many research and evaluations are going on to include haptics in commercial and research prototype RMIS system. Nevertheless those systems which include haptics mostly provide only force feedback, with limited reliability. Some researchers have also developed tactile feedback systems for RMIS, but some of these implementations are still technologically limited since tactile feedback inherently requires spatially distributed sensing and display of tactile information. An example of the interaction between devices and operators in a RIMS scenario is reported in Fig. 2.

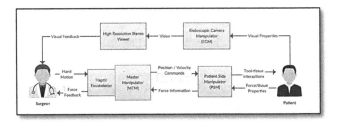

Fig. 2. Information flow in RMIS with haptic feedback.

The main challenges of Haptics in RMIS is the need of haptic techniques and sensors on the user and patient sides to acquire haptic information [16–18]. These sensors need to be very small to be fitted with the current surgical tools without affecting the manoeuvrability and dexterity of the tool itself. Commercially available force sensors are useful in measuring forces and torques produced during teleoperation. However, the size of these sensors has to be minimized to allow its use in the surgical environment. Apart from constraints in size and geometry, bio-compatibility and sterilization are other demanding constraints.

Some researchers have created specialized grippers with force sensors attached to the jaws. An ideal option would be estimating the forces applied indirectly without using force sensors on the gripper. The other challenge is the haptic display used to convey the information to the surgeon. Kinesthetic or force feedback system provides resolved force to the hand via force feedback devices. However, the fidelity of such force feedback devices is limited due to the dynamics force created by higher inertia and friction that are difficult to account or to measure. Accurate force feedback requires also a set of accurate dynamic models of the master and patient side manipulator to guarantee the stability of the system and the transparency of the force feedback. The displayed force feedback can also be affected by time delays due to the computational time and the delay of the transmission.

Even though, force feedback appears to be enough in many surgical procedures, tactile information such as contact location, finger-pad deformation, and pressure distribution can be necessary particularly during palpation. Therefore, the addition of tactile, haptic devices could also improve the operation procedure.

Another approach is using sensory substitution methods such as audio feedback, visual and graphical feedback or other forms like vibrotactile display [18].

Visually observing the tissue properties during the motion of the surgical instrument can also be used as feedback. However, such systems should be designed carefully not to distract the surgeon's view of the patient.

2.1 The Da Vinci Research Kit (DVRK)

2.1.1 Overall Configuration

The DVRK is a research platform from Intuitive Surgical: it is used to enhance collaborative research and development of new technologies for RMIS.

At the Antal Bejczy Center for Intelligent Robotics, Obuda University, a DVRKT system is available; the system is made of the following components (Fig. 3):

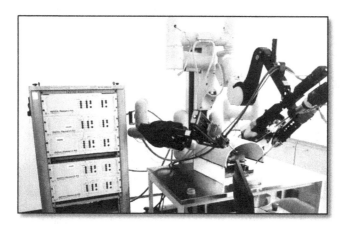

Fig. 3. The DV Research Kit (DVRKT) at Antal Bejczy Center for Intelligent Robotics.

- two Master Tool Manipulators (MTMs)
- two Patient Side Manipulators (PSMs)
- one High-Resolution Stereo Viewer (HRSV)
- one foot pedal tray and an hardware interface between the two consoles
- one Endoscopic Camera Manipulator (ECM)
- one Control Electronic System which is based on IEEE-1394 FPGA boards and Quad Linear Amplifier (QLA).

An overarching telerobotic software is available in order to control the DVRKT. This software is based on the Open Source Robotic Operative System (R.O.S.). It has different functional layers, namely the Hardware Interface (I/O), the Low-Level Control (e.g. PID), the High-Level Control, the Teleoperation system and, finally, the Application. Computer Assisted Intervention Systems (Cisst) libraries and Surgical Assistant Workstation (SAW) are used. The Low-Level Control layer consists of the PID joint controllers (one for each manipulator). The High-Level Control is provided by two components that are specific for the da Vinci MTM and PSM. These provide the forward and inverse kinematics, the trajectory generation, and the gripper control. They also manage the state transitions for the Da Vinci manipulators, such as the homing (MTM and PSM), the engaging the sterile adapter plate (PSM), and the engaging the instrument (PSM). The Teleoperation layer is provided by two instances of a general-purpose SAW component that each connect one MTM to one PSM. Finally, the Application layer is provided by a console application with HRSV that emulates the master console environment of the DVRKT (Fig. 4).

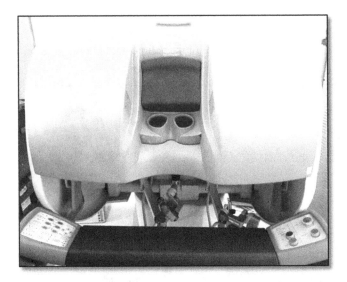

Fig. 4. The DVRKT HRSV console and master manipulators.

2.1.2 Gripper and Tool Configuration & Software Configuration

A variety of different and multi-purpose tools are available for the DVRKT. In this application we will focus on one of the most commonly used tool, the Endowrist. This gripper, as it is shown in Fig. 1, is a 4 DOF surgical tool, which is commonly used by Da Vinci operators. The tool is composed of tendons and pulley, which allows to orient the gripper around different rotational axes. The tendon actuation of the Endowrist introduces some non-linearities, which cause some challenges while modelling and controlling the device.

The R.O.S. software which is available to control the DVRKT provides a set of libraries and utilities. Thanks to these libraries, communication between different robot control processes in one computer or across multiple computers are available: in this study, the position sensing and force feedback controllers are developed as ROS topics that publish the robot state in ROS messages and accept commands by subscribing to ROS messages. An overview of the block diagram of the sensing and control software is reported in Fig. 2. Figure 5 also shows the implementation of the software and its visualizer.

2.2 Force Estimation and Control

Dynamic control of robotic manipulator and haptic devices may be performed via Impedance and Admittance control [19]. Impedance and Admittance Haptic devices interaction control are the most popular type of control system. In the Impedance Control, changes in position are used as an input to compute the output forces; similarly, in the Admittance Control a measured force is used as an input affecting the position and causing a change of the position.

Assuming to implement an Admittance Controller on the DVRKT means that a force sensor has to be fitted on the tip of the DVRK slave tools. However, as it was reported in the Sect. 1 (Introduction), embedding force sensors on a DVRKT tool is not easily achievable due to multiple requirements which involve the size, the biocompatibility, and the need of being able to sterilize the tool before the surgical procedure.

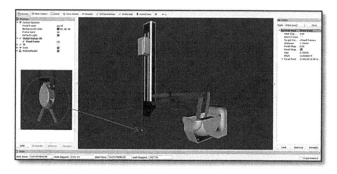

Fig. 5. The DVRK simulation environment under R.O.S. with the RViz 3D visualizer.

On the other side, an Haptic device based on implementing the Impedance Controller should have an intrinsic low friction and inertia. Such a device should be also back-driveable to minimize the dynamic distortion vs. the user's perception. Such a type of Haptic device can be used in applications requiring low force and torques; moreover, these devices have quite a simple design and low cost. For surgical robots with low mass and inertia, the change in desired and actual position of the patient side robot (i.e. where the desired task is a target position of the master manipulator) can be used to display forces which are applied to the environment. However, the reliability of such systems depends on the occurring dynamic and forces. For teleoperated surgical robots, such as the DVRKT, the master manipulator links have relatively large inertial values, in addition, most of the inertial parameter's are not precisely known. This uncertainty makes the impedance haptic feedback quite challenging. Finally, implementing impedance control for force feedback directly from the master DVRKT manipulator is difficult and therefore the role (and need for) an external force feedback device is critical.

The goal here is to develop a technique which uses the change of the position and velocity of the slave gripper in order to compute a proportional amount of force feedback which can be then displayed to the end-user of the DVRKT by means of a haptic exoskeleton.

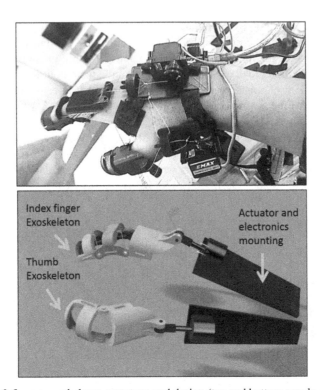

Fig. 6. The 2-fingers exoskeleton prototype and design (top and bottom panels, respectively).

2.3 Design of the Exoskeleton

A two-finger exoskeleton has been designed in order to be coupled with the DVRKT. The exoskeleton has been designed via 3D modelling software and then manufactured through a 3D printing process via extrusion: it is made of Acrylonitrile Butadiene Styrene (ABS) material and equipped with 2 servomotor which are physically connected to the elements of the inter-distal and distal phalanges of the index and thumb through a tendon-driven mechanism. The device is shown in Fig. 6. Details about the design, the sensors & actuators, and the tendon mechanism and kinematics are reported in [20].

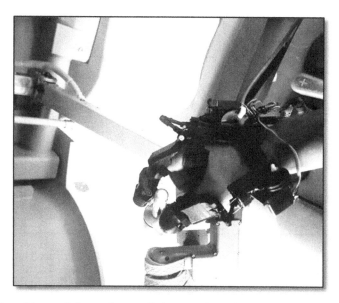

Fig. 7. Setting of the exoskeleton when applied to an end-user interacting with the DVRKT patient side manipulators.

2.4 Design of the Controller

Given the aforementioned exoskeleton, we are looking for providing the DVRKT operator with the perception and feeling of grasping. An object, which is gripped between the index finger and thumb should be emulated with a force feedback matching the grip force occurring on the DVRK tool's end effector, i.e. the Endowrist (Fig. 1). Figure 7 shows the setting of the exoskeleton when applied to an end-user interacting with the DVRKT Patient Side Manipulators.

In order to achieve this, the DVRKT and Exoskeleton control system should be designed as a bilateral control system, which receives position commands from the slave robot and reflects the interaction forces on the haptic device.

To this aim, an Impedance control algorithm has been applied for force control of the haptic interface that is coupled with the master robot. During operation, the operator moves the master-haptic interface generating position commands, the impedance between the operator and the haptic interfaces varies dynamically. If the impedance parameters and the dynamics of the master robot are precisely known, a control algorithm can be developed based on the dynamic model of the robot. However, this approach is challenging to implement mainly because of the uncertainty of the dynamic model and parameter variations. The other factor is that the forces that need to be displayed and replicated on the user side are very small compared to the occurring forces of the robot dynamic. In addition, a small positional error can cause a very high force, which results in damaging the user or the robot itself.

Impedance control algorithms monitor the contact forces by controlling the position of the manipulator and using the desired impedance, since the impedance defines the

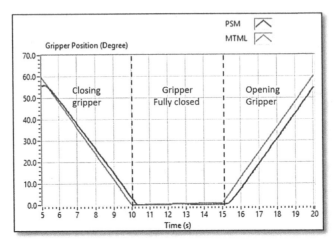

Fig. 8. PSM and MTML profiles under tele-manipulation of the PSM gripper (blue and red lines, respectively). (Color figure online)

relationship between the gripping force and the gripper velocity. For precise operation, the force due to the dynamics (i.e., inertia, friction, and gravity) must be adequately compensated, so that the operator only feels the contact and sliding force of the tool-tissue interaction. Various studies have been done on defining the contact model, the contact stability and performance [21–23]. These researches mainly focused on simplifying the dynamics of the master robot and on compensating the error induced by the simplification [19, 24, 25].

In this paper the haptic feedback is provided through an external exoskeleton device and, therefore, the dynamics of the master robot can be considered as transparent vs. the slave device. During operation, the end-user moves the MTM while grasping the MTM gripper. These movements are tracked and used to compute the control commands of the PSM.

The process is replicated under the R.O.S. environment and a simulation is performed. In the simulation, a PD controller is used to track the position of MTM joint and to implement a control effort, which actuates the PSM motors so that the PSM smoothly follows the MTM position. The linear position of the PSM tools is controlled as it follows:

$$F_{PSM} = K_p \cdot (x_{MTM} - x_{PSM}) - K_d \cdot \dot{x}_{PSM} \tag{1}$$

Where F_{PSM} is the control force effort, x_{MTM} is the position of the MTM, and x_{PSM} is the position of the PSM tool. The control gains are set to be automatically tuned by ROS PID autotune for smooth tracking and stability.

Similarly, the orientation of the PSM tool, including the gripper, is controlled as it follows:

$$\tau_{PSM} = K_p \cdot (\vartheta_{MTM} - \vartheta_{PSM}) - K_d \cdot \dot{\vartheta}_{PSM} \tag{2}$$

Where τ_{PSM} is the control torque effort, ϑ_{MTM} is the angle of the MTM wrist, and ϑ_{PSM} is the angle of the PSM wrist.

2.5 Design of the Gripper Controller

In absence of force feedback, the DVRKT slave gripper simply follows the motion of the DVRKT master gripper and - when an object gets in contact with the environment - such an object is grasped. In this work, a reverse control should be also applied, such as the master follows the motion (i.e. the position and the velocity) of the slave. Thus, our controller uses a PID controller τ_{exo} to generate an input torque effort for the exoskeleton, which is coupled with the master gripper manipulator.

First, let us consider a forward control of the slave gripper by the master. As shown in Fig. 8, when the master gripper is closing or opening, the slave gripper follows the master. The MTM position is used as setpoint (desired value of the controller) whereas the PSM position is used as a state (the actual value of the controlled motion), control effort is estimated based on the error (e) calculated from the difference of PSM and MTM gripper position. It holds:

$$e_x = \vartheta_{MTM} - \vartheta_{PSM}$$
$$\dot{e}_x = \dot{\vartheta}_{MTM} - \dot{\vartheta}_{PSM} \tag{3}$$

where ϑ_{MTM} is the angle of the MTM gripper, and ϑ_{PSM} is the angle of the PSM gripper; $\dot{\vartheta}_{MTM}$ is the angular speed of the MTM gripper, and $\dot{\vartheta}_{PSM}$ is the angular speed of the PSM gripper. While the gripper is closing, it holds $e_x > 0$; on the contrary, when the gripper is opening, it holds $e_x < 0$. However, when the object is gripped by the PSM tool, a significant error is introduced, and the PSM will not be able to follow the MTM anymore.

Considering a linear relationship between the deformation of the grasped object and the applied force applied, the error is proportional to the stiffness of the grasped object. Therefore, an error threshold value $e_{x\,threshold}$ is set to estimate the force and torque that should be applied by the exoskeleton. If $e_x > 0$ and $e_{x\,threshold} > e_x$, then the gripper is in contact with an object. Finally a torque τ_{effort} should be applied by the exoskeleton to restrict the movement of the fingertip thereby reducing the error between the MTM and the PSM gripper positions.

$$\tau_{effort} = K_p \cdot e_x + D_p \cdot \dot{e}_x + I_p \int_0^t e_x dt \tag{4}$$

Where τ_{effort} is the commanded torque to the exoskeleton motors and the gains depends on the stiffness and damping parameters of the grasped object. The K_p, Dp and Ip values have to be chosen in order to allow a successful grasping under different load conditions while preserving its stability. This mapping allows the end-user piloting the PSM gripper while applying different amounts of grip force to the object.

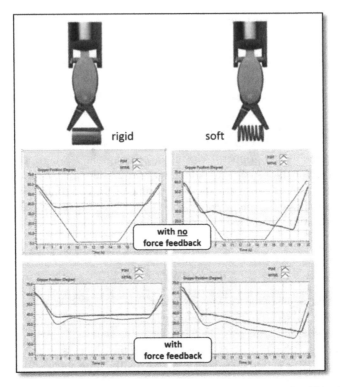

Fig. 9. Force-feedback tele-operation of the MTM and PSM Gripper (red and blue lines, respectively): positions *with* and *without* force feedback (top and bottom panels) for rigid and soft objects (left and right panels) are reported. (Color figure online)

3 Results

A solid and rigid object, as well as a soft components were considered: performed simulation uses both a rigid object and a spring object to mimic different scenarios in which the DVRKT is gripping a body tissue. The dynamic behaviour of the tissue with respect to the external applied forces and torques were modelled as a spring-damper system. According to [201], the desired impedance can be designed through the stiffness parameter, Kd, and the damping parameter, Dd. The motor position in the joint coordinates system can be also controlled by using a PD controller such as:

$$F_m = -K_d \cdot (x - x_s) - D_d \cdot \dot{x} \qquad (5)$$

where x_s is the desired position.

Preliminary practical tests were conducted to test the reliability of the system. The communication between the controller and the exoskeleton was handled via USB. Mbed ROS serial node subscribes to the control effort node, and the motor control map the control effort in the range of the maximum and minimum torque needed to actuate the motor. R.O.S. packages were also integrated to test the force feedback and the efficiency of the PID controller algorithms. ROS control nodes and topics used for both the DVRK virtual simulation and the exoskeleton controller were implemented. A DVRK PSM node publishes its time-varying setpoint to the PID controller node which applies corrections via the control effort topic of the exoskeleton controller. The DVRK MTML node also publishes the current value of the MTM position to the state topic. The simulation plots the MTM and PSM gripper positions as shown in Fig. 9.

4 Conclusion and Discussion

In this paper, a novel approach for using a 3D printed exoskeletons as a force feedback device in the DVRKT tele-operated system has been presented. The study was developed in the context of current literature where it was observed that many haptic studies on grip force control are still focusing on cutaneous feedback and not so much on kinesthetic feedback. It is still under discussion how the absence of force feedback on these applications may increase the difficulty of performing remote handling and object manipulation. Many studies have shown, in fact, that a simple force feedback (e.g. providing feedback of the grip) can significantly improve the transparency in robotic-assisted surgery and RMIS. The grip force feedback, in fact, can be employed to enhance surgeons perception of the mechanical properties of the tissue during a RMIS surgical procedure.

In the proposed system of this work we define a single point of contact of the haptic interface in order to display forces to the operator, where these forces mimic the mechanical properties of the tissue getting in contact with the end-effector of the robot (Fig. 9). Even if this is a preliminary integration study, it is important to notice that other studies have also shown that users tend to apply more grip forces in the absence of haptic feedback. Therefore, a proportional amount of force feedback can help these users to reduce their effective gripping force on the patient side. While grasping objects, people may then be able to adjust and fine tune their grip force according to the effective load of force. This result clearly helps in providing enough gripping force and prevent the tissue from being damaged and the tool from slipping. It also avoids damaging the organs due to an excessive force which can also increase the stress and fatigue of the surgeon.

Future works may include a study of the effect of the force feedback when using exoskeleton on the accuracy and time that is needed to complete surgical training procedures. The ergonomic advantage and disadvantages of such haptic feedback systems also needs to be furtherly studied and developed. Psychophysics experiments should also be conducted to analyze the effect of this approach compared to cutaneous feedback and visual feedback only [26]. Further studies must also be completed using teleoperation scheme which uses force sensors at the slave manipulator to support a comparison with the position control methods.

Acknowledgments. We thank all staff of the Department of Mathematics and Computer Science, Liverpool Hope University and of the Antal Bejczy Center for Intelligent Robotics, Obuda University for their valuable support.

This work was presented in thesis form in fulfilment of the requirements for the PhD in Robotics of the student A.M. Tadesse from the Robotics Laboratory, Department of Mathematics & Computer Science, Liverpool Hope University.

References

1. Seibold, U., Kubler, B., Hirzinger, G.: Prototype of instrument for minimally invasive surgery with 6-axis force sensing capability. In: Proceedings of the 2005 IEEE International Conference on Robotics and Automation. ICRA 2005, pp. 496–501. IEEE (2005)
2. Intuitive Surgical. Intuitive | da Vinci Surgical Instruments | EndoWrist (2019). https://www.intuitive.com/products-and-services/da-vinci/instruments. Accessed 28 Feb 2019
3. De, S., Rosen, J., Dagan, A., Hannaford, B., Swanson, P., Sinanan, M.: Assessment of tissue damage due to mechanical stresses. Int. J. Robot. Res. 26(11-12), 1159–1171 (2007)
4. Santos-Carreras, L., Hagen, M., Gassert, R., Bleuler, H.: Survey on surgical instrument handle design: ergonomics and acceptance. Surg. Innov. 19(1), 50–59 (2012)
5. Tholey, G., Desai, J.P., Castellanos, A.E.: Force feedback plays a significant role in minimally invasive surgery: results and analysis. Ann. Surg. 241(1), 102 (2005)
6. Horeman, T., Rodrigues, S.P., Jansen, F.-W., Dankelman, J., van den Dobbelsteen, J.J.: Force measurement platform for training and assessment of laparoscopic skills. Surg. Endosc. 24(12), 3102–3108 (2010)
7. Botden, S.M.B.I., Torab, F., Buzink, S.N., Jakimowicz, J.J.: The importance of haptic feedback in laparoscopic suturing training and the additive value of virtual reality simulation. Surg. Endosc. 22(5), 1214–1222 (2008)
8. King, C.-H., et al.: Tactile feedback induces reduced grasping force in robot-assisted surgery. IEEE Trans. Haptics 2(2), 103–110 (2009)
9. Koehn, J.K., Kuchenbecker, K.J.: Surgeons and non-surgeons prefer haptic feedback of instrument vibrations during robotic surgery. Surg. Endosc. 29(10), 2970–2983 (2015)
10. Johansson, R.S., Westling, G.: Roles of glabrous skin receptors and sensorimotor memory in automatic control of precision grip when lifting rougher or more slippery objects. Exp. Brain Res. 56(3), 550–564 (1984). https://doi.org/10.1007/BF00237997
11. Macefield, V.G., Häger-Ross, C., Johansson, R.S.: Control of grip force during restraint of an object held between finger and thumb: responses of cutaneous afferents from the digits. Exp. Brain Res. 108(1), 155–171 (1996)
12. Nowak, D.A., Hermsdörfer, J., Glasauer, S., Philipp, J., Meyer, L., Mai, N.: The effects of digital anaesthesia on predictive grip force adjustments during vertical movements of a grasped object. Eur. J. Neurosci. 14(4), 756–762 (2001)
13. Pacchierotti, C., Chinello, F., Malvezzi, M., Meli, L., Prattichizzo, D.: Two finger grasping simulation with cutaneous and kinesthetic force feedback. In: Isokoski, P., Springare, J. (eds.) EuroHaptics 2012. LNCS, vol. 7282, pp. 373–382. Springer, Heidelberg (2012). https://doi.org/10.1007/978-3-642-31401-8_34
14. Minamizawa, K., Kajimoto, H., Kawakami, N., Tachi, S.: A wearable haptic display to present the gravity sensation-preliminary observations and device design. In: Euro-Haptics Conference, 2007 and Symposium on Haptic Interfaces for Virtual Environment and Teleoperator Systems. World Haptics 2007. Second Joint, pp. 133–138. IEEE 2007
15. Westebring-van der Putten, E.P., van den Dobbelsteen, J.J., Goossens, R.H., Jakimowicz, J.J., Dankelman, J.: The effect of augmented feedback on grasp force in laparoscopic grasp control. IEEE Trans. Haptics 3(4), 280–291 (2010)
16. Li, M., et al.: Using visual cues to enhance haptic feedback for palpation on virtual model of soft tissue. Med. Biol. Eng. Comput. 53, 1177–1186 (2015). https://doi.org/10.1007/s11517-015-1309-4
17. Wurdemann, H.A., et al.: Mapping tactile information of a soft manipulator to a haptic sleeve in RMIS. In: 3rd Joint Workshop on New Technologies for Computer/Robot Assisted Surgery (CRAS 2013) (2013)

18. Li, M., et al.: Using visual cues to enhance haptic feedback for palpation on virtual model of soft tissue. Med. Biol. Eng. Comput. **53**(11), 1177–1186 (2015)
19. Hogan, N.: Adaptive control of mechanical impedance by coactivation of antagonist muscles. IEEE Trans. Autom. Control **29**(8), 681–690 (1984)
20. Tadesse, A.M.: Development of wearable haptic devices with integrated hand tracking systems for virtual reality interactions. Ph.D. Dissertation, Supervisor: E. L. Secco. DoS: D. Reid. Liverpool Hope University (2019)
21. Adams, R.J., Hannaford, B.: A two-port framework for the design of unconditionally stable haptic interfaces. In: IROS, pp. 1254–1259 (1998)
22. Edward Colgate, J., Michael Brown, J.: Factors affecting the z-width of a haptic display. In: Proceedings of the 1994 IEEE International Conference on Robotics and Automation 1994, pp. 3205–3210. IEEE (1994)
23. Millman, P.A., Stanley, M., Edward Colgate, J.: Design of a high performance haptic interface to virtual environments. In: Virtual Reality Annual International Symposium 1993, pp. 216–222. IEEE. (1993)
24. Lasky, T.A., Hsia, T.C.: On force-tracking impedance control of robot manipulators. In: Proceedings of the 1991 IEEE International Conference on Robotics and Automation 1991, pp. 274–280. IEEE (1991)
25. Jung, S., Hsia, T.C.: Neural network impedance force control of robot manipulator. IEEE Trans. Ind. Electron. **45**(3), 451–461 (1998)
26. Maereg, A.T., Nagar, A., Reid, D., Secco, E.L.: Wearable vibrotactile haptic device for stiffness discrimination during virtual interactions. Front. Robot. AI **4**, 42 (2017)

Wearable Technologies and Smart Measurement

Evaluating the Requirements of Digital Stress Management Systems: A Modified Delphi Study

Kim Janine Blankenhagel$^{(\boxtimes)}$, Miriam Linker, and Rüdiger Zarnekow

Technical University Berlin, Straße des 17. Juni 135, 10623 Berlin, Germany
k.blankenhagel@tu-berlin.de

Abstract. Stress is a major health problem in this century, and it is associated with adverse health consequences. Its prevention and management are a great challenge, and only a minority of the affected persons receive treatment. New digital technologies offer opportunities to provide effective psychological interventions to address the negative consequences of occupational stress. However, the knowledge of the importance of different functions and features of digital stress management systems remains largely unexplored. This work closes that research gap by conducting a Delphi study, in which 20 experts prioritized requirements in three rounds. The purpose of the present study is to enable developers of digital stress management systems (DSMS) to profitably select and use functions and characteristics of those systems, taking into account the available resources. Thus, the aim is to find DSMS that better counteract excessive stress. Finally, 82% of all requirements meet the consensus threshold.

Keywords: Digital stress management systems · Burnout prevention · eHealth

1 Introduction

Burnout is a major public health issue due to the generally elevated levels of stress and its growing complexity in the professional context [1]. Stress can be caused by work-related factors, such as excessive workload, or through individual sources, for example, work-family conflicts [2]. Long-term stress is not only associated with an increased risk of burnout but also with other mental disorders and somatic problems such as cardiovascular disease [3]. Undoubtedly, stress and the associated health consequences lead to high direct and indirect costs incurred by both employers and the society due to healthcare costs, lower productivity, and absenteeism [2]. Nevertheless, the rate of participation in conventional preventive services is low, and face-to-face stress reduction interventions require excessive human resource allocations and suffer time conflict issues [4]. At the same time, the technological capability to mine, interpret, and respond to a large amount of data for promoting the welfare of human subjects is growing [5]. Therefore, research continues to focus on the use of digital technologies. They are promising in terms of acceptability, effectiveness, and economic sustainability to support stress management and reduce the negative consequences of work-related stress [4]. In addition to adequate physical exercise, the ability to cope with stress is one of the most important factors in

G. M. P. O'Hare et al. (Eds.): MobiHealth 2019, LNICST 320, pp. 229–248, 2020.
https://doi.org/10.1007/978-3-030-49289-2_18

preventing burnout [6]. The term preventive digital stress management systems (DSMS), as defined in this article, encompasses coping strategies for the preservation of mental, physical, and social health. The aim is to reduce stress caused by work-related pressure and contribute to finding a healthy balance. DSMS are mainly provided in the digital form (derived from [7]). Currently, there are only a few DSMS on the market (e.g., applications on smartphones). Moreover, there are also certain initial studies dealing with the effectiveness and moderating factors of DSMS [8–10].

However, in general, the market is commercially driven, and the importance of the different functions and features of DSMS are poorly represented in the existing research. In order to close this gap, we conducted a Delphi study with 20 experts who prioritized the requirements for DSMS in three rounds. The obtained list of requirements was developed by the authors in 2018 using 15 semi-structured qualitative interviews. This list is the foundation for the present study. The purpose is to first confirm the requirements and then to enable developers of DSMS to profitably select and use the functions and characteristics, keeping in mind the available resources. Thus, the aim is to develop DSMS that better counteract excessive stress.

The Delphi study design is a suitable method for the present prioritization because it structures the necessary communication processes well and can produce a well-founded consensus due to its mixture of questionnaires and controlled opinion feedback.

2   Background

DSMS usually aim to reduce the symptoms of work-related stress, thereby increasing the wellbeing of users [11]. They provide new ways to feel, think, and act in stressful situations to reduce stressors, improve reactions to stressors, or mitigate the physiological or psychological effects of stress [2]. They focus on teaching different techniques to cope with stress [12] and differ in terms of various aspects, such as delivery, intervention content, length, or scope [10]. Often, DSMS are delivered in sessions over several weeks, whereby there are short systems (such as 2-week interventions); in contrast, some are also delivered over months or years [10]. In general, the interventions and exercises focus on an individual level and comprise meditation, mindfulness, breathing, and relaxation techniques, biofeedback, time management, and other cognitive behavioral elements [2, 13]. There are two types of systems, which differ in guidance. Guided interventions have some kind of human support, such as e-mail reminders or counselor support, whereas unguided ones have no support or only technical support [2].

The effectiveness of psychological and psychotherapeutic health interventions provided via the internet is frequently studied, and their results are promising [10]. Whether these findings can be transferred to DSMS and internet interventions can also be effective in prevention in the field of stress remains little studied and no conclusive evidence of effectiveness is available. A few analyses have been performed to examine the effectiveness of DSMS in comparison to a group on waiting list, which show a significant reduction of stress [3, 11, 14, 15]. Moreover, comparisons with a no-treatment group [16] or to an attention group [17] indicate the effectiveness of DSMS too. Elena Heber and Wasantha Jayawardene explored related research, and both of the meta-analyses demonstrate positive effects of DSMS [4, 10]. As many relevant parameters, such as type and length of the interventions, usage of guidance, outcomes, measurements, or settings, vary in the studies, the results are not quite comparable and generalizability is difficult to assess [2, 18]. Furthermore, the effects of individual interventions of DSMS are mostly unexplored, sample sizes of the trials are often small, and the measurement of stress as a success control is often carried out solely through self-assessments (e.g., Perceived Stress Scale) rather than through objective methods, such as biomarkers (e.g. cortisol levels). It is striking that DSMS are often tested on groups, constituting people with relevant symptoms in a stressful period of life (e.g., healthcare professionals who have higher burnout, depression, and suicide rates) [13–15, 18–20]. Thus, from the perspective of a universal preventive stress setting, no conclusions can be drawn regarding people in their everyday life with lower stress levels. In addition, studies analyze outcomes such as stress, perceived stress, depression, etc. after a short time of using DSMS [10, 12, 19, 20]. Change in stress management, attitudes, and behavior are fundamental basic psychological processes, which may take a long period to manifest. Therefore, study periods may not be enough to cover long-term effects, and the first research results should be interpreted with care.

In summary, there is insufficient knowledge available of what makes DSMS successful in reducing stress and preventing burnout. Thus, we aim to bridge the research gap by prioritizing the requirements of DSMS.

3   Methods

This analysis is based on an explorative study conducted in 2018, replacing the first phase of a typical Delphi study. As it provides an underlying list of requirements, the study is crucial and described in more detail below. Afterward, an in-depth description of the methodical approach of this study is presented.

3.1   Preliminary Study

The requirements for DSMS were derived from a qualitative interview study and its analysis [21]. As the body of knowledge lacks assessment, interpretation patterns, and action orientations as well as the identification of individual perspectives, semi-structured, guideline-based interviews were chosen as a suitable methodology to identify the requirements. In order to better understand the specificity of the DSMS application, the interviews were conducted from four different perspectives (health insurance companies, care providers, the private sector, and users). The interview partners were selected according to Flickl following case selection using a qualitative sampling plan, in order to include a targeted selection of particularly meaningful cases [22]. The employed interview guideline was based on the principles established by Döring and Bortz and was deductively derived from the literature [23]. The interviews were analyzed as per the qualitative content analysis presented by Mayring, utilizing a software for qualitative analysis (MaxQDA) [24]. The requirements identified from the interviews were aggregated and coded, rule-based, on a developed coding guide, which defined the characteristics of the individual categories. The interview material was cross-validated, and the Cohen's Kappa coefficient was determined to be 0.85 [21]. Table 1 collates all the requirements.

Table 1. Underlying Requirements

ID	Requirement
1	Consecutive, adaptive, small-step goals; behavioral goals derived from health goals
2	Reminder functions to goals, open exercises or other mature interactions; individually configurable
3	Short interaction times (about 5-15 min per day); quick check-in, clear structure and menu navigation, overviews
4	Simple and intuitive usability, fun to use
5	Hidden content, only a few technical terms
6	Highly personal and clear everyday relevance
7	Everyday suitability and high wearing comfort
8	Clear presentation of cause and effect relationships
9	High individualization including personal on-boarding, individual configuration options and tailoring to the user
10	Support to identify stressors and derive appropriate measures
11	Measurement of stress level
12	Customization to specific user situations
13	High autonomy; proactive construction
14	Feedback functions in acute stress situations and effectiveness of implemented measures and exercises; reports on medium- to long-term trends in stress levels
15	Diary or documentation function
16	Continuous measurements of heart rate variability and respiratory rate
17	Analysis of vocal pitch, muscular tension in the neck area and skin resistance
18	At least one stress-measuring functionality is available and transformed into an understandable main metric; detailed drill down capabilities for stress levels
19	Detection of deviations from the normal pattern
20	Adaption of stress monitoring over time
21	Interventions include exercises in psychological self-education
22	Interventions include exercises for self-reflection
23	Interventions include exercises to build up anti-stress resources
24	Interventions are scientifically driven
25	Possibility of integration of a doctor, psychotherapist, or medical professional
26	Adequate overview function for a supervising physician
27	Profound data concept regarding data security and data protection

(continued)

Table 1. (*continued*)

ID	Requirement
28	Encapsulated and encrypted storage and processing of users data
29	Anonymous and aggregated data transmission
30	Transparency and information regarding data usage
31	Raw data material available in a machine-readable and structured format; possibility of deletion
32	Integration of artificial intelligence for individualization
33	High mobility; offline use
34	Compatibility and integration with other applications

Finally, a total of 34 requirements in the domains of Human Centricity, Medicine, and Technology were determined, which are mainly non-functional. Therefore, it can be assumed that aspects of user-friendliness and the method of implementation are of great importance for the success of DSMS. As equivalent DSMS that meet all the requested requirements can be highly complex and very expensive, this study focused on validation and prioritization.

3.2 Follow-up Study

We used the established method of a Delphi study; it is based on the concept of pooled intelligence intended to enhance individual judgments and capture the collective opinion of experts [25]. Due to the incomplete state of knowledge about prioritization of the requirements of DSMS, we considered the Delphi study a suitable research tool to augment unanimity in opinions. Delphi studies that use ranking have been widely used in information systems research to develop group consensus regarding the relative importance of issues, particularly in health sciences [26–28]. The literature does not present a consistent definition of the method, but it is possible to define particular features characterizing its nature. It is an instrument for the improved recording of group opinions, the basic concept being the use of expert knowledge to solve problems in several iterations. The process is characterized by the addition of anonymous feedback regarding the general opinion of all experts after each round [29]. The averages produced in the decision-making processes of expert groups prove to be better than the averages of individual expert responses [30]. Furthermore, compared to other methods of forming opinions in groups (e.g., focus groups), the Delphi method neutralizes the influence of dominant opinion leaders (e.g., by reason of their authority, personality, reputation, etc.) due to its anonymity [31]. The involvement of experts and the use of a formalized questionnaire are further characteristics of Delphi studies [29]. As we have already derived the requirements of DSMS in the context of a previous qualitative study, the open-ended initial phase of a traditional Delphi process has been omitted in the present study, and this is, therefore, to be considered a modified Delphi study.

Figure 1 demonstrates the methodical approach, which is presented in detail below.

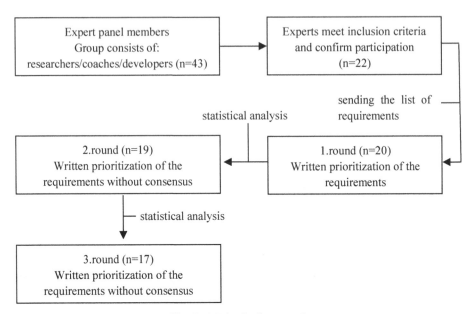

Fig. 1. Methodical approach

Expert Panel Selection. Initially, we recruited experts who are highly familiarized with the combination of stress management and digital services. In order to cover different perspectives, we asked experts to participate in the study who are active researchers, coaches/consultants, and developers. Scientists were selected according to their research activities and publications in the field of digital stress management, coaches and consultants according to their orientation and popularity, and developers according to their proximity with the topic. In total, we contacted 43 experts by telephone and e-mail as well as provided an information sheet regarding the research team, the content, the objective, and the proposed duration of the study. In addition, we asked the selected experts to self-assess their expert status in terms of stress management and digital health services by classifying them into four categories (low, average, high, very high) as compared to other experts in their field. As the level of knowledge of the expert panel is a critical success factor in Delphi studies [29], we only included experts in the study if they rated their expert knowledge as high or very high.

There is disagreement in the literature regarding the optimal scope of a Delphi expert group. According to Woudenberg, a panel size of three people is considered too small [32], and Brooks prefers a maximum of 25 experts [33]. Even though larger panels generally reduce any possible biases, in an experiment on the necessary panel size, Duffield showed that the results of two different groups (n = 16 versus n = 34) are in agreement by 92% [34]. On this basis, we aimed for a group of 15–25 experts. A total of 22 experts pledged their participation at the end of the recruitment phase.

Round 1. We conducted the first round of the Delphi study in October 2018. In order to reduce costs, time, and effort and avoid geographical boundaries, we conducted the study digitally. The experts received the list of 34 requirements via e-mail and were asked to prioritize each requirement. In addition, open comment fields were provided. The scale consisted of the four classic categories listed below:

"Must":   The requirement is absolutely essential.
"Should":   The requirement should be met but is not absolutely essential.
"Could":   The requirement could be met if a more valuable requirement did not interfere.
"Won't":   The requirement should not be met

Out of the participants, 20 experts returned the prioritized list on time, and their replies were included in the evaluation.

The objective of the study was to build consensus among the expert group on the importance of individual requirements for effective and successful DSMS. Therefore, we defined the following two essential criteria for reaching consensus, and both had to be met:

1. 70% of all experts select the same category.
2. The interquartile range (IQR) is less than or equal to one.

With the two criteria, we ensured that consensus can only be reached if a clear majority of the experts had the same opinion (Criterion 1) and if the answers were little scattered (Criterion 2: 75% of all answers fluctuate between two categories at most). After the first round, we evaluated all the questionnaires, calculated the mean, mode, relative frequency, and interquartile range. Requirements that fulfilled both criteria were removed from the process as a consensus had already been reached. At the end of the first round, 15 of the 34 requirements were endorsed by the experts, and the remaining 19 did not meet the threshold.

Round 2. Subsequently, we sent a revised list of requirements to the same experts in a second round. In this round, only those requirements were sent that did not fulfill the previous criteria for consensus. In addition, we visually presented the results of the first round in general and also informed each expert of his own answer. The total distribution was represented by circles of different colors and sizes. They comprised the three categories "more than 40%...," "20–40%...", or "less than 20% of all experts chose the respective category." Then, we again asked the experts for another set of prioritizations, considering the general opinion, and received a total of 19 completed questionnaires at the end of the deadline. Afterward, we evaluated them in the same way as the first round. Overall, consensus was reached on 11 out of the 19 requirements.

Round 3. The third round included a repeated revision of the requirement list by excluding the requirements that had gained consensus previously. We again asked the experts to prioritize the remaining requirements and invited them to explain their choice if it differed from the general group perspective. From the participants, 17 experts participated in the third round, and consensus was reached on 2 of the remaining 8 requirements. Since the difference between the second and third rounds was negligible, we did not expect any further movements in a potential fourth round; thus, we completed the study.

4 Results

The participants in round 1 of the modified Delphi study self-identified as one of the following: coach (n = 9, 45%), developer of DSMS (n = 6, 30%), or researcher (n = 5, 25%). The proportions of the genders were almost at par (11 males, 9 females). Lastly, 70% of all participants reported very high expert status in both stress management and digital health services.

Table 2 anonymously lists the characteristics of all the participating experts from round 1.

Table 2. Expert characteristics

ID	Background	Gender	Expert level – stress management	Expert level – digital health services
1	Developer		High	Very high
2	Researcher	Female	Very high	Very high
3	Developer	Male	High	Very high
4	Developer	Male	High	Very high
5	Coach	Male	Very high	Very high
6	Coach	Male	Very high	High
7	Coach	Female	Very high	High
8	Coach	Female	High	High
9	Researcher	Male	Very high	Very high
10	Researcher	Male	Very high	Very high
11	Coach	Female	Very high	Very high
12	Developer	Female	Very high	Very high
13	Researcher	Female	Very high	Very high
14	Coach	Male	Very high	High
15	Coach	Male	Very high	Very high
16	Developer	Female	Very high	Very high
17	Coach	Female	High	High
18	Researcher	Male	High	High
19	Coach	Female	Very high	Very high
20	Developer	Male	Very high	Very high

4.1 Results of Round 1

The prioritization from the first round resulted in 15 requirements with consensus. Overall, it is especially striking that the requirements with meta-level and conceptual characteristics reached consensus (e.g., 1, 7, 12, 26). In contrast, concrete requirements about implementation resulted in less consensus (e.g., 2, 16, 21–23). This indicates that experts agree on the importance of basic design issues, but that the importance of several functions leads to different opinions and still offers potential for discussion. In the following three sections we present the results of all 15 requirements with consensus in the first round.

Requirements with the Prioritization "Must" (n = 9). In total, 9 out of 15 requirements were classified as essential for successful DSMS. This includes the idea that DSMS should incorporate multi-purpose, adaptive, small-scale goals in order to create positive incentives for the user and motivate them (Requirement 1). Without exception, all coaches selected the category "Must." Their work requires an excellent understanding of the areas of goal setting and motivation. Therefore, their clear prioritization robustly confirms that setting appropriate goals also plays an important role in the context of digital systems and should definitely be implemented. Across all participating groups, 86% chose the category "Must". Thus, this requirement meets the consensus threshold (IQR = 0).

Furthermore, the experts agree that DSMS processing times should be very short (Requirement 3). The fast pace of (work) life today explains the increasing importance of time requirements. People who suffer from stress are willing to use a DSMS only if they can operate it quickly. This understanding is particularly pronounced among developers (all of them marked the category "Must"). With regard to sustainable utilization, simple and intuitive usability as well as fun to use (Requirement 4) are also essential requirements according to expert ratings. The consideration of a clear, everyday reference and high everyday suitability of DSMS are also highly important requirements (Requirements 6 and 7), and it should be ensured that any intervention is scientifically proven (Requirement 24). There is agreement among the participating experts that DSMS must have a strong data protection concept (Requirement 27) and must inform the user transparently and comprehensively about the use of the data (Requirement 30). Both requirements found 100% consensus among the researchers as well as among the developers. The provision of the raw data material in a machine-readable and structured format as well as the possibility of deletion are also very high priorities for the experts (Requirement 31).

Requirements with the Prioritization "Should" (n = 3). The experts consider a high degree of individualization (Requirement 9) of the DSMS to be preferable but not absolutely necessary. Tailoring to individual users' needs can be implemented, for example, by employing a software that gets to know the user, identifies his stressors, and supports him with personalized instructions and exercises. The answers of the coaches and researchers are all located in the two highest evaluation categories. Moreover, with a total of 74% agreement between all of the experts on "Should," Requirement 9 narrowly achieved the consensus criteria. With an interquartile range of 0, one check mark at "Could" (developer) and none at "Won't," we assume that the "Should" prioritization tends to be of higher importance. In addition to tailoring the system to a person, an individual adaption to the user's environment is also considered desirable by the experts (Requirement 12). It should be possible to disable or individually configure the interaction with the DSMS adapted to the circumstances of personal everyday life.

Among the researchers, there is absolute agreement on the prioritization of "Should," but the opinion among the developers is incoherent. This distribution can be traced to an increased degree of difficulty in implementation, thereby leading to disagreement or rather uncertainty among the developers. Furthermore, high autonomy as well as a proactive structure of the DSMS (Requirement 13) are seen as a "Should" requirement for appropriate application by the experts.

Requirements with the prioritization "Could" (n = 3). The experts agree that the measurement of stress levels on the basis of voice analysis, muscular tension in the neck area and skin resistance (Requirement 17) has a low priority and should only be done if there are available resources left after the implementation of more important requirements. Expert 02 comments that

"reliable and suitable stress detection [with the mentioned technique] is not yet satisfactorily possible."

Due to the abstract nature of the symptom stress, its measurability is generally difficult and the experts believe that voice analyses, measurement of skin resistance as well as muscular tensions should be given low priority. No one selected the category Must, but two experts selected the category Won't. Similarly, the experts rate the involvement of medical specialists and the provision of overviews for physicians (Requirements 25 and 26) as low on importance. Because DSMS are designed to reduce excessive stress and prevent burnout, they are naturally preventive and take effect before the onset of a disease. Therefore, the focus is on self-management and the integration of physicians does not seem necessary.

Table 3 contains all of the requirements with a consensus after round 1, and also specifies the mean, mode and interquartile ranges.

Table 3. Requirements with consensus in round 1

Requirement	Mean	Mode	IQR
Must:			
6	3.9	4	0
30	3.89	4	0
27	3.85	4	0
4	3.8	4	0
1	3.75	4	0
3	3.7	4	0.5
24	3.65	4	1
7	3.6	4	0.5
31	3.63	4	1
Should:			

(*continued*)

Table 3. (*continued*)

Requirement	Mean	Mode	IQR
9	3.16	3	0
13	3	3	0
12	2.9	3	0
Could:			
26	2.35	2	0.5
25	2.15	2	0
17	2	2	0

Must ≙ 4, Should ≙ 3, Could ≙ 2,
Won't ≙ 1

4.2 Results of Round 2

The prioritization in the second round resulted in 11 requirements gaining consensus. Overall, the experts agree on the topics of stress measurement and the design of exercises (e.g., 11, 18, 21).

Requirements with the Prioritization "Must" (n = 8). The experts evaluate individually configurable reminder functions for goals, open exercises, or other interactions with the system (Requirement 2) as crucial features. In addition, a clear presentation of cause and effect relationships (Requirement 8) is highly important due to the motivating effect. For example, after a completed exercise, the DSMS visualizes the reduced stress levels and emphasizes the casual link. The developers particularly consider this presentation to be very important (100% chose the category "Must"), whereas the researchers and coaches vary between "Must" and "Should," with more focus on "Must".

Furthermore, it is very important that DSMS provide functions that support the identification of the user's stressors and, if necessary, derive appropriate measures to reduce stress (Requirement 10). In the same vein, the measurement of stress (Requirement 11) constitutes a basic function because it is suitable for drawing conclusions about possible stressors. This logic matches expert ratings, because Requirement 11 reaches consensus with the prioritization "Must." Both coaches and developers evaluate the two related requirements (10 and 11) similarly. Only the opinion of the researchers is slightly more inconsistent. In addition, agreeing on the great importance of measuring stress levels, the experts also consider the translation of the stress levels measured into an understandable metric and its detailed breakdown (for example, subdividing stress into low-, medium-, and high-stress phases or specifying the duration of the stress phase) to be essential (Requirement 18). With a relative frequency of 79% and an interquartile range of 1, this requirement meets the consensus threshold. Only the coaches express a few different opinions, and Expert 17 comments:

"The measurement and presentation of stress levels could be also counterproductive, because the affected person is confronted directly with having a very high level of stress."

In conclusion, the experts consider stress measurement as a meaningful and profitable functionality, although it cannot be ruled out that in individual cases, the existing stress load of the user may be further aggravated by its measurement and presentation.

Both the psycho-educative and educational interventions (Requirement 21) and reflective exercises (Requirement 22) are must-have requirements. The mean values indicate that the provision of reflective interventions is of a little more importance than psychoeducational ones (mean of 3.79 versus 3.68). The field of self-reflection includes exercises for better body perception (body scan), increased awareness and sensitization, as well as self-observation exercises. The present prioritization emphasizes that in addition to several new tracking functions, the stimulation of self-reflection also is vital in the area of digital systems. Expert 08 states:

"People should also get a feeling for their body and intuition again and learn this through self-reflection and questioning."

After the second round, the technical requirement for anonymous and aggregated data transmission (Requirement 29) also achieves the prioritization "Must". As 86% of the experts with a very high level knowledge of digital health technologies chose the "Must" category (among those with high expert status, it is only 40%) and because Requirement 29 necessitates deep technical understanding, the distribution indicates very high importance. If data transmission is not necessary, Expert 01 alternatively recommends that applications can work on a smartphone in a completely encapsulated way, including data processing, so that personalized systems can be implemented.

Requirements with the Prioritization "Should" (n = 1). The requirement of adapting the stress-measuring monitoring element to development over time and period of use (Requirement 20) reaches the prioritization of "Should." Therefore, it is desirable to offer frequent learning opportunities at the beginning of usage to quantify and evaluate one's own stress levels and identify the stressors. Afterward, medium- to long-term trends of stress development gain spotlight rather than the cause-effect relationships and individual situations.

Requirements with the Prioritization "Could" (n = 2). The detection of deviations from normal behavior (for example, the user only stays in the office and hardly ever leaves it) has a lower priority among the experts (Requirement 19). This suggests that such deviations can either not be sufficiently causally attributed to stress or that they provide little profitable information. Moreover, the possibility of integrating data and results from other applications (e.g., pedometer) into the DSMS (Requirement 34) is granted lower priority. Without exception, all answers are located in the two categories "Should" and "Could," whereby the experts with very high expert status in terms of digital health services tend more toward "Could" compared to those with high expert status (75% versus 66%).

Table 4 contains all the requirements with consensus after round 2 as well as specifies the mean, mode, and interquartile ranges.

Table 4. Requirements with consensus in round 2

Requirement	Mean	Mode	IQR
Must:			
22	3.79	4	1
2	3.68	4	1
18	3.68	4	1
21	3.68	4	1
8	3.67	4	1
10	3.63	4	1
11	3.58	4	1
29	3.58	4	1
Should:			
20	2.79	3	0
Could:			
34	2.26	2	1
19	2.21	2	0

Must $\triangleq$ 4, Should $\triangleq$ 3, Could $\triangleq$ 2, Won't $\triangleq$ 1

4.3 Results of Round 3

In general, the third round showed only a few changes in the overall opinion and yielded two more requirements with consensus.

Requirements with the Prioritization "Must" (n = 2). The participating experts agree that in addition to providing psycho-educative and reflective exercises, those for building up anti-stress resources (Requirement 23) are also of utmost importance for improving the balance of stress periods and recreation (examples are resource analysis or time management). DSMS offering a high degree of mobility (Requirement 33) is also considered extremely important. Thus, they should be accessible on a smartphone or other devices that can be carried every day and used any time. Furthermore, a higher flexibility can be achieved if the application is available offline as well.

Table 5 presents all the requirements with consensus after round 3 and specifies the mean, mode, and interquartile ranges.

Table 5. Requirements with consensus in round 3

Requirement	Mean	Mode	IQR
Must:			
23	3.71	4	1
33	3.53	4	0

Must ≙ 4, Should ≙ 3, Could ≙ 2,
Won't ≙ 1

5 Discussion

After the three Delphi rounds, 28 of the 34 requirements reached the consensus threshold. Among them, not a single requirement was labeled with "Won't," so the requirements derived from the previous study can be all confirmed.

Figure 2 visualizes the development of the prioritization of the requirements over the three rounds. The inner circle refers to the first round, followed by the outward second, and finally the outermost third round. The requirement number is located in the middle of each circle.

Although the experts in the second round agree that DSMS should measure stress levels either way (see Fig. 2, Requirement 11/18: "Must"), there seems to be a strong disagreement on the suitable method of stress measurement. Requirements 15–17 present possible methods of stress measurement, with lower preference ("Could" prioritization) given to voice analyses, measurement of skin resistance, and muscular tension (Requirement 17). There is no consensus on the importance of diary and documentation functions (Requirement 15), which can be used in a broad sense to quantify stress levels. The answers range from "Must" to "Could" at this point. Moreover, the experts do not reach consensus on the continuous measurement of pulse, heart rate variability, and respiratory rate (Requirement 16). However, looking at the development of the prioritization over the three rounds, one sees an increasing focus on the categories of "Must" and "Should." In general, the results suggest that the measurement of pulse, heart rate variability, and respiratory rate is the most relevant method of stress measurement; however, the significance is not sufficient due to the prevailing disagreement. This can be attributed to the fact that stress is abstract compared to other diseases, thus rendering its measurement difficult. This uncertainty is also reflected in the market, as a lot of DSMS have not yet integrated stress measurement or only a rudimentary one, if any.

With respect to the interaction between the user and the system, it is noteworthy that although the experts agree in the second round that the reminder functions on goals, exercises, or other interactions are considered essential (Requirement 2), there is no consensus on the importance of feedback in acute stress situations (Requirement 14). Thus, it can be concluded that organizational reminders are really desired, but the importance of those in health-related content is unclear. There are hardly any recommendations on this concern in the literature either. Because all the check marks for Requirement 14 are located in the categories "Must" and "Should" in the last round, we can suppose that feedback functions are generally considered useful in acute stress situations. Some

Requirements with the prioritization **Must**				
transparency regarding data usage	strong personal and everyday relevance	goals	profound data concept	simple usability, fun to use
short interaction times	everyday suitability	available data	scientifically based interventions	identifying stressors
stress-measuring functionality	psychological self-education	self-reflection	reminders	measurement of stress level
anonymous, aggregated data transmission	cause and effect relationships	high mobility	exercises to build up anti-stress resources	

Requirements with the prioritization **Should**			
high autonomy	high individualization	customization to the specific user situation	adaption of stress monitoring over time

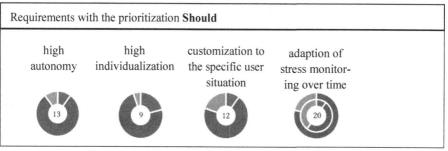

Fig. 2. Results

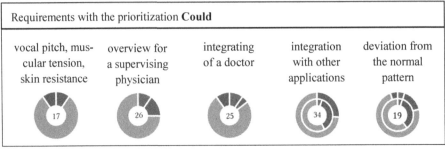

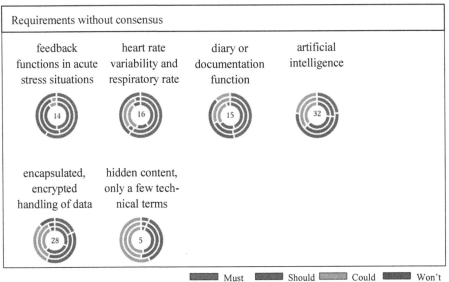

Fig. 2. (*continued*)

experts state that it is better not to present any feedback directly in the stress situation itself but with a slight delay. This minimizes the risk of aggravating the stress level due to the given notification, whereas the user can more easily reflect on the stress-inducing situation afterward.

Furthermore, there is no agreement on how important it is to use only hidden content in a playful way and with few technical terms. On the one hand, healthy people without cognitive impairments comprise the DSMS target group, and a facilitation of interventions is usually not necessary. Thus, Requirement 5 can be a low priority. Conversely, users of DSMS often have heavy workloads and little free time, which necessitates a presentation of easily understandable content, as per Requirement 5. On an average, it is prioritized by the experts with the value of 2.5.

By already agreeing in the first round on the "Should" prioritization for Requirements 9 and 12, the experts highlight that an individual tailoring of the DSMS to the user and his environment is desirable. In order to implement it, the use of artificial intelligence (Requirement 32) would basically be conceivable. However, this aspect does not reach any consensus. The mixed responses can be attributed to the fact that artificial intelligence is a promising but new technology which is not yet mature for a wide range of applications. Expert 10 comments regarding the Requirement 32:

> *"Should, not must. It's very complicated with AI and it requires extremely much data to be correct."*

Further annotations from the experts suggest that working with artificial intelligence has great potential and is promising for the future. Expert 13 states:

> *"There is no doubt that AI is the future."*

In sum, the results of the Delphi study reveal that strong motivational elements (Requirement 1, 2, 4, 8) and the conditions of usage (Requirement 3, 6, 7) are crucial to successful DSMS. This gives priority to the user first and emphasizes that DSMS are being developed for healthy people, who possibly do not feel such symptoms as compared to those who are already suffering from a condition like burnout. Therefore, great attention should be paid to motivational aspects so that preventive programs, such as DSMS, are used permanently.

In addition, the three types of DSMS exercises (Requirements 21–23) are also validated and given high priority. This aligns with the previous study, in which all the interviewed participants (health insurance companies, care providers, users, and the private sector) recommended their availability. These are also strongly addressed and examined in the literature [10, 11, 20]. Furthermore, the high prioritization of goalsetting (Requirement 1, "Must" prioritization in the first round) is consistent with findings from the literature [8, 35]. On the other hand, it is notable that everyday suitability (Requirement 7) and scientific evidence of offered interventions (Requirement 24) were already given extremely high importance in the first round, but these aspects are hardly considered in the literature. This underlines that some of the requirements identified in the preliminary study and prioritized in this study remain little known to date.

Some results of this study do not align with the literature. The experts consider the integration of other digital systems or external stakeholders, such as physicians, of little importance, although research has proven that guided interventions are more effective than unguided ones [10]. This can be attributed to a poor cost-benefit ratio of guidance or to the visionary focus of the experts on successful self-management and the well-empowered user.

In conclusion, a focus on the key features of DSMS, such as providing appropriate measurement methods and interventions to reduce excessive stress and its motivating presentation, is far more important than the integration of multiple additional functions.

6 Limitations and Future Work

There were several limitations to this study. There was a risk of ambiguity and conditional statements provided with the list of requirements. The experts may have interpreted the statements differently, and this could lead to a distortion in the results. In order to minimize this risk to the greatest extent possible, explanations of several of the requirements were also provided to the experts.

Although we executed a considerable search to identify experts, it is possible that some areas of expertise, geographic regions, and disciplines were not as well represented as others. For example, the experts only came from Europe and the United States, with a special focus on Germany. Thus, the findings may have limited the generalizability to other countries and regions, where the culture, handling of stress, or the work environment are very likely to be different. Another potential limitation of the study is that we only employed a panel of experts rather than the users themselves.

The knowledge presented by the experts in this study can be accessed by users who wish to test DSMS and directly report their findings and experience. Moreover, the additional involvement of employers as a further stakeholder group would be of interest, as they are closely related to the stress-causing source of burnout.

Furthermore, it will be beneficial to run comprehensive validations to evaluate the upcoming costs and the equipment required.

7 Conclusion

This article confirms and prioritizes the given list of requirements for DSMS. After the three rounds of this Delphi study, 82% of all the requirements had reached consensus. The experts agree that the offering of psycho-educative and reflective exercises as well as those to build up anti-stress resources must be given high priority.

In addition, DSMS should provide reminder functions, goal setting features, and stress measurement methods. A clear reference to everyday life and high suitability for everyday use as well as high mobility are also vital characteristics. Some of those less important ones are, in the experts' opinion, the involvement of medical professionals, the possibility to integrate other applications into the DSMS, and the use of some specific stress measurement methods (voice analyses, skin resistance, muscular tensions). Overall, the study demonstrates that there is strong agreement on the importance of individual functions and features for successful DSMS. The results support developers in profitably selecting and using functions and characteristics for better DSMS in order to counteract excessive stress. We believe that the improvement of DSMS is an effective way to reach more working individuals with psychological interventions in order to reduce stress and help strike a healthy balance. This could be important from both public health and societal perspectives.

References

1. Möltner, H., Leve, J., Esch, T.: Burnout-Prävention und mobile Achtsamkeit: Evaluation eines appbasierten Gesundheitstrainings bei Berufstätigen (Burnout Prevention and Mobile Mindfulness: Evaluation of an App-Based Health Training Program for Employees). Gesundheitswesen (Bundesverband der Ärzte des Öffentlichen Gesundheitsdienstes (Germany)) **80**(3), 295–300 (2018)
2. Kuster, A.T., Dalsbø, T.K., Luong Thanh, B.Y., Agarwal, A., Durand-Moreau, Q.V., Kirkehei, I.: Computer-based versus in-person interventions for preventing and reducing stress in workers. Cochrane Database Syst. Rev. **8**, CD011899 (2017)

3. Ly, K.H., Asplund, K., Andersson, G.: Stress management for middle managers via an acceptance and commitment-based smartphone application. A randomized controlled trial. Internet
   Interv. **1**(3), 95–101 (2014)
4. Jayewardene, W.P., Lohrmann, D.K., Erbe, R.G., Torabi, M.R.: Effects of preventive
   online mindfulness interventions on stress and mindfulness: A meta-analysis of randomized
   controlled trials. Prev. Med. Rep. **5**, 150–159 (2017)
5. Pisani, A.R., et al.: Human Subjects Protection and Technology in Prevention Science:
   Selected Opportunities and Challenges. Prev. Sci. Official J. Soc. Prev. Res. **17**(6), 765–778
   (2016)
6. Walter, U., Krugmann, C.S., Plaumann, M.: Burn-out wirksam prävenieren? Ein system-
   atischer Review zur Effektivität individuumbezogener und kombinierter Ansätze (Preventing burnout? A systematic review of effectiveness of individual and combined approaches).
   Bundesgesundheitsblatt, Gesundheitsforschung, Gesundheitsschutz **55**(2), 172–182 (2012)
7. Günthner, A., Batra, A.: Stressmanagement als Burn-out-Prophylaxe (Prevention of burnout
   by stress management). Bundesgesundheitsblatt, Gesundheitsforschung, Gesundheitsschutz
   55(2), 183–189 (2012)
8. Billings, D.W., Cook, R.F., Hendrickson, A., Dove, D.C.: A web-based approach to managing
   stress and mood disorders in the workforce. J. Occup. Environ. Med. **50**(8), 960–968 (2008)
9. Ebert, D.D., Lehr, D., Heber, E., Riper, H., Cuijpers, P., Berking, M.: Internet- and mobile-
   based stress management for employees with adherence-focused guidance: efficacy and
   mechanism of change. Scand. J. Work Environ. Health **42**(5), 382–394 (2016)
10. Heber, E., et al.: The benefit of web- and computer-based interventions for stress: a systematic
    review and meta-analysis. J. Med. Internet Res. **19**(2), e32 (2017)
11. Jonas, B., Leuschner, F., Tossmann, P.: Efficacy of an internet-based intervention for burnout:
    a randomized controlled trial in the German working population. Anxiety Stress Coping **30**(2),
    133–144 (2017)
12. Ahtinen, A., et al.: Mobile mental wellness training for stress management: feasibility and
    design implications based on a one-month field study. JMIR mHealth and uHealth **1**(2), e11
    (2013)
13. Pospos, S., et al.: Web-based tools and mobile applications to mitigate burnout, depression,
    and suicidality among healthcare students and professionals: a systematic review. Acad. Psy-
    chiatry **42**(1), 109–120 (2018). The Journal of the American Association of Directors of
    Psychiatric Residency Training and the Association for Academic Psychiatry
14. Amutio, A., Martínez-Taboada, C., Delgado, L.C., Hermosilla, D., Mozaz, M.J.: Acceptability
    and effectiveness of a long-term educational intervention to reduce physicians' stress-related
    conditions. J. Continuing Educ. Health Prof. **35**(4), 255–260 (2015)
15. Allexandre, D., Bernstein, A.M., Walker, E., Hunter, J., Roizen, M.F., Morledge, T.J.: A
    web-based mindfulness stress management program in a corporate call center: a randomized
    clinical trial to evaluate the added benefit of onsite group support. J. Occup. Environ. Med.
    58(3), 254–264 (2016)
16. Lange, A., van de Ven, J.-P., Schrieken, B., Smit, M.: 'Interapy' Burn-out. Prävention und
    Behandlung von Burn-out über das Internet. Verhaltenstherapie **14**(3), 190–199 (2004)
17. Morledge, T.J., et al.: Feasibility of an online mindfulness program for stress management
    – a randomized, controlled trial. Ann. Behav. Med. Publ. Soc. Behav. Med. **46**(2), 137–148
    (2013)
18. Heber, E., Lehr, D., Ebert, D.D., Berking, M., Riper, H.: Web-based and mobile stress man-
    agement intervention for employees: a randomized controlled trial. J. Med. Internet Res.
    18(1), e21 (2016)
19. Hintz, S., Frazier, P.A., Meredith, L.: Evaluating an online stress management intervention
    for college students. J. Couns. Psychol. **62**(2), 137–147 (2015)

20. Hasson, D., Anderberg, U.M., Theorell, T., Arnetz, B.B.: Psychophysiological effects of a web-based stress management system: a prospective, randomized controlled intervention study of IT and media workers ISRCTN54254861. BMC Public Health **5**, 78 (2005)

21. Blankenhagel, K.J., Theilig, M.-M., Koch, H., Witte, A.-K., Zarnekow, R.: Challenges for preventive digital stress management systems - identifying requirements by conducting qualitative interviews. In: Proceedings of the 52nd Hawaii International Conference on System Sciences 2019, pp. 3810–3819 (2019)

22. Flick, U.: Qualitative Sozialforschung. Eine Einführung. In: 8th edn. Rororo Rowohlts Enzyklopädie, vol. 55694. Rowohlts Enzyklopädie im Rowohlt Taschenbuch Verlag, Reinbek bei Hamburg (2017)

23. Döring, N., Bortz, J.: Forschungsmethoden und Evaluation in den Sozial- und Humanwissenschaften, 5th edn. Springer, Heidelberg (2016). https://doi.org/10.1007/978-3-642-41089-5

24. Mayring, P.: Qualitative Inhaltsanalyse. Grundlagen und Techniken. 12th edn. Beltz Pädagogik. Beltz, Weinheim (2015)

25. de Villiers, M.R., de Villiers, P.J.T., Kent, A.P.: The Delphi technique in health sciences education research. Med. Teach. **27**(7), 639–643 (2005)

26. Efstathiou, N., Ameen, J., Coll, A.-M.: A Delphi study to identify healthcare users' priorities for cancer care in Greece. Eur. J. Oncol. Nurs. Official J. Eur. Oncol. Nurs. Soc. **12**(4), 362–371 (2008)

27. Zelmer, J., van Hoof, K., Notarianni, M., van Mierlo, T., Schellenberg, M., Tannenbaum, C.: An assessment Framework for e-Mental health apps in canada: results of a modified Delphi process. JMIR mHealth uHealth **6**(7), e10016 (2018)

28. Keeney, S., Hasson, F., McKenna, H.P.: The Delphi Technique in Nursing and Health Research. Wiley-Blackwell, Chichester (2011)

29. Häder, M., Häder, S.: Die Delphi-Technik in den Sozialwissenschaften. VS Verlag für Sozialwissenschaften, Wiesbaden (2000)

30. Okoli, C., Pawlowski, S.D.: The Delphi method as a research tool. An example, design considerations and applications. Inf. Manag. **42**(1), 15–29 (2004)

31. Skinner, R., Nelson, R.R., Chin, W.W., Land, L.: The Delphi method research strategy in studies of information systems. CAIS **37**, 31–63 (2015)

32. Woudenberg, F.: An evaluation of Delphi. Technol. Forecast. Soc. Chang. **40**(2), 131–150 (1991)

33. Brooks, K.W.: Delphi technique. Expanding applications. North Central Assoc. Q. **53**(3), 377–385 (1979)

34. Duffield, C.: The Delphi technique A comparison of results obtained using two expert panels. Int. J. Nurs. Stud. **30**(3), 227–237 (1993)

35. Ebert, D.D., et al.: Efficacy and cost-effectiveness of minimal guided and unguided internet-based mobile supported stress-management in employees with occupational stress: a three-armed randomised controlled trial. BMC Public Health **14**, 807 (2014)

Preliminary Assessment of a Smart Mattress for Position and Breathing Sensing

Lucia Arcarisi[1], Carlotta Marinai[1], Massimo Teppati Losè[1], Marco Laurino[2], Nicola Carbonaro[1,3], and Alessandro Tognetti[1,3(✉)]

[1] Department of Information Engineering, University of Pisa, Pisa, Italy
alessandro.tognetti@unipi.it
[2] Institute of Clinical Physiology, National Research Council, Pisa, Italy
[3] Research Center "E. Piaggio", University of Pisa, Pisa, Italy

Abstract. Sleep is a one of the most important activity for maintaining the health and well-being of each subject. In order to monitor continuously the quality of sleep of the general population in non-invasively way, we developed an innovative sensorized "smart" mattress (SmartBed). SmartBed is equipped with sensors to detect environmental and subject-related information. In particular, SmartBed is equipped with accelerometers and a sensing textile matrix able to detect the distribution of pressures of a subject laying on the mattress. The purpose of this work is to demonstrate how the sensing textile matrix is not only able to detect how the subject is positioned on the mattress over time, but also it allows to detect other physiological parameters and in particular the subject's respiratory activity. In this work, we show that: (i) the sensing textile matrix allows a precise position detection; (ii) it is possible to extract accurately the respiratory frequency from the sensing textile matrix by using a specifically tailored algorithm. In conclusion, the sensors integrated in SmartBed make possible to detect important information (position and respiratory activity) to determine the quality of a subject's sleep in a robust, accurate and non-invasive way.

Keywords: Sleep analysis · Sensing mattress · Smart textile · Breathing monitoring

1 Introduction

Individual experience of insufficient or inadequate sleep is one of the most common health problems. About 65% of the Italian population report generic disorders during the night, while 10% suffers from pathological disorders related to poor sleep [1]. These subjects often report drowsiness during the day, absenteeism at work and reductions in performance. Inadequate sleep may become the cause of accidents even on the road. Furthermore, insomnia can lead to more complex pathologies [2] not only of a metabolic nature (such as diabetes or dyslipidemia) and cardiovascular diseases (such as myocardial infarction or hypertension), but also cognitive and psychopathological (such as depression and anxiety disorders). Currently, through polysomnography it is possible to

© ICST Institute for Computer Sciences, Social Informatics and Telecommunications Engineering 2020
Published by Springer Nature Switzerland AG 2020. All Rights Reserved
G. M. P. O'Hare et al. (Eds.): MobiHealth 2019, LNICST 320, pp. 249–255, 2020.
https://doi.org/10.1007/978-3-030-49289-2_19

evaluate the quality of sleep of patients [3]. Unfortunately, polysomnography is highly invasive, and the lack of comfort prevents the subject from sleeping in a natural situation and does not allow a measurement that reflects reality. For all these reasons the development of a systematic, preventive, personalized and non-invasive method for the analysis of sleep is particularly important.

To overcome these limits, we aim at developing a smart-bed [4]: a sensing and intelligent mattress that can collect and process physiological data (heart rate, breathing rate), environmental parameters, movements and positions of the patient.

As a relevant subsystem of the smart bed we have designed a sensing textile, integrated in the mattress, able to detect the distribution of pressures when a subject is laying on the bed. The pressure signals obtained can be used to detect the subject position and movements and extract the subject breathing rate. This work is focused on a preliminary assessment of the pressure sensing matrix in the detection of subject position and respiratory frequency. We discuss the sensor structure, the signal acquisition methodology, the recognition of subject position and the possible solutions to determine the patient's respiratory activity.

2   Materials and Methods

2.1   Pressure Sensing Matrix

We have developed the pressure sensing matrix, designed to map the pressures exerted by a person's body in terms of position coordinates and intensity, by employing an array of piezoresistive sensors, inspired by [5]. Each individual transducer consists of a piezoresistive textile capable of modifying the electrical properties when a deformation is applied. The material is composed of a single solution from colloidal particles of conductive (for example carbon black) dispersed in a matrix polymer.

For the realization of the sensor related to a single mattress (190×90 cm), a surface of about 125×75 cm was built based on a matrix of 15×13 sensing areas, where 15 are

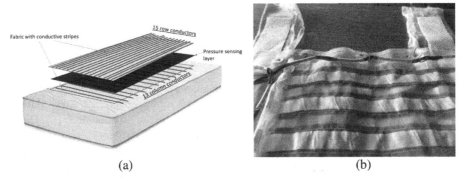

(a)   (b)

Fig. 1. a) Inner layer of CARBOTEX 03-82 (black layer, currently crawled in the direction of the lines); external PET layers with conductive stripes of row (15) and column (13) arranged orthogonally between them. **b)** Internal layer of CARBOTEX 03-82 cut into strips (black part); horizontal row and vertical column conductive tracks (silver parts) sewn onto the PET layer.

horizontal rows and 13 vertical columns, with equally spaced detection areas. With this design, positions of the head and feet are not considered. The pressure-sensitive layer is a conductive fabric (CARBOTEX 03-82 of SEFAR AG), while for the upper and lower layers a PET fabric was used, again from SEFAR AG and designed following our specifications, in which equidistant metallic strips are integrated (see Fig. 1 and Fig. 1b). The described detection architecture introduces parasitic resistances in directions transversal to the conductive strips, which create relevant cross-talk in the measurement. For this reason, we decided to cut the pressure-sensitive layer also into strips, in the direction identified by the lines (see Fig. 1b).

2.2 Data Acquisition

As indicated above, the crossing of a line (with index i) and a column (with index j) forms the sensitive element of the structure: the sensing area (taxel). By feeding the specific i-th row with a voltage and reading the voltage value on the j-th column, it is possible to measure the resistance of the identified element (i, j). Repeating the operation for all the combinations of row and column, the data of all the sensitive surface are obtained. This was achieved thanks to an Arduino Mega 2560 board and a protoboard that implements a voltage divider for reading. The board has 16 analog inputs and 54 digital inputs; then, to set the connection, the 15 lines have been connected to the digital inputs (imposing 3 V) and the 13 columns to the analog inputs. Through the Arduino IDE development environment, it was possible to program the card and perform the reading; the latter, for the elimination of any noise, is followed by a simple arithmetic average, every 10 acquisitions.

2.3 Subject Position

We have developed a Matlab Grafical User Interface that display the acquired resistance value as a false color image. Processing was performed using the MATLAB environment. Using a Master-Slave approach, the Matlab application was used as master, while the Arduino board worked as slave: the Matlab environment ask the data by writing a predefined code on the serial port and, in response, the Arduino board sends a complete reading on the same serial (the resistance value of the 195 sensing areas). Data are then saved to be processed off-line. This type of communication allows to manage the sending and receiving of data and therefore to control the sampling frequency (fc = 4 Hz). Once the vector has been received, the distribution of the pressures for each sensing area is displayed. A linear interpolation was used to improve the overall quality of the image.

2.4 Breathing Detection

The main objective is to detect the respiratory act and the frequency associated with it. These, in fact, are parameters of fundamental importance within the sleep analysis, not only to hypothesize the phase but also to identify possible sleep apnea. Finally, the last purpose was to understand how the subject position influences the accuracy of breathing detection.

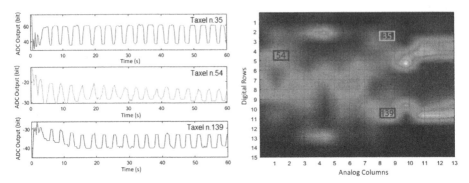

Fig. 2. Periodic trend of the three sensing areas found by visual inspection, test in deep breathing; (Right) Image of the subject in supine position and identification of significant sensing area

By acquiring the signal and performing a visual analysis we observed that certain sensing areas show a periodic trend coherent with breathing activity (see Fig. 2).

For the determination of the respiratory frequency we developed a Fourier transform based procedure (FFT algorithm in Matlab).

3   Results

3.1   Position

Different subjects lay down on the mattress and assumed different typical sleeping positions, in the following pictures we report the reconstructed interpolated. It is possible to notice how some specific areas of the subject can be easily recognized (Fig. 3).

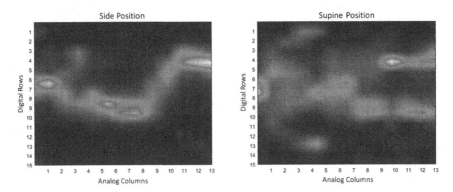

Fig. 3. Image of subject lying in different positions

3.2   Respiration

We acquired data from subjects lying on the mattress versus a ground truth (breathing cannula with a NTC-3950 termistor).

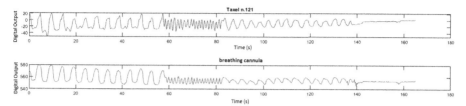

Fig. 4. Trend over time of a significant sensing area and of the cannula; demonstration of the significance of the smart-bed signal.

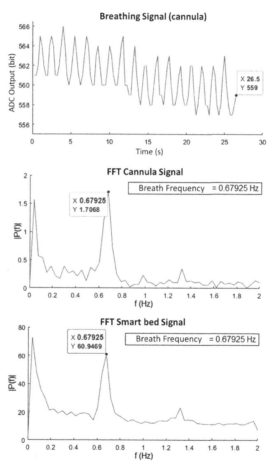

Fig. 5. Rapid breathing pattern in supine position; FFT from the cannula signal and from the sensing mattress, as can be verified the peak values of the first harmonics coincide; in the box the value of the respiratory frequency extracted from the algorithm.

In a first experiment (see the comparison of Fig. 4), the tests were conducted according to the following pattern: deep breathing for 60 s, fast for 30 s, normal for 60 s and finally apnea for 15–30 s; in the supine and prone positions.

By using the FFT based algorithm, we made a first attempt was to demonstrate that the sensing mattress had the ability to identify the patient's respiratory rate (always comparing it to the ground-truth) in time slots in which breathing variable. Subsequently, we investigated the performance in the four possible lying positions (supine, prone and from the side). To prove that the mattress could determine the respiratory rate, the subjects were asked to breathe with a constant frequency, in the range of 60 s for deep and normal breathing, 30 s for the fast and about 15 s for the 'apnea; in all positions. As regards the Fourier analysis, performed on the sensing area, very promising results have been obtained by performing the sum of the modules of the Fourier transforms of each sensing areas in the considered time period. All the respiratory modalities have been correctly recognized (i.e. the peaks of the first harmonic coincide for ground truth and mattress). Considering the different lying positions, the least reliable results are those in which the subject is lying on his side. An explanatory image is shown in Fig. 5.

Following these investigations, other tests were conducted with a total duration of about 165 s, in which the patients' respiratory rate was variable; therefore the subjects were asked to breathe in the following way: deeply for 60 s, quickly for 30 s, normally for 60 s and in apnea for the remaining time. The calculation of the FFT, in this case, was determined with a more complex algorithm in which it is calculated on mobile time windows of 30 s, within the entire test period (always 165 s). The choice of the width of the floating window must be adapted to the total duration of the experiment. In our case, we choose a 30 s time window. From the results obtained it can be seen that the

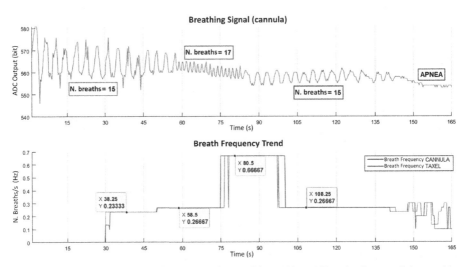

Fig. 6. Analysis related to a subject in a supine position; (Above) Respiration trend detected by the thermistor and n. breaths corresponding to each mode; (Bottom) Trend of respiratory rate over time with values highlighted for each phase; as you can see the values of the respiratory frequencies coincide between the smart-bed and the cannula, reflecting reality.

smart-bed, using the algorithm developed, appropriately recognizes the respiratory rate in almost all positions (on the side there is the greatest probability of error), while, as regards respiratory modalities, apnea (for the choice of the 30 s window) and occasionally normal breathing are more difficult to identify. Fig. 6 shows an explanatory image of the analysis.

4   Conclusions

In this work, we investigated the capability of detecting the position and breath of subject on a sensing mattress to perform a non-invasive sleep analysis.

Future developments include the improvement of algorithms, in part already implemented, for the best apnea capture and for solving problems related to the side position. For the purposes of greater accuracy in the results, it could be advantageous: to use thresholds on the peaks relating to the FFT signals to eliminate spurious identifications of the respiratory frequencies, perform a moving average with an adaptive window (at present only one version is available with a constant window) on the data deriving from the sensorized mattress that would reduce the noise in apnea acquisitions.

Acknowledgements. LAID project is co-funded by Tuscany POR FESR 2014-2020 (DD 3389/2014 call 1). We would to thank all our industrial partners: Materassificio Montalese S.P.A, EB Neuro S.P.A and BP Engineering S.P.A.

References

1. Terzano, M.G., et al.: Studio Morfeo: insomnia in primary care, a survey conducted on the Italian population. Sleep Med. **5**(1), 67–75 (2004)
2. Leger, D., Guilleminault, C., Bader, G., Levy, E., Paillard, M.: Medical and socio-professional impact of insomnia. Sleep **25**(6), 625–629 (2002)
3. Douglas, N.J., Thomas, S., Jan, M.A.: Clinical-value of polysomnography. Lancet **339**(8789), 347–350 (1992)
4. Laurino, N.C.M., Menicucci, D., Alfi, G., Gemignani, A., Tognetti, A.: A smartbed for non-obtrusive physiological monitoring during sleep: the LAID project. In: Mobihealth 2019 (2019, in press)
5. Zhou, B., Lukowicz, P.: Textile pressure force mapping. In: Schneegass, S., Amft, O. (eds.) Smart Textiles. Human–Computer Interaction Series, pp. 31–47. Springer, Cham (2017). https://doi.org/10.1007/978-3-319-50124-6_3

Preliminary Investigation on Band Tightness Estimation of Wrist-Worn Devices Using Inertial Sensors

Masayuki Hayashi$^{(\boxtimes)}$, Hiroki Yoshikawa, Akira Uchiyama, and Teruo Higashino

Osaka University, Osaka, Japan
{m-hayashi,h-yoshikawa,uchiyama,higashino}@ist.osaka-u.ac.jp

Abstract. Nowadays, wearable devices enable us to collect biological data from a massive number of people. However, the reliability of the collected data varies due to various factors such as band tightness and incorrect attachment. In this paper, we investigate the band tightness estimation by using an inertial sensor of a wrist-worn device. First, we analyze the relationship between the band tightness and the data reliability through a preliminary experiment. Then, we design the band tightness estimation as a classification problem based on frequency domain features. The evaluation results show the effectiveness of the frequency domain features, achieving the accuracy of 81.7% for the 3-class band tightness classification.

Keywords: Wrist-worn device · Inertial sensor · Machine learning · Tightness estimation

1 Introduction

With the recent rapid spread of wearable sensors, it has become possible to easily collect various biological data. For example, a wrist-worn device called empatica E4[1] enables us to obtain heart rate, sweating level (Electrodermal Activity), and skin temperature. Also, by using an earphone sensor called cosinuss° One[2], heart rate and tympanic temperature (core temperature) can be recorded on a smartphone. Such biological data is expected to be used in various situations such as healthcare and sports [1].

In our research group, we have been developing a framework to construct big biological data using wearable devices from a massive number of participants. We assume they use various wearable sensors such as wrist-worn devices, chest heart rate devices, and ear-worn devices depending on their preference to collect their biological data in various environments such as gyms, parks, etc. as shown in

---

[1] https://www.empatica.com/en-int/research/e4/.

[2] https://www.cosinuss.com.

G. M. P. O'Hare et al. (Eds.): MobiHealth 2019, LNICST 320, pp. 256–266, 2020.
https://doi.org/10.1007/978-3-030-49289-2_20

Fig. 1. In such scenarios, we seldom assume that the participants wear the devices correctly because they wear the devices by themselves without enough knowledge. Even participants with the knowledge about the correct use of the devices may wrongly wear them by accident. Moreover, a wrist-worn device may slightly move on the wrist due to exercise, which results in the looseness. Obviously, the diversity of the appropriateness of the device attachment leads to the different reliability of the measured data. Therefore, the reliability of the collected biological data is non-uniform, which becomes a serious problem when we analyze the big data. In fact, many researchers and analysts have to start with data cleansing [2] since this problem is actually very common in big data analysis.

However, if we are able to know the reliability of the collected data at the time of data collection, it can be widely used for various purposes. For example, we may simply filter the data with low reliability before analysis. Furthermore, if we can detect the low reliability in real-time, we may send notifications to the subjects to check the device attachment. Based on the above idea, in this paper, we investigate band tightness estimation using inertial sensors by focusing on wrist-worn devices. To mitigate the effect of noise, many researchers have worked on noise filtering in the wearable sensing. For example, Refs. [4,5] propose methods to remove outliers of inter-beat (RR) interval (RRI). Also, Ref. [6] leverages the ECG (Electrocardiogram) patterns to calculate RRI. Ref. [3] filters the effect of body movement by focusing on the characteristic of Photoplethysmography (PPG) sensors. However, in spite of the continuous effort by many researchers and developers, commercial off-the-shelf (COTS) wrist-worn devices cannot detect the slight difference of the band tightness without special sensors such as strain gauges.

Therefore, our goal is to estimate the band tightness for COTS wrist-worn devices. We firstly investigate the relationship between the band tightness and the reliability of the measured heart rate through preliminary experiment. Then, we design a method to estimate band tightness based on machine learning by using the inertial sensor of the wrist-worn device. Our key idea is that different band tightness causes differences in vibration of the wrist-worn devices along with the arm movement. To capture the vibration difference, we employ frequency domain features extracted by FFT (Fast Fourier Transform).

To investigate the performance of our band tightness estimation, we collected data from two subjects with different band tightness in jogging. The result indicates that the frequency domain features are more effective than the others, supporting the appropriateness of our key idea. Overall, we have confirmed that our method can estimate the band tightness (i.e. *Loose*, *Medium*, and *Tight*) with accuracy of 81.7%, highlighting the usefulness of the inertial sensor for the band tightness estimation.

2   Preliminary Experiment on Band Tightness

2.1   Experiment Settings

To investigate the relationship between the band tightness and the quality of the heart rate measurement, we collected real data from one subject with five

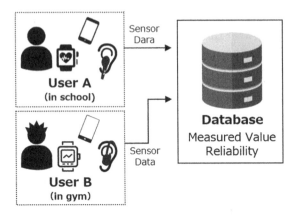

Fig. 1. Overview of Biological data collection platform

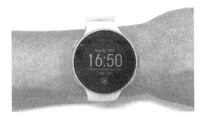

Fig. 2. Wrist-worn device: Polar Vantage V

levels of tightness. We used Polar Vantage V shown in Fig. 2 as a wrist-worn device. We note that Polar Vantage V is more tolerant to noise due to wrist movement since it employs a sophisticated sensor fusion technique by using a touch sensor, a 3-axis accelerometer, and multiple PPG sensors [7]. The subject jogged for two minutes for each tightness level. In total, we collected 10-min data with five tightness levels. We define the tightness level as shown in Table 1 according to the wrist size of the protruding bump of the wrist bone. We note that we attached an inertial sensor TSND151 to Vantage V as shown in Fig. 3 because it does not provide APIs to access to the raw inertial measurements. We set the sampling rate of TSND151 to 1,000 Hz for both of the 3-axis acceleration and the 3-axis angular velocity. For the ground-truth, we used a Holter monitor FM160 manufactured by Fukuda Denshi.

2.2   Result

Band Tightness and Heart Rate. Figure 4 shows the heart rates measured by the wrist-worn device and the Holter monitor. We see that the heart rate measured by the wrist-worn device is close to the Holter monitor in *Very Tight* and *Tight*. The peak and the trend are still similar in *Medium* tightness although we also see the difference slightly larger than *Very Tight* and *Tight*. However,

Table 1. Definition of band tightness

Tightness	Band length (0 cm = wrist size)
Very Tight	+1.0 cm
Tight	+1.5 cm
Medium	+2.0 cm
Loose	+2.5 cm
Very Loose	+3.0 cm

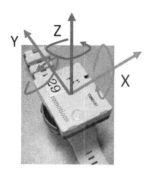

Fig. 3. Inertial sensor attached onto Vantage V

the difference between the wrist-worn device and the Holter monitor is clearer in *Loose* and *Very Loose*.

The result indicates that the band tightness is closely related with the reliability of the heart rate measurement. Especially, the measurement reliability is obviously low when the band is loose. Therefore, we conclude that the band tightness is one of the key indices to know the data reliability.

Band Tightness and Wristband Vibration. To investigate the cause of the low reliability when the band is loose, we analyze the relationship between the band tightness and the measurement of the wristband inertial sensor (i.e. 3-axis acceleration and 3-axis angular velocity). Specifically, we first analyze the variances of the inertial measurement because different band tightness may lead to different vibration of the wrist-worn device. Figure 5 shows the variances of the acceleration and the angular velocity in *Tight*, *Medium*, and *Loose*. The variances are calculated for a sliding window with a 10-s width and one-second slide step. We see some difference between different band tightness. The angular velocity of y-axis shows relatively clear difference between *Tight* and *Loose*. However, the variances cannot completely capture the differences between different tightness.

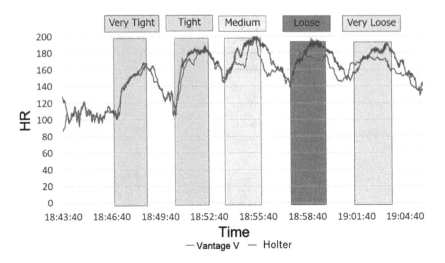

Fig. 4. Band tightness and heart rate

The vibration of the wrist-worn device is quite small compared to the arm motion during exercise. To separate the vibration due to the arm motion and the other factors, we apply Fast Fourier Transform (FFT) to the acceleration and the angular velocity. Figure 6 shows a frequency spectrum of the y-axis angular velocity in *Tight*. The clear peak around 1.5 Hz is close to the frequency of the arm motion. Actually, the vibration due to the other factors appears in the higher frequency. Figure 7 shows the scaled frequency spectrum for each band tightness. We see that the spectrum of *Loose* contains more high frequency components than *Tight*. Also, the peaks of the higher frequency appear around the frequencies of the integral multiple of 1.5 Hz (i.e. the arm motion frequency). This is because the arm motion causes the small vibration.

From the above observation, we have confirmed that the acceleration and the angular velocity of the wrist-worn device are useful for the band tightness estimation. In the following Sect. 3, we design the band tightness estimation method by using machine learning.

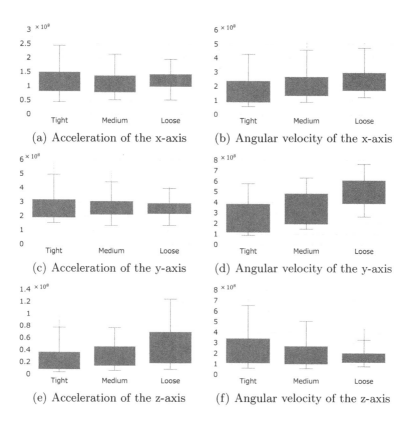

Fig. 5. Variances of acceleration and angular velocity

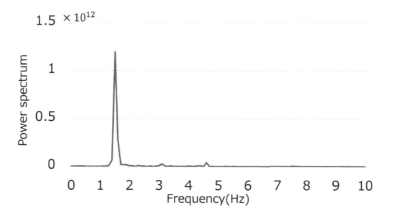

Fig. 6. Frequency spectrum of Y-axis angular velocity (*Tight*)

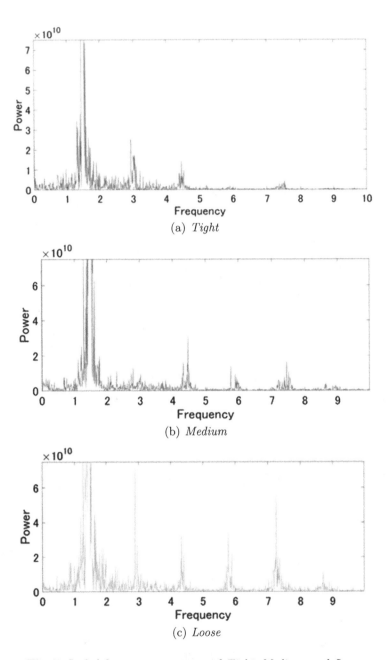

(a) *Tight*

(b) *Medium*

(c) *Loose*

Fig. 7. Scaled frequency spectrum of *Tight*, *Medium*, and *Loose*

3 Band Tightness Estimation

In our preliminary experiment, *Very Tight* and *Very Loose* are extreme conditions which seldom occur in the real environment. Therefore, in this paper, we focus on the other tightness categories: *Tight*, *Medium*, and *Loose*. Then, we design the band tightness estimation as classification based on machine learning using the acceleration and the angular velocity of the wrist-worn device.

Table 2. Feature candidates

Component (3-axes)	Feature
Acceleration	Mean, Median, Max, Variance
Angular velocity	Mean, Median, Max,Variance
Frequency component of acceleration	Mean, Median, Max, Variance
Frequency component of angular velocity	Mean, Median, Max, Variance

Table 2 lists the features used in the classification. We set a sliding window with the width of W and the slide step of one second for feature extraction. According to the result of the preliminary experiment, we also use the frequency domain features. First, we define the frequency f_1 due to the arm motion as the highest peak between 0 and 2.0 Hz. Then, we define the i-th frequency component f_i as $i f_1$ ($i = 2 \ldots 10$). Finally, we extract features of f_i from the frequency spectrum between $[f_i - 0.5, f_i + 0.5]$ Hz. In total, we extract 264 features as candidates. We further apply feature selection based on the feature importance determined by Decision Tree algorithm.

4 Evaluation

4.1 Settings

We collected the jogging data from two males aged 20's. For each session of data collection, each subject configured the tightness to *Loose*, *Medium*, and *Tight* and jogged two minutes for each tightness. We collected four sessions from one of the subjects and two sessions from the other subject on different days and/or times. We note that we did not control any motions such as arm swing styles.

We conduct one-session-out cross-validation for evaluation. For the parameter settings, we use the window width $W = 10$ s unless otherwise stated. We compared SVM (Support Vector Machine), KNN (K-Nearest Neighbors), LR (Logistic Regression), and RF (Random Forest) for machine learning algorithms. In the following evaluation, we have used the best feature set for each algorithm.

4.2   Result

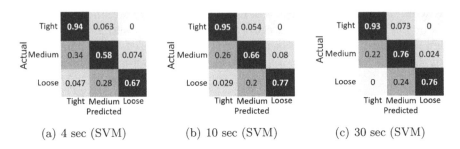

(a) 4 sec (SVM)   (b) 10 sec (SVM)   (c) 30 sec (SVM)

Fig. 8. Effect of window size W

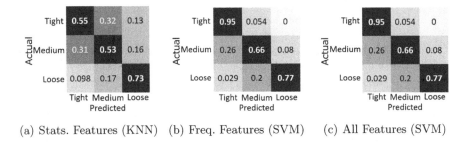

(a) Stats. Features (KNN)   (b) Freq. Features (SVM)   (c) All Features (SVM)

Fig. 9. Confusion matrices of different feature sets

Effect of Window Size. The window size W is closely related with the real-timeness of the band tightness estimation. To see the effect of W, Fig. 8 shows the confusion matrices of different window size W. In all the cases, SVM performed the best for the machine learning algorithm.

We see that the accuracy increases with the increase of the window size. From the result, we have confirmed a larger window size is effective for the classification. However, we need to consider the trade-off between realtimeness and the classification accuracy.

Feature Comparison. Figure 9 shows the confusion matrices of different feature sets. To see the effect of frequency features, we have compared the classification performance of statistical features, frequency features, and all features. We define the statistical features as those except frequency features.

We note that the best machine learning algorithms are different for the different feature sets. KNN is the best for the statistical feature set while SVM is the best for the other feature sets. The classification by the statistical feature

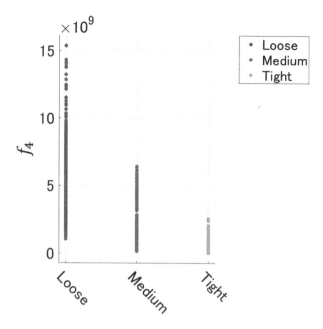

Fig. 10. Overlap of feature value

set achieves the accuracy of 60.3% while the classification by the frequency feature set shows the accuracy of 79.3%. Also, the result using all the features is equivalent to that based on the frequency feature set. This result indicates the effectiveness of the frequency features for the band tightness estimation. However, the accuracy of *Medium* is relatively low due to the confusion between the neighboring classes. To further investigate the cause of the low accuracy, Fig. 10 shows the distributions of the frequency feature f_4. The distributions of *Medium* and the other classes overlap to some extent, which is the main reason of the low accuracy. To improve the performance, we may further analyze the tiny movement of the wrist-worn device precisely.

5   Conclusion

In this paper, we investigate the design of the band tightness estimation using an inertial sensor of a wrist-worn device. Our key design is the frequency domain features based on the key observation that different band tightness causes difference in vibration of the wrist-worn devices. The evaluation results show the effectiveness of our design, achieving the accuracy of 81.7% for 3-class tightness classification.

Our future work includes further evaluation by collecting more data samples. We are also planning to investigate other factors related with the reliability of the biological data.

Acknowledgment. This paper is partially supported by Innovation Platform for Society 5.0 from Japan Ministry of Education, Culture, Sports, Science and Technology.

References

1. Pantelopoulos, A., Bourbakis, N.G.: A survey on wearable sensor-based systems for health monitoring and prognosis. IEEE Trans. Syst. Man Cybern. Part C (Appl. Rev.) **40**(1), 1–12 (2010)
2. Saha, B., Srivastava D.: Data quality: the other face of big data. In: Proceedings of 2014 IEEE 30th International Conference on Data Engineering, pp. 1294–1297 (2014)
3. Fukushima, H., Kawanaka, H., Shoaib, Md.B., Oguri, K.: Estimating heart rate using wrist-type photoplethysmography and acceleration sensor while running. In: Proceedings of 2012 Annual International Conference of the IEEE Engineering in Medicine and Biology Society, pp. 2901–2904 (2012)
4. Eguchi, K., Aoki, R., Shimauchi, S., Yoshida, K., Yamada, T.: RR interval outlier proceeding for heart rate variability analysis using wearable ECG devices. Adv. Biomed. Eng. **7**, 28–38 (2018)
5. Salai, M., Vassányi, I., Kósa, I.: Stress detection using low cost heart rate sensors. J. Healthcare Eng. **2016** (2016)
6. Nakano, M., Konishi, T., Izumi, S., Kawaguchi, H., Yoshimoto, M.: Instantaneous heart rate detection using short-time autocorrelation for wearable healthcare systems. In: Proceedings of 2012 Annual International Conference of the IEEE Engineering in Medicine and Biology Society, pp. 6703–6706 (2012)
7. POLAR: How optical heart rate monitoring works with polar precision prime[TM] — polar blog.https://www.polar.com/blog/optical-heart-rate-monitoring-polar-precision-prime/. Accessed 14 Jul 2019

Artificial Intelligence at the Edge in the Blockchain of Things

Tuan Nguyen Gia[1], Anum Nawaz[1,2], Jorge Peña Querata[1(✉)],
Hannu Tenhunen[1], and Tomi Westerlund[1]

[1] Turku Intelligent Embedded and Robotic Systems (TIERS) Group,
Department of Future Technologies, University of Turku, Turku, Finland
{tunggi,jopequ,hatenhu,tovewe}@utu.fi
[2] Shanghai Key Laboratory of Intelligent Information Processing,
School of Computer Science, Fudan University, Shanghai, China
nanum18@fudan.edu.cn
https://tiers.fi

Abstract. Traditional cloud-centric architectures for Internet-of-Things applications are being replaced by distributed approaches. The Edge and Fog computing paradigms crystallize the concept of moving computation towards the edge of the network, closer to where the data originates. This has important benefits in terms of energy efficiency, network load optimization and latency control. The combination of these paradigms with embedded artificial intelligence in edge devices, or Edge AI, enables further improvements. In turn, the development of blockchain technology and distributed architectures for peer-to-peer communication and trade allows for higher levels of security. This can have a significant impact on data-sensitive and mission-critical applications in the IoT. In this paper, we discuss the potential of an Edge AI capable system architecture for the Blockchain of Things. We show how this architecture can be utilized in health monitoring applications. Furthermore, by analyzing raw data directly at the edge layer, we inherently avoid the possibility of breaches of sensitive information, as raw data is never stored nor transferred outside of the local network.

Keywords: Blockchain · Edge computing · AI · Edge AI · E-health · U-health · IoT · Internet of Things · ECG monitoring · ECG feature extraction · Ubiquitous health · Ethereum

1 Introduction

With an increasing ubiquity of connected devices penetrating smart homes, smart cities, smart factories or smart farms, the Internet of Things (IoT) is generating vast amounts of data [1,2]. However, many challenges related to IoT data ownership, security, privacy, and information sharing still remain [3–6]. The increasing integration of third-party services into IoT applications further

G. M. P. O'Hare et al. (Eds.): MobiHealth 2019, LNICST 320, pp. 267–280, 2020.
https://doi.org/10.1007/978-3-030-49289-2_21

increases the risk of security vulnerabilities and cyber attacks [7]. Even with the-state-of-the-art encryption methods, the IoT presents a non-negligible threat to users' privacy and personal data security [8]. While the IoT was born with the boom in cloud computing, in recent years distributed computing approaches are extending its potential [9–16]. The edge and fog computing paradigms aim at migrating computational load towards the edge of the network. Data is processed at the local network level or radio access point station and only important information is transmitted over the network. For example, raw ECG data can be processed at a smart gateway for extracting important ECG features such as heart rate, P and T waves. Depending on the applications, raw data or processed data is stored at distributed edge storage. Edge approaches allow for reduced latency and more efficient use of both network and computational resources, but they also raise additional security considerations and requirements [17].

Blockchain technology has seen increasing penetration in multiple technological areas in the last decade [18], since its first introduction as part of the Bitcoin stack [19]. A blockchain platform can be seen a public and distributed digital data ledger that allows nodes to record proof of integrity and is unalterable a posteriori. Blockchain enables a decentralized manner of sharing data, and an immutable record of transactions, among other benefits. Compared to a centralized infrastructure, such as most cloud-based IoT Systems, blockchain technology has the advantage of allowing end-users or devices to exchange information, data and their assets directly without any intermediate third parties involved in the process while securing data integrity [20]. With these advantages, blockchain can be a suitable candidate to deal with some existing security challenges in many applications [21]. For instance, blockchain can be leveraged as a trading platform between data producers (i.e., the end-devices in an IoT system or the edge gateway where sensor node data is being analyzed and processed), and data consumers or (i.e., third-party applications or end-user applications) [22].

The integration of blockchain technology into the IoT has drawn growing attention of the research community in recent years. Significant efforts have been devoted to propose secured approaches which utilize blockchain technology to secure M2M transactions in the IoT [23]. An important part of the works to date is focused on either secure access policies, such as the direct connection between end-users and smart home appliances [24], or secure machine-to-machine communication [25]. Although these approaches can indeed provide high levels of security to IoT platforms [26], their integration within edge-assisted remote and real-time monitoring applications is not deeply investigated in those works.

In this paper, we present an architecture for the Blockchain of Things that integrates artificial intelligence at the edge (Edge AI) algorithms for efficient and secure information management and privacy protection in healthcare applications. The presented system architecture extends our previous work [27], and it is illustrated in Fig. 1. We also discuss further the potential of this application in various fields. The proposed architecture secures IoT data integrity with a distributed platform based on the Ethereum blockchain and utilizes Edge AI for computational offloading at the fog and edge layer. Integrating fog and

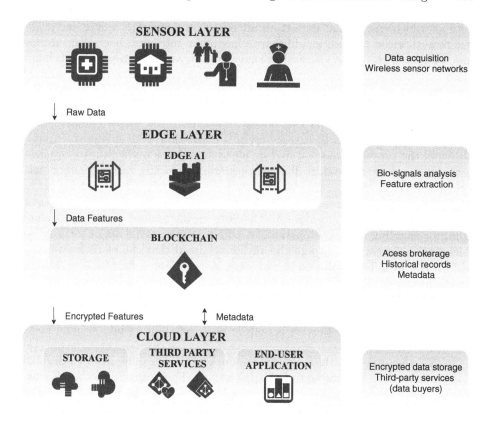

Fig. 1. Proposed system architecture

edge computing creates new opportunities for enhanced peer-to-peer security and authorized access [28, 29].

The rest of this paper is organized as follows. Section 2 overviews previous works in the use of blockchain technology in the IoT, the Edge AI paradigm and the use of blockchain for healthcare applications. Section 3 then introduces the system architecture, and outlines the benefits of integrating Edge AI with blockchain for different applications in the IoT. Section 4 presents the experimental data and results. Finally, Sect. 5 concludes the work and lays out future work directions.

2   Related Work

In the healthcare IoT domain, it is often recommended that patients should have the ability to access their own health data. Nonetheless, the data should be consistent, protected and unaltered over time by any third parties or patients themselves [30, 31]. Therefore, it is necessary to have a high level of security methods which ensure that data transmitted over a network is secure and available to authorized parties, in addition to having an integrity check that ensures immutability of the data. Many efforts have been devoted to propose blockchain-based methods to improve security, transaction speed, and avoid fraud control in healthcare.

In [32], the authors introduced and discussed different access policies to protect the privacy of private patient's data. In addition, the authors implemented deep learning algorithms to extract useful information from private raw data. Although the proposed method and its algorithms focus on healthcare applications, they can be applied in different scenarios including cases in larger perspectives.

In [33], the authors presented a blockchain-based approach for sharing patient data within a network. In addition, the authors introduced a consensus algorithm for enabling data interoperability. Different measurements of security on blockchain were carried out and the authors claimed that the blockchain-based method is a promising solution for avoiding or overcoming problems in sharing private health data.

In [34], the authors introduced a blockchain-based method for proffering a proof of predefined endpoints in clinical trials. They claimed that applying blockchain methods can provide a high level of reliability while keeping costs low.

In [35], the authors introduced a framework which has a modified traditional blockchain method for suiting to IoT applications. The proposed method is suitable for resource-constrained devices while it maintains a high level of privacy and security. The framework ensures that transactions over a blockchain network are more anonymous and secure.

In [36], Simic *et al.* showed that it is feasible to apply blockchain into healthcare IoT systems to protect data transmitted over a network. The authors have examined several possibilities of utilizing smart contracts for healthcare IoT systems. They claimed that a combination of blockchain and IoT can benefit different distributed applications.

In [37], Pham *et al.* presented a remote health monitoring system utilizing blockchain. In this system, bio-signal sensor nodes collect and filter patient data. The useful information extracted from the collected data is written into blockchain. In case of abnormalities, the extracted information is written immediately to blockchain and a push notification is triggered to inform medical doctors.

3 Protecting Data Privacy with the Ethereum Blockchain

As compared to the original blockchain platform developed for the bitcoin by Satoshi Nakamoto [19], the Ethereum platform provides the Ethereum Virtual Machine (EVM) which is fully autonomous in terms of its system execution by using smart contracts. Smart contracts are scripts with predefined terms and conditions for system transactions. This peer-to-peer (P2P) distributed ledger relies on its miner nodes. Miner nodes act as validator nodes for every new transaction block, which are created within certain time intervals. In general, a single transaction block is a combination of a header block and a data block. The data block stores the hash of the processed and analyzed data, while the header contains the hash of previous and current blocks, metadata, timestamp and a short characterization of the data. If another user or a third party service wants to access or exchange data, the header data characterization description can be utilized to see the details of the data block before the transaction is carried out. The data itself is stored encrypted in a cloud storage solution or in the device itself if the capacity is enough.

The proposed system architecture is illustrated in Fig. 1 and it consists of three layers. First, the data generation layer, which consists of sensors and actuators without any computational layer. These sensors and actuators depend on mining nodes which will collect data from these devices. Sensor and actuators merely communicate with one miner node which can be used as a gateway to transfer their data to other gateways or cloud servers. Bluetooth low energy (BLE) or Wi-Fi is often used this layer. BLE uses less energy whilst Wi-Fi can transmit a larger data packet size and offer higher bandwidth. Second, the network layer, where P2P networking is used in this private ethereum network for communication and data transfer. The distributed ledger topologies are defined on this layer. Different topologies like side chains, shard chains, off-chains can be used to handle scarce computing-devices issues and scalability. Smart contracts or scripts run to handle all the processes in a network. Finally, the third layer is the application layer. Smart applications of the IoT consists of a wide range of use-cases like smart homes, smart industries, digital medical and many more. To access these systems, end-users, third parties or control centers need to join the network first and then request data via the ethereum network.

3.1   Application Areas

In this section, we give an overview of potential applications for the proposed architecture. We outline the benefits and trade-offs of integrating our proposed platform in different IoT domains. We cover the areas of smart homes, smart cities, industrial applications, connected vehicles with vehicle-to-vehicle (V2V) and vehicle-to-everything (V2X) communication, and ubiquitous health.

A common problem of IoT devices in all application areas is their security vulnerabilities in terms of (1) third-party access and control, (2) unauthorized use of data, and (3) leakage of raw data. While previous works have studied the problem of protecting access to these devices by integrating blockchain technology extensively, we will focus on the benefits of the proposed for ensuring that data from sensor nodes is only accessed by authorized third parties, and that raw data is never made available to these parties through processing at the local network level and before inclusion in the blockchain. Furthermore, the blockchain provides an immutable record of all data requests from third parties.

Smart Home IoT Providers

In the smart home domain, an increasing number of industrial players are introducing a variety of commodities, from voice assistants to smart fridges. However, these are not exempt from security vulnerabilities [38], and many of them suppose a serious threat to privacy in users' homes. Previous works have been focusing on using blockchain for securing access and control of smart home appliances. This can significantly reduce the risk of having a spy inside our homes [39]. However, while communication between third-party services is secured, the use of data gathered by these devices is still being controlled by third-parties.

A smart gateway, which can replace a traditional home Wi-Fi router, serves as a bridge between sensor nodes and cloud storage or third-party applications, and at the same time the smart gateway can be utilized to deploy deep learning analysis and other AI processing which cannot run directly on resource-constrained devices. Moreover, because the processed data is only stored locally or encrypted in cloud storage, all data access requests are stored in the blockchain and therefore access to data is not managed by an external party but by smart gateways directly.

Cybersecurity in Open Smart Cities

The concept of Smart City mostly relies on IoT. A city is considered to be *smart* when it uses large amounts of IoT sensor data to efficiently improve the management of its assets and resources [40]. Another key aspect of smart cities is openness. By making public all or part of the IoT data that is gathered, city administrators can engage citizens, local business and large enterprises equally to develop new products and services based on the data. This benefits both the city management team and the involved parties, with a positive effect on the city's economy. In this case, however, it is essential to have a proper methodology for both sharing data with third parties and ensuring that public datasets are not misused.

With the implementation of the proposed architecture, administrators can have full control and monitor the access of third parties of this data. Moreover, transaction fees and data prices in the ethereum blockchain within the proposed solution can be used to naturally control the amount of data that each external user is accessing. In summary, our proposed solution not only provides a secure and safe way of distributing IoT data gathered around the city to external users or developers, but it also provides a base for edge computing and local network analysis and processing. By managing to which level the data is processed in edge gateways, which information is processed in the gateways, and which information or raw data is available to external applications.

Modular Smart Factories in Industry 4.0

The fourth industrial revolution, or Industry 4.0, has promised to develop more agile, modular and smart manufacturing environments where traditional production lines are replaced by automated and intelligent lines in which individual products can be customized *on the fly* [41]. The process towards Industry 4.0

requires the integration of the IoT in industrial environments and the installation of IoT sensor suites and actuators. This will allow managers to gather vast amounts of data and be able to adjust the manufacturing process dynamically to improve its efficiency.

Although autonomous machines and robots are heavily used in smart factories, they cannot replace humans completely. In some parts of a production chain, tight cooperation between machines and humans is unavoidable. Therefore, it is required that smart factories must guarantee a high safety level for humans working with autonomous machines. A method for enhancing situational awareness via intercommunication between everything can be applied in smart factories to address the target. In detail, a machine such as co-robot communicates and obtains useful information from other machines or even humans. For instance, a machine in a room can get a position and gesture of engineering who is walking in an adjacent room and is likely to come close to it. Based on both the received information and the data collected by the machine itself, it is able to forecast potential safety-critical situations and react in real-time to avoid accidents. In such a system, latency and security are essential because a piece of incorrect information provided by the third party or delayed information can cause a serious consequence. Therefore, smart factories need an advanced secured architecture which can guarantee a trusted intercommunication between machines and human with low latency.

Internet of Vehicles, V2V, and V2X

Nowadays, the number of connected vehicles is increasing significantly due to their benefits such as improving energy efficiency, reducing travelling time, or avoiding car accidents. The concept of connected vehicles often refers to a number of communication protocols used to connect the driver with other objects. For instance, communication in connected vehicles can be categorized into a vehicle to infrastructure (V2I), vehicle to vehicle (V2V), vehicle to Cloud (V2C), vehicle to pedestrian (V2P) and, in general, vehicle to everything (V2X) communication. In these scenarios, security is essential because incorrect or modified data introduced in the system by untrusted third parties can cause serious consequences such as a car accident or even death. Conventional security methods which need a central control system may not be completely suitable for some of the connected vehicles because those methods can cause an increase in communication latency. In such vehicle systems, real-time data and reaction are required. The proposed solution is a potential candidate for such real-time connected vehicle systems as it can provide high levels of security while the latency does not increase. With the proposed architecture, data related to other vehicles on a street can be exchanged directly with a connected vehicle through edge gateways in the near infrastructure. Moreover, the Edge AI opens multiple possibilities for computational offloading [42, 43]. The benefits of our proposed architecture are in the control of the use of private vehicle data by third parties. In the V2X scenario, these can be other vehicles (V2V) or infrastructure around the road (V2I) (Fig. 2).

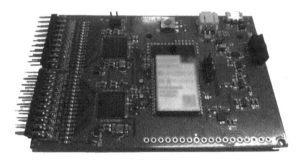

Fig. 2. Sensor node

Ubiquitous Health

Privacy and private health data must be carefully protected because leaked information can cause serious consequences. For instance, the leakage information such as health status can be used for hijacking purposes or spreading false rumors which causes money and mental damages. It is required that remote and real-time health monitoring systems must ensure a high level of security. Nonetheless, there are still many challenges of security issues in these systems. Blockchain can play an important role in improving a security level in these systems [27]. By combining blockchain with artificial intelligence at the edge of the network, a system can provide end-to-end protection to users' privacy. First, sensitive raw data is processed at the local network level, and therefore the risk of raw data being leaked is eliminated. With the blockchain utilized to manage an access to processed data and features, end-users can have full control over their data while allowing third-party applications to have access only the information that has been processed already.

4   Experiment and Results

In order to test the feasibility of the proposed architecture, and the possibilities for deployment and real-time execution, we have targeted a use case of ECG feature extraction and arrhythmia detection with convolutional neural networks (CNN). We have used a complete remote health monitoring IoT-based system utilizing blockchain and edge/fog computing. However, in this paper, we just focuses on edge gateways which have been used for deploying the advanced algorithms such as ECG feature extraction and arrhythmia detection with CNN. Other parts of the system have been discussed in detail in our previous papers [12,44,45].

4.1   Sensor Node

In this paper, ECG is collected by our multi-channel ECG sensor node which will be described in detail in another work. The sensor node is able to collect

Table 1. Loading time of the different Arrythmia classification requirements

	Execution time
Loading numerical libraries	960 ms
Loading tensorflow and keras	1478 ms
Loading trained model	6683 ms
ECG feature extraction	150 ms
Arrythmia classification	849 ms

Table 2. Blockchain transaction average execution times

	Average execution time
Ethereum transaction request	17 ms
New data block creation	10 s

16-channel ECG signals with high resolutions (i.e., each channel can collect from 125 samples/s to 1000 samples/s). Then, depending on the requirements of each application, the data can be pre-processed and kept intact before being sent to a smart Edge gateway via BLE or Wi-Fi. In this paper, raw ECG data is collected from the sensor node with a sampling rate of 250 samples/s per channel and sent to a smart Edge gateway via Wi-Fi. The collected data is not processed at the sensor node because it is difficult or even not feasible to run heavy computation methods (e.g., ECG feature extraction based on wavelet transform) at the sensor node [46–48]. Instead the data will be processed at the Edge gateway which is capable of running heavy computations while fulfilling latency requirements [49]. The data rate of 250 samples/s can fulfill the requirements of common ECG data quality standards [50]. In general, BLE is preferred over Wi-Fi because BLE consumes much less energy than Wi-Fi for a similar transmissions. However, BLE cannot be chosen for this case because BLE cannot support this large data rate (i.e., about 3 Mbps for up to 12 channels in each sensor node) [51].

4.2 Gateway

The edge gateways used in our system are Raspberry Pi 3B+ single-board computer (1.4 GHz quad-core processor, 1 GB SRAM, BLE, Wi-Fi). The operating system running at the gateway is Ubuntu. The gateway is able to store different data and information such as parameters used for algorithms and temporary health data. The parameters are often kept intact and they are only modified by a system administrator. The gateway can reserve 20 GB for storing temporary health data. Raw data is not stored but only the extracted features. If the storage is near its full capacity, then part of the data is encrypted and transferred to cloud-based storage solutions. All the services (e.g., ECG feature extraction) run on the gateway. In our experiments, the Pi runs ECG feature extraction adapted from [52], while a deep learning based arrhythmia classification model

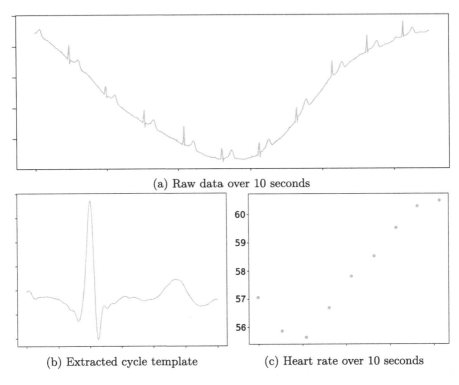

(a) Raw data over 10 seconds

(b) Extracted cycle template   (c) Heart rate over 10 seconds

Fig. 3. Results of the data analysis at the edge gateway.

adapted from [53] is deployed in the as well. The Pi was used in order to prove the viability and effectiveness of the proposed architecture. If more computational resources are required, then this can be replaced by any other hardware capable of running Ubuntu.

4.3   Performance

To initialize the system, a private ethereum network is created, generating authority and transaction accounts. The first step is to configure a new genesis file to build the first block of the custom ethereum network. Smart contracts were written in solidity and tested by using Remix IDE. We have analyzed the execution times of the feature extraction, arrhythmia detection and blockchain requests in order to assess the possibilities of real-time operation. The execution times of the different processes are shown in Tables 1 and 2. The feature extraction and arrhythmia classification processes deployed in this use case are single-threaded and therefore executed within a single core. As the Raspberry Pi 3B+ has 4 cores, it is possible to concurrently execute the analysis of two sensor nodes in parallel together with other background processes. The analysis of ECG data is made in batches of 10 s, where an average ECG cycle template is extracted and the heart rate and other features are calculated.

An example of the raw and processed data is shown in Fig. 3. Then, the template is utilized for arrhythmia classification.

The loading times required for loading numerical libraries, the deep learning libraries Tensorflow and Keras, and the trained model are shown in Table 1. Taking these into account, we deploy the model in the edge gateway in a way that the required libraries and the deep learning model are only loaded every time the gateway is rebooted. Transaction requests time in the ethereum network was 17 ms as average while using public Wi-Fi. Miner nodes take 10 s as average to create a new data block.

In summary, since the analysis is carried out every 10 s, a single Raspberry Pi 3B+ board is able to handle multiple sensor nodes connected via Wi-Fi or Bluetooth. We can safely assume that around 8 sensor nodes can be handled in real-time without reaching the maximum level of performance and therefore allowing for uncertainties in the measurements.

After data processing, the extracted features are encrypted with AES-256 [54,55] and stored in a third party storage solution. A custom distributed storage solution can be employed instead if tighter control of the data storage is required. Then, metadata including device ID and type of data are stored in the blockchain through the execution of a series of smart contracts.

5   Conclusion and Future Work

We have utilized a blockchain-based architecture for managing data security and integrity in IoT applications, and improved it by integrating Edge AI techniques to enhance the applications' security and protect users' privacy further. This is of particular interest for mission-critical and data-sensitive applications such as health monitoring applications in the IoT. We have implemented our proposed approach using ECG sensor nodes and a Raspberry Pi Model 3B+ as an edge gateway. The gateway ran a full ethereum node and processed ECG data in real-time with feature extraction and arrhythmia detection algorithms deployed. We show that real-time computation with arrhythmia classification is possible with multiple nodes, and the analysis part utilizes more computation resources than a typical ethereum deployment.

In future work, we will further integrate how the AI algorithms are executed together with the smart contracts in an ethereum network. In addition, we will extend the current system to a larger number of applications in the domain of ubiquitous health monitoring and others.

References

1. Al-Fuqaha, A., et al.: Internet of Things: a survey on enabling technologies, protocols, and applications. IEEE Commun. Surv. Tutor. 17(4), 2347–2376 (2015)
2. Gia, T.N., et al.: Edge AI in smart farming IoT: CNNs at the edge and fog computing with lora. In: IEEE AFRICON-2019 (2019)

3. Moosavi, S.R., et al.: Session resumption-based end-to-end security for healthcare Internet-of-Things. In: 2015 IEEE CIT, pp. 581–588. IEEE (2015)
4. Gubbi, J., et al.: Internet of Things (IoT): a vision, architectural elements, and future directions. Future Gener. Comput. Syst. **29**(7), 1645–1660 (2013)
5. Moosavi, S.R., et al.: Sea: a secure and efficient authentication and authorization architecture for IoT-based healthcare using smart gateways. Procedia Comput. Sci. **52**, 452–459 (2015)
6. Moosavi, S.R., et al.: End-to-end security scheme for mobility enabled healthcare Internet of Things. Future Gener. Comput. Syst. **64**, 108–124 (2016)
7. Fernandes, E., et al.: Security analysis of emerging smart home applications. In: 2016 IEEE Symposium on Security and Privacy (SP), pp. 636–654 (May 2016)
8. Apthorpe, N., Reisman, D., Feamster, N.: A smart home is no castle: privacy vulnerabilities of encrypted IoT traffic. arXiv preprint arXiv:1705.06805 (2017)
9. Ali, M., et al.: Intelligent autonomous elderly patient home monitoring system. In: ICC 2019–2019 IEEE International Conference on Communications (ICC), pp. 1–6. IEEE (2019)
10. Gia, T.N., et al.: Edge AI in smart farming IoT: CNNs at the edge and fog computing with lora (2019)
11. Dastjerdi, A.V., Buyya, R.: Fog computing: helping the Internet of Things realize its potential. Computer **49**(8), 112–116 (2016)
12. Gia, T.N., et al.: Energy efficient fog-assisted iot system for monitoring diabetic patients with cardiovascular disease. Future Gener. Comput. Syst. **93**, 198–211 (2019)
13. Ali, M., et al.: Autonomous patient/home health monitoring powered by energy harvesting. In: GLOBECOM 2017–2017 IEEE Global Communications Conference, pp. 1–7. IEEE (2017)
14. Sarker, V.K., et al.: A survey on lora for IoT: integrating edge computing. In: 2019 Fourth International Conference on Fog and Mobile Edge Computing (FMEC), pp. 295–300. IEEE (2019)
15. Queralta, J.P., et al.: Edge-AI in lora-based health monitoring: fall detection system with fog computing and LSTM recurrent neural networks. In: 2019 42nd International Conference on Telecommunications and Signal Processing (TSP), pp. 601–604. IEEE (2019)
16. Metwaly, A., et al.: Edge computing with embedded AI: thermal image analysis for occupancy estimation in intelligent buildings. In: INTelligent Embedded Systems Architectures and Applications, INTESA@ESWEEK 2019. ACM (2019)
17. Roman, R., Lopez, J., Mambo, M.: Mobile edge computing, fog et al.: a survey and analysis of security threats and challenges. Future Gener. Comput. Syst. **78**, 680–698 (2018)
18. Conoscenti, M., Vetró, A., De Martin, J.C.: Blockchain for the Internet of Things: a systematic literature review. In: 2016 IEEE/ACS 13th International Conference of Computer Systems and Applications (AICCSA), pp. 1–6 (November 2016)
19. Nakamoto, S.: Bitcoin: a peer-to-peer electronic cash system. White Paper (2008)
20. Shafagh, H., et al.: Towards blockchain-based auditable storage and sharing of IoT data. In: Proceedings of the 2017 on Cloud Computing Security Workshop, CCSW 2017, pp. 45–50. ACM, New York (2017)
21. Huh, S., Cho, S., Kim, S.: Managing IoT devices using blockchain platform. In: 2017 19th International Conference on Advanced Communication Technology (ICACT), pp. 464–467. IEEE (2017)
22. Novo, O.: Blockchain meets IoT: an architecture for scalable access management in IoT. IEEE Internet Things J. **5**(2), 1184–1195 (2018)

23. Tang, B., et al.: A hierarchical distributed fog computing architecture for big data analysis in smart cities. In: Proceedings of the ASE BigData & SocialInformatics 2015, p. 28. ACM (2015)

24. Dorri, A., et al.: Blockchain for IoT security and privacy: the case study of a smart home. In: 2017 IEEE International Conference on Pervasive Computing and Communications Workshops (PerCom Workshops), pp. 618–623. IEEE (2017)

25. Christidis, K., Devetsikiotis, M.: Blockchains and smart contracts for the Internet of Things. IEEE Access **4**, 2292–2303 (2016)

26. Kshetri, N.: Can blockchain strengthen the Internet of Things? IT Prof. **19**(4), 68–72 (2017)

27. Nawaz, A., et al.: Edge AI and blockchain for privacy-critical and data-sensitive applications. In: The 12th International Conference on Mobile Computing and Ubiquitous Networking (ICMU) (2019)

28. Ndibanje, B., Lee, H.-J., Lee, S.-G.: Security analysis and improvements of authentication and access control in the Internet of Things. Sensors **14**(8), 14786–14805 (2014)

29. Bahga, A., Madisetti, V.: Internet of Things: A Hands-on Approach. VPT, New York (2014)

30. Li, M., Yu, S., Ren, K., Lou, W.: Securing personal health records in cloud computing: patient-centric and fine-grained data access control in multi-owner settings. In: Jajodia, S., Zhou, J. (eds.) SecureComm 2010. LNICST, vol. 50, pp. 89–106. Springer, Heidelberg (2010). https://doi.org/10.1007/978-3-642-16161-2_6

31. Mandl, K.D., et al.: Public standards and patients' control: how to keepelectronic medical records accessible but private. BMJ **322**(7281), 283–287 (2001)

32. Mamoshina, P., et al.: Converging blockchain and next-generation artificial intelligence technologies to decentralize and accelerate biomedical research and healthcare. Oncotarget **9**(5), 5665 (2018)

33. Peterson, K., et al.: A blockchain-based approach to health information exchange networks. In: Proceedings of NIST Workshop Blockchain Healthcare, vol. 1, pp. 1–10 (2016)

34. Irving, G., Holden, J.: How blockchain-timestamped protocols could improve the trustworthiness of medical science. F1000Research **5**, 22 (2016)

35. Dwivedi, A.D., et al.: A decentralized privacy-preserving healthcare blockchain for IoT. Sensors **19**(2), 326 (2019)

36. Simić, M., et al.: A case study IoT and blockchain powered healthcare. In: International Conference on Engineering and Technology (ICET-2017) (June 2017)

37. Pham, H.L., Tran, T.H., Nakashima, Y.: A secure remote healthcare system for hospital using blockchain smart contract. In: 2018 IEEE Globecom Workshops (GC Wkshps), pp. 1–6. IEEE (2018)

38. Apthorpe, N., et al.: Spying on the smart home: privacy attacks and defenses on encrypted IoT traffic. arXiv preprint arXiv:1708.05044 (2017)

39. Hernandez, G., et al.: Smart nest thermostat: a smart spy in your home. Black Hat USA, pp. 1–8 (2014)

40. Albino, V., Berardi, U., Dangelico, R.M.: Smart cities: definitions, dimensions, performance, and initiatives. J. Urban Technol. **22**(1), 3–21 (2015)

41. Lasi, H., et al.: Industry 4.0. Bus. Inf. Syst. Eng. **6**(4), 239–242 (2014)

42. Qingqing, L., et al.: Edge computing for mobile robots: multi-robot feature-based lidar odometry with FPGAs. In: The 12th International Conference on Mobile Computing and Ubiquitous Networking (ICMU) (2019)

43. Qingqing, L., et al.: Visual odometry offloading in Internet of vehicles with compression at the edge of the network. In: The 12th International Conference on Mobile Computing and Ubiquitous Networking (ICMU) (2019)
44. Gia, T.N., et al.: Fog computing approach for mobility support in Internet-of-Things systems. IEEE Access **6**, 36064–36082 (2018)
45. Jiang, M., et al.: IoT-based remote facial expression monitoring system with sEMG signal. In: 2016 IEEE Sensors Applications Symposium (SAS), pp. 1–6. IEEE (2016)
46. Gia, T.N., et al.: Fog computing in healthcare Internet of Things: a case study on ECG feature extraction. In: 2015 IEEE CIT, pp. 356–363. IEEE (2015)
47. Palacios-Enriquez, A., Ponomaryov, V.: Feature extraction based on wavelet transform using ECG signal. In: 2013 International Kharkov Symposium on Physics and Engineering of Microwaves, Millimeter and Submillimeter Waves, pp. 632–634. IEEE (2013)
48. Gia, T.N., et al.: Fog computing in body sensor networks: an energy efficient approach. In: Proceedings of IEEE International Body Sensor Networks Conference (BSN), pp. 1–7 (2015)
49. Gia, T.N., et al.: Customizing 6LoWPAN networks towards Internet-of-Things based ubiquitous healthcare systems. In: 2014 Norchip, pp. 1–6. IEEE (2014)
50. Steinberg, C., et al.: A novel wearable device for continuous ambulatory ECG recording: proof of concept and assessment of signal quality. Biosensors **9**(1), 17 (2019)
51. Sarker, V.K., et al.: Portable multipurpose bio-signal acquisition and wireless streaming device for wearables. In: 2017 IEEE Sensors Applications Symposium (SAS), pp. 1–6. IEEE (2017)
52. Carreiras, C., et al.: BioSPPy: biosignal processing in Python, 2015. Accessed Aug 2019
53. Jun, T.J., et al.: ECG arrhythmia classification using a 2-D convolutional neural network. arXiv preprint arXiv:1804.06812 (2018)
54. Dhaou, I.B., et al.: Low-latency hardware architecture for cipher-based message authentication code. In: 2017 IEEE International Symposium on Circuits and Systems (ISCAS), pp. 1–4. IEEE (2017)
55. Gia, T.N., et al.: Low-cost fog-assisted health-care IoT system with energy-efficient sensor nodes. In: 2017 13th International Wireless Communications and Mobile Computing Conference (IWCMC), pp. 1765–1770. IEEE (2017)

Continuous Wellness Tracking with Firstbeat – Usability, User Experience, and Subjective Wellness Impact

Timo Partala[✉], Laura Saar, Minna Männikkö, Maarit Karhula, and Tuulevi Aschan

South-Eastern Finland University of Applied Sciences, Patteristonkatu 3, 50100 Mikkeli, Finland

{timo.partala,laura.saar,minna.mannikko,maarit.karhula,
tuulevi.aschan}@xamk.fi

Abstract. Current wellness technologies are capable of monitoring wellness related parameters even 24 h a day for multiple days. The aim of the current research was to study the usability, user experience, and wellbeing impact of the wellness analysis Firstbeat, which is based on continuous measurement of heart rate variability (HRV) and user activity. 42 persons in working life participated in an intervention study, in which their wellbeing was continuously monitored for 3–7 days and they received a detailed wellness report and a personal plan for improvement. In a follow-up questionnaire, the participants reported good usability and user experience for the system, as well as significantly reduced stress and increased self-esteem, while no significant changes were observed in the other measured aspects related to subjective wellbeing. The results suggest that the usage of continuous wellness measurement systems using electrodes in the chest area, such as Firstbeat, can be experienced positively by their users. Further research is needed on effective methods for utilizing the rich information from the measurements in achieving lasting positive changes in lifestyle.

Keywords: Wellbeing · Wellness technology · Firstbeat · Heart Rate Variability · Usability · User experience

1 Introduction

With recent technological advances, continuous wellness measurements have become feasible for prolonged periods of time, while still preserving good measurement accuracy. As many commercially available wellness technologies can provide valid measurements, the focus of research has shifted to also include issues such information presentation, user experience, user acceptance, motivating the user, and wellness impacts of the technology. Given the large worldwide potential of wellness technology, the number of studies focusing on these issues from the user's perspective is still relatively small.

Previous studies of heart rate monitors and activity trackers have reported both positive and negative user experiences. For example, Preusse et al. [1] found and analyzed various different usability and user acceptance related challenges with commonly used

© ICST Institute for Computer Sciences, Social Informatics and Telecommunications Engineering 2020
Published by Springer Nature Switzerland AG 2020. All Rights Reserved
G. M. P. O'Hare et al. (Eds.): MobiHealth 2019, LNICST 320, pp. 281–293, 2020.
https://doi.org/10.1007/978-3-030-49289-2_22

activity trackers. In contrast, Karapanos et al. [2] presented examples of how activity trackers can support positive user experiences, by better supporting the users' psychological needs. For example, they can enhance the feelings of autonomy by providing people more control of their exercising or relatedness by connecting family members to joint healthy activities. Meyer et al. [3] recently found that high levels of usability and comfort were associated with the usage of clip, wristband, and mobile app based activity trackers by the users. Oh and Lee [4] identified both positive and negative user experience issues related to existing activity trackers and other quantified self technologies. The identified issues were related to user input, design, sharing and privacy, data visualization, and data accuracy, among other things.

Ahtinen et al. [5] studied using common heart rate monitors in exercising from a user experience perspective. Their results suggested relatively good usability, but only moderate motivating impact for exercising. The findings by Ehmen et al. [6] indicate fairly high acceptance and qualitative user experience in response to two popular wellness systems using heart rate monitor belts. However, their participants also reported a number usability problems related to both systems. An early version of the Firstbeat wellness analysis using heart rate variability and activity tracking was also found to be time-consuming and expensive by mobile workers [7]. In addition, sleep sensing devices (based on both heart rate monitoring and accelerometers) have been found to provide useful and objective feedback that is beneficial to their users [8].

The subjective wellness impacts of modern heart rate variability based wellness technologies such as the Firstbeat system have not been extensively studied. Instead, the focus has been on the validation of the technology in measuring, for example, stress and recovery, as well as in utilizing those measures in scientific studies (see Sect. 2.3). The aim of this study was to report experiences of a wellness intervention utilizing the Firstbeat wellness analysis, which is based on continuous measurements of heart rate variability and user activity. Specifically, the aim was to study usability, user experience, and subjective wellbeing impact of the analysis and its technological solution in a sample of people in working life. We were particularly interested in understanding user experiences related to continuous wellness measurements over multiple days, and whether it is possible to obtain lasting positive effects on subjective wellbeing by means of a single wellness intervention.

2   Method

2.1 Participants

The participants were 42 volunteers (30 females and 12 males) participating actively in working life during the study. The average age of the participants was 44.3 years (range 27–65 years). 24 participants had a lower or higher university degree and 18 participants did not have a university degree. 35 participants were employees and seven participants were entrepreneurs in organizations participating in our wellness related projects. The organizations were: a bank, an accounting office, two mass transit companies, a media company, a municipal organization, an advertising agency, a beauty salon, a child welfare organization, an engineering company, and several micro companies represented by their entrepreneurs. All the participants were geographically from Finland, and all the materials, instructions, and questionnaires were delivered in the native language of the participants (Finnish). As an incentive, the participants received the wellness analysis and a personal plan for improvement free of charge.

The 42 participants included in the final data analysis reported that they used the Firstbeat system successfully and that they did not use any other wellness technologies during the intervention period. 31 participants chose the most common Firstbeat measurement period of three days and 11 participants chose an optional longer measurement period of 4–7 days. On average, the participants used the measurement technology for 3.5 days. The average time between receiving the report and personal plan from the intervention and filling in the follow-up questionnaire was 44.7 days. Previous studies on wellness technologies (e.g. [5]) report positive effects lasting for several weeks, and the current study also aimed at investigating the possible lasting effects of the intervention by aiming the evaluation period (time before the follow-up questionnaire) at 4–8 weeks.

2.2 Procedure

The implementation of the study was carried out within two projects at South-Eastern Finland University of Applied Sciences. Both projects aimed at studying methods for improving the wellbeing of employees and entrepreneurs of the participating companies by using wellness technology. The researchers and authors of this paper were completely independent of Firstbeat technologies. The goal of the Firstbeat intervention was to give the project participants tools for improving their own wellbeing through improved wellness related self-knowledge.

An information session was organized in each company, in which volunteer participants from each company were given detailed instructions for carrying out the analysis successfully, including the placement of the electrodes. In case of micro companies with only one participant, the same information was provided in a personal meeting. All the participants were told that their participation is fully voluntary and information from the wellness measurements, as well as information from the follow-up questionnaire is treated confidentially. The information from the wellness measurements was to only visible to participants themselves and the wellness specialist, who organized the study and gave personal feedback to participants.

Shortly after the measurements were carried out, group meetings (employees) or personal meetings (entrepreneurs) were organized to help the participants in interpreting their results and setting personal goals in order to improve their well-being. The participants received their wellness reports using encrypted e-mail or on paper before the meetings. In the meetings, the participants were presented with basic information about autonomic nervous system (e.g. the functions of the sympathetic and parasympathetic nervous system), heart rate variability, the importance of exercise, and the various analyses presented in their Firstbeat reports were explained in detail. Finally, the participants received personal advice in setting their wellness goals according to the Firstbeat method, described in the next section.

2.3   The Firstbeat Wellness Analysis

The Firstbeat wellness analysis aims at providing meaningful physiological information that helps people improve their overall well-being and performance. It is based on heart rate variability (HRV) and motion sensor measurements. The analysis and the measurement technology is based on more than 15 years of development. The system is used by many organizations worldwide to improve the wellbeing of their personnel and it has also been used in numerous scientific physiological studies to study stress and recovery, as well as physical activity, oxygen intake, and energy expenditure [e.g. 9, 10].

Heart rate variability has been shown to be associated with stress and recovery. Generally, a low variability in heartbeats indicates that the body is under stress from, for example, exercise or psychological events. In contrast, a higher variability in heartbeats usually means that the body has a strong ability to tolerate stress or is recovering from prior stress. By accurately measuring HRV it possible to gain an understanding of the state of the autonomic nervous system at any given moment. The Firstbeat Bodyguard 2 measurement device used in the Firstbeat wellness analysis has been shown to provide an accurate method for long term HRV monitoring during daily life [11].

The package given to each participants contained the Firstbeat Bodyguard 2 measuring device, two leaflets of instructions, and disposable electrodes (Fig. 1). The participants were also given plenty of extra electrodes (in addition to those pictured below) to be able to replace them more than once per day, if necessary. The Firstbeat wellness system uses an electrocardiogram (ECG) with two electrodes to produce the heart rate variability measurements. The electrode attached to the recording device was placed on the right side of the body just beneath the collar bone. The second electrode was placed on the rib cage on the lower left side of the body. The measurement and recording started

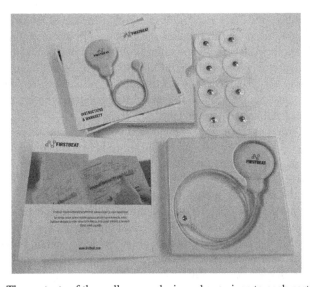

Fig. 1. The contents of the wellness analysis package given to each participant.

automatically after both electrodes were attached to the body. The device also included a motion sensor to estimate the amount of exercise and energy expenditure.

The system included a loadable battery with a battery life of at least six days and a recording capacity of about 20 days of wellness data. The weight of the system was 24 g. Its sampling resolution in measuring heart rate variability was 1000 Hz. The resolution of the motion sensor was 12.5 Hz. The battery of the device could be loaded by connecting the measurement unit of the device to a standard USB port of a computer. The USB connection was also used to transfer the data stored on the device for the Firstbeat software.

When the participants started using the analysis, they received an e-mail with a link to the Firstbeat startup questionnaire. They were asked to give a self-evaluation related to their exercise, eating, alcohol consumption, stress, recovery, sleeping, health, and wellbeing. They also received a link to a web diary, which they could use on their computers or smart phones. For each measurement day, they were instructed to mark their work periods, sleeping periods, exercise periods, and any other meaningful activities, as well as any medicine taken and doses of alcohol consumed.

The Firstbeat measurement device is intended to be worn day and night except when it would come into contact with water. Typically, the participants of the current study removed the devices once a day for a short period when they took a shower and replaced the electrodes. The participants were instructed to use the wellness analysis for at least one rest day – or a less stressful working day – and two working days, which is the standard procedure for a Firstbeat analysis.

After they had completed the measurement period, the participants received a full Firstbeat wellness report (2018 version) with at least seven pages. The first page of the report repeated the participant's answers in the self-evaluation questionnaire. On pages two to four (for a three day measurement), the results from the wellness analysis were presented separately for each day of measurement. Each page presented the amount and percentage of stress, recovery, and physical exercise periods during the day. In addition, a timeline of stress, recovery, and physical activity periods was presented augmented with the participant's diary notes. Furthermore, the following information was provided: amount of recovery during work; amount and quality of recovery during sleep (Fig. 2); length of light, moderate, and vigorous physical activity; energy expenditure; and steps taken during the day. Overall scores on a scale of 0–100 were also presented for balance of stress and recovery, restorative effect of sleep (Fig. 2), and positive health effects of exercise.

On page five, a summary over the whole measurement period was presented. It included a timeline of stress, recovery, and physical activity during the whole measurement period. Daily scores and overall scores (0–100) over the whole measurements period were also presented for balance of stress and recovery, recovery during sleep, and health effects of exercise. A summary view of exercise and energy expenditure was also presented. Finally, an overall wellness score (0–100) was presented taking into account all the measured wellness aspects.

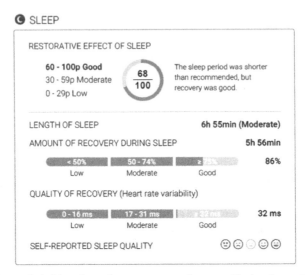

Fig. 2. A sample infobox from the report presenting an analysis of one night's sleep.

On page six they, together with a wellness specialist, set personal goals for improving their well-being by choosing from sixteen predefined goals related to stress management, sleep and recovery, exercise, and nutrition (e.g. "I will attempt to go to bed early enough to get enough sleep"). They also had a possibility to define their own personal goals. A sample report in English is available on Firstbeat website [12].

2.4 Questionnaire

The main research method for collecting data from the participants concerning the wellness intervention was an electronic questionnaire. It consisted of three main methods: System Usability Scale, AttrakDiff2, and a subjective wellbeing questionnaire.

On the first page on the questionnaire, the general instructions for the questionnaire were presented to the participant. The participant was instructed to input his/her participant number sent in an invitation e-mail by the researcher, who conducted the wellness analysis. On the second page of the questionnaire, the participant was asked to report demographic information and information related to the usage of the wellness measurement device. Specifically, the participant was asked to report his/her gender, age, education level from six alternatives, profession, occupation, and whether they work as an employee or an entrepreneur. Moreover, the participants reported the number of days they used the device to record their wellness parameters and the numbers of days passed since they read the report and made their personal plans.

System Usability Scale. The widely used System Usability Scale (SUS) method was used as the method for evaluating the perceived usability of the Firstbeat system. On the third page of the questionnaire the participant was asked to complete SUS in its original form using a 1–5 Likert scale as suggested by Brooke [13]. At the end of the page, the participants also had a possibility to give qualitative comments about the usability of the Firstbeat system and the usability problems they encountered.

AttrakDiff2. On page four of the questionnaire, the AttrakDiff2 method suggested by Hassenzahl [14] was used as the method to study user experiences. The four central concepts of Hassenzahl's user experience model were studied using seven-point semantic differential scales. The concepts were: pragmatic quality (quality of use from a task-oriented perspective), hedonic quality: identification (how well the system allows the user to relate to it), hedonic quality: stimulation (how well the system fulfills the stimulation needs of the user), and attractiveness (overall impression and judgement of the system). Each concept was studied using seven scales, thus the number of scales in the questionnaire was 28. The participants also had a possibility to give qualitative comments about the user experience of the system.

Subjective Wellbeing Questionnaire. On page five, the aim was to examine the subjective wellbeing effects of the current intervention briefly, yet as holistically as possible. A brief questionnaire probing 15 central aspects of subjective wellbeing was constructed for the purposes of the current study. Many of the concepts were taken from the wellness related concepts of WHOQOL-BREF [15], which is a cross-culturally validated quality of life assessment. Drawing from the self-determination theory and studies highlighting psychological needs and emotions as important correlates of subjective wellbeing [16–19], further wellbeing related concepts were identified for the questionnaire.

Each statement on page five of the questionnaire began with: "After using the Firstbeat system and reading the report – when compared to time before using the system – I have felt…" and the statements ended with the endings presented in Table 1 below. Each

Table 1. The wellbeing aspects in the study and the corresponding statement endings.

Wellbeing aspect	Statement ending
Physical health	…myself physically healthy
Bodily pain	…physical pain
Sleep quality	…that I sleep well
Stress	…myself stressed
Autonomy	…that my actions are autonomous
Competence	…that I can successfully complete different tasks and projects
Relatedness	…that I have positive social relationships
Self-esteem	…that I have high self-esteem
Positive emotions	…positive emotions such as joy, pride, or interest
Negative emotions	…negative emotions such as worry, sadness, or anxiety
Meaningful life	…that I lead a purposeful and meaningful life
Optimism	…that I am optimistic about the future
Active lifestyle	…that my lifestyle is active
Energy	…myself energetic
Depression	…myself depressed

statement was studied using a 1–7 scale with the following anchors: 1 = less than before – 4 = as much as before – 7 = more than before. In addition, the participants could leave any free-form qualitative comments about the wellness aspects of the intervention.

2.5 Data Analysis

Data from SUS was analyzed according to the original instructions [13] including reverse scoring, and calculating an overall score from 0 to 100. The results were interpreted using the adjective scale suggested by Bangor et al. [20]. The results from the AttrakDiff2 questionnaire using seven point semantic differential scales were transferred to a scale from −3 to 3, displayed visually and averaged by the four user experience components in Hassenzahl's model [14]. For the wellbeing data, one sample t-tests were used to determine statistically, whether the ratings for the different subjective wellbeing related aspects differed significantly from the middle point of the scale, which suggested that no change in relation to the wellbeing related aspect has taken place.

3   Results

3.1 Usability

The average SUS score for the Firstbeat wellness analysis was 76.7 (range 45–100). According to the adjective scale for SUS developed by Bangor et al. [20], this result indicated 'good' usability. More specifically, the score was between what is typically perceived as 'good' (mean 71.4) and 'excellent' (mean 85.5).

3.2 User Experience

The results for the AttrakDiff2 components studying different aspects of user experience are presented in Fig. 3. The averaged user experience ratings were on the positive side of the scale for all four concepts, and there were no significant differences between the means.

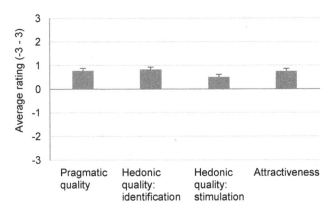

Fig. 3. Mean ratings and standard errors of the means for the central user experience concepts.

The detailed results from all of the AttrakDiff2 scales are presented in Fig. 4. Almost all of the single ratings were on the positive side of the scale, however, the system was seen as a bit technical and also quite a bit undemanding instead of being able to provide positive challenge. When giving this rating, the participants were possibly thinking of the easy usability of the system instead of the challenge posed by the analysis as a whole (e.g. the measurement started automatically when the electrodes were attached). Positive adjectives associated with the system included: good, motivating, novel, professional, and presentable.

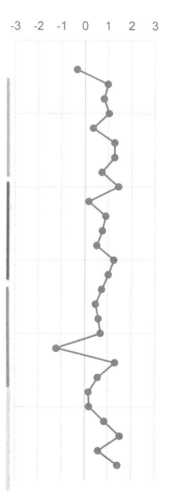

-3 -2 -1 0 1 2 3

Technical – Human
Complicated – Simple
Impractical – Practical
Cumbersome - Straightforward
Unpredictable - Predictable
Confusing - Clearly structured
Unruly – Manageable
Isolating - Connective
Unprofessional - Professional
Tacky – Stylish
Cheap - Premium
Alienating - Integrating
Separates me - Brings me closer
Unpresentable – Presentable
Conventional – Inventive
Unimaginative - Creative
Cautious - Bold
Conservative - Innovative
Dull - Captivating
Undemanding - Challenging
Ordinary - Novel
Unpleasant - Pleasant
Ugly - Attractive
Disagreeable – Likeable
Rejecting - Inviting
Bad - Good
Repelling – Appealing
Discouraging – Motivating

Fig. 4. Mean ratings for the 28 AttrakDiff2 scales (colors indicate components of user experience: green = pragmatic quality; blue = hedonic quality, identification; light blue = hedonic quality, stimulation; yellow = attractiveness). (Color figure online)

3.3 Subjective Wellbeing

The results from the subjective wellbeing questionnaire are presented in Table 2 below (scale: 1 = less than before – 4 = as much as before – 7 = more than before).

Table 2. Mean ratings and standard errors of the means for the different aspects of subjective wellbeing.

Wellbeing aspect	Mean (SEM)
Physical health	4.02 (.09)
Bodily pain	3.93 (.06)
Sleep quality	4.10 (.15)
Stress	3.71 (.11)
Autonomy	4.00 (.11)
Competence	4.10 (.10)
Relatedness	4.07 (.06)
Self-esteem	4.19 (.09)
Positive emotions	4.17 (.10)
Negative emotions	3.88 (.10)
Meaningful life	4.21 (.12)
Optimism	4.17 (.11)
Active lifestyle	4.19 (.12)
Energy	4.12 (.10)
Depression	3.83 (.12)

The statistical analysis revealed that the participants evaluated that they have felt significantly less stressed after using the system and reading the report than before usage ($t = 2.6$, $p = .012$). The participants also rated their self-esteem as higher after the intervention than before it ($t = 2.0$, $p = .044$). The other ratings did not differ significantly from the center point of the scale (suggesting no significant changes).

3.4 Qualitative Comments

The qualitative comments gathered in the questionnaire were largely in line with the quantitative results. There were no major usability problems highlighted by the users. Single comments were given about skin irritation with the electrodes, lack of indication when the device is fully loaded, and the usability of making diary entries.

The qualitative comments for the wellbeing effects of the system included a variety of different comments ranging from being aware of the wellness aspects to be improved, but not making any changes in lifestyle, to putting the set goals into action and noticing wellness improvements. Thus, there seemed to be a lot of variation in the participants' reactions to the results and the goals set at the end of the analysis.

4 Discussion

In the current study, usability, user experience, and subjective wellbeing impact were measured in response to an intervention implemented using the Firstbeat wellness system. In a working life sample of participants, the results suggested good usability for the system, as it received a SUS score of 76.7 out of 100. The results also suggested above average user experience in all measured aspects: pragmatic quality, hedonic quality (identification), hedonic quality (stimulation), and attractiveness. Thus, system was evaluated to have a good balance of hedonic and pragmatic qualities (self-orientation and task-orientation) [14]. Finally, the participants reported reduced subjective stress and higher self-esteem after the wellness intervention. Stress-related visualizations form a central part of the Firstbeat report, and the current results suggest that the participants of the current study were indeed able to use that information to reduce their stress levels in practice. However, it should be noted that the results suggested no significant changes for 13 of the 15 studied aspects related to subjective wellbeing.

Many previous studies [e.g. 1, 5–7] have pointed out usability barriers in the adoption of wellness technology, especially in technologies utilizing physiological wellness measurements. The current results suggest that Firstbeat has been successful in avoiding any major usability problems, and the minimalistic user interaction is simple enough for users in a working age population. Regarding user experience, the current results are in line with [6], who reported positive user experiences for heart rate monitor belts. The current results suggest that continuous mobile wellness measurements – even if they use electrodes, which are somewhat invasive and in constant physical contact with the user – can be well accepted by their users and even evoke a positive user experience.

On the other hand, the reported changes in subjective wellbeing were relatively small and only some of the participants reported making relevant changes in lifestyle based on the results. These results highlight the difficulty of translating wellness related awareness and goal setting into behavior that actually enhances holistic wellbeing. Consolvo et al. [21] divide design efforts of wellness technology into four chapters: collecting behavioral data, providing self-monitoring feedback, supporting goal-setting, and moving forward. The first three chapters have been mainly well considered in the design of the Firstbeat system, while the greatest challenges seems to be in achieving changes in the users' lifestyles and lasting improvements in wellbeing. Continuous wellness measurements can provide accurate information, but plain awareness of one's physiological state or setting goals may not be enough for achieving lasting effects [22].

Consolvo et al. [21] suggested that moving forward in wellbeing includes, for example, assessing the user's progress, and supporting the user over her lifespan. These could also be key elements in the context of continuous well-being measurements and the Firstbeat system. Possible topics for future research include studying the patterns of using the Firstbeat system over a longer period of time, when the use is initiated by the user her/himself. In addition, effective persuasive technologies [23] could be applied in addition to the Firstbeat analysis with the goal of achieving more positive changes in wellbeing related experiences and behavior.

The limitations of the current study should also be discussed. The participants of the current study were on average middle-aged and participating in working life, thus the results are not directly generalizable to other groups, for example, students or the elderly. The participants also come from a limited geographical region in Finland, in other regions there might be different cultural factors affecting the perceptions of the system. Finally, within the limits of the current research it was possible to carry out a single wellness intervention and study the usage of one wellness analysis and the related technological solution. Thus, it was not possible to make comparisons between different systems or study possible benefits of recurrent use of the Firstbeat analysis.

Overall, the current results provide a clear picture about the wellness intervention studied. The results confirm that it is possible for users to be monitored for even about 24 h per day by a wearable device measuring heart rate variability and activity, and still have positive user experiences related to the technology. The participants of the current intervention also reported significantly reduced stress and improved self-esteem after the intervention. The assessment of user progress and long-term support [21], as well as persuasive technology [23] may be key additions to the Firstbeat approach on the road towards even more effective and holistic improvements in wellbeing.

Acknowledgments. The authors would like to thank all the companies and individuals who participated in the current study. This research was carried out within three projects. The DIDIVE and Tiedosta projects were funded by Häme and South Savo Centres for Economic Development, Transport and the Environment from the European Social Fund (projects S20895 and S20924), respectively. The Smart Well-being and Food Services for the Future project was funded by the Regional Council of South Savo from the European Regional Development Fund (project A72562).

References

1. Preusse, K.C., Mitzner, T.L., Fausset, C.B., Rogers, W.A.: Older adults' acceptance of activity trackers. J. Appl. Gerontol. **36**(2), 127–155 (2017)
2. Karapanos, E., Gouveia, R., Hassenzahl, M., Forlizzi, J.: Wellbeing in the making: peoples' experiences with wearable activity trackers. Psychol. Well-Being **6**(1), 1–17 (2016). https://doi.org/10.1186/s13612-016-0042-6
3. Meyer, J., Fortmann, J., Wasmann, M., Heuten, W.: Making lifelogging usable: design guidelines for activity trackers. In: He, X., Luo, S., Tao, D., Xu, C., Yang, J., Hasan, M.A. (eds.) MMM 2015. LNCS, vol. 8936, pp. 323–334. Springer, Cham (2015). https://doi.org/10.1007/978-3-319-14442-9_39
4. Oh, J., Lee, U.: Exploring UX issues in quantified self technologies. In: Proceedings of Eighth International Conference on Mobile Computing and Ubiquitous Networking (ICMU 2015), pp. 53–59 (2015)
5. Ahtinen, A., Mäntyjärvi, J., Häkkilä, J.: Using heart rate monitors for personal wellness – the user experience perspective. In: Proceedings of Engineering in Medicine and Biology Society (EMBS 2008), pp. 1591–1597 (2008)
6. Ehmen, H., Haesner, M., Steinke, I., Dorn, M., Gövercin, M., Steinhagen, E.: Comparison of four different mobile devices for measuring heart rate and ECG with respect to aspects of usability and acceptance by older people. Appl. Ergon. **43**(3), 582–587 (2012)
7. Hyrkkänen, U., Vartiainen, M.: Heart rate variability measurements in mobile work. In: Eriksson-Backa, K., Luoma, A., Krook, E. (eds.) WIS 2012. CCIS, vol. 313, pp. 60–67. Springer, Heidelberg (2012). https://doi.org/10.1007/978-3-642-32850-3_6
8. Ravichandran, R., Sien, S.W., Patel, S.N., Kientz, J.A., Pina, L.R.: Making sense of sleep sensors: how sleep sensing technologies support and undermine sleep health. In: Proceedings of the Human Factors in Computing Systems (CHI 2017), pp. 6864–6875 (2017)

9. Föhr, T., et al.: Physical activity, heart rate variability–based stress and recovery, and subjective stress during a 9-month study period. Scandinavian J. Med. Sci. Sports **27**(6), 612–621 (2017)
10. Hallman, D.M., Ekman, A.H., Lyskov, E.: Changes in physical activity and heart rate variability in chronic neck–shoulder pain: monitoring during work and leisure time. Int. Arch. Occup. Environ. Health **87**(7), 735–744 (2013). https://doi.org/10.1007/s00420-013-0917-2
11. Parak, J., Korhonen, I.: Accuracy of Firstbeat Bodyguard 2 beat-to-beat heart rate monitor. White paper by Firstbeat Technologies Ltd. https://assets.firstbeat.com/firstbeat/uploads/2015/11/white_paper_bodyguard2_final1.pdf. Accessed 2 Sept 2019
12. Firstbeat Technologies: Firstbeat Lifestyle Assessment, Full Report. https://www.firstbeat.com/wp-content/uploads/2015/09/Lifestyle-Assessment-2016-full-report.pdf. Accessed 2 Sept 2019
13. Brooke, J.: SUS-A quick and dirty usability scale. In: Jordan, P.W., Thomas, B., Weerdmeester, B.A., McClelland, I.L. (eds.) Usability Evaluation in Industry, pp. 189–194. Taylor and Francis, London (1996)
14. Hassenzahl, M.: The interplay of beauty, goodness, and usability in interactive products. Hum. Comput. Interact. **19**(4), 319–349 (2004)
15. Whoqol Group: Development of the World Health Organization WHOQOL-BREF quality of life assessment. Psychological medicine **28**(3), 551–558 (1998)
16. Partala, T., Kallinen, A.: Understanding the most satisfying and unsatisfying user experiences: emotions, psychological needs, and context. Interact. Comput. **24**(1), 25–34 (2012)
17. Partala, T., Saari, T.: Understanding the most influential user experiences in successful and unsuccessful technology adoptions. Comput. Hum. Behav. **53**, 381–395 (2015)
18. Ryan, R.M., Deci, E.L.: Self-determination theory and the facilitation of intrinsic motivation, social development, and well-being. Am. Psychol. **55**(1), 68–78 (2000)
19. Sheldon, K.M., Elliot, A.J., Kim, Y., Kasser, T.: What is satisfying about satisfying events? Testing 10 candidate psychological needs. J. Pers. Soc. Psychol. **80**(2), 325–339 (2001)
20. Bangor, A., Kortum, P., Miller, J.: Determining what individual SUS scores mean: adding an adjective rating scale. J. Usability Stud. **4**(3), 114–123 (2009)
21. Consolvo, S., Klasnja, P., McDonald, D.W., Landay, J.A.: Designing for healthy lifestyles: design considerations for mobile technologies to encourage consumer health and wellness. Found. Trends Hum. Comput. Interact. **6**(3–4), 167–315 (2014)
22. Miyamoto, S.W., Henderson, S., Young, H.M., Pande, A., Han, J.J.: Tracking health data is not enough: a qualitative exploration of the role of healthcare partnerships and mHealth technology to promote physical activity and to sustain behavior change. JMIR mHealth uHealth **4**(1), 1–12 (2016)
23. Orji, R., Moffatt, K.: Persuasive technology for health and wellness: state-of-the-art and emerging trends. Health Inform. J. **24**(1), 66–91 (2018)

Developing a Novel Citizen-Scientist Smartphone App for Collecting Behavioral and Affective Data from Children Populations

Christos Maramis[1]([⊠]), Ioannis Ioakimidis[2], Vassilis Kilintzis[1],
Leandros Stefanopoulos[1], Eirini Lekka[1], Vasileios Papapanagiotou[3], Christos Diou[3],
Anastasios Delopoulos[3], Penio Kassari[4], Evangelia Charmandari[4],
and Nikolaos Maglaveras[5]

[1] Department of Medicine, Aristotle University of Thessaloniki, Thessaloniki, Greece
{chmaramis,billyk,lekka}@med.auth.gr, lstefano@auth.gr
[2] Department of Biosciences and Nutrition, Karolinska Institutet, Huddinge, Sweden
Ioannis.Ioakimidis@ki.se
[3] Department of Electrical and Computer Engineering, Aristotle University of Thessaloniki,
Thessaloniki, Greece
{vassilis,diou}@mug.ee.auth.gr, adelo@eng.auth.gr
[4] Biomedical Research Foundation, Academy of Athens, Athens, Greece
peniokassari@gmail.com, echarmand@med.uoa.gr
[5] Department of Industrial Engineering and Management Sciences, Northwestern University,
Evanston, USA
nikolaos.maglaveras@northwestern.edu

Abstract. The paradigm of citizen-science, i.e., scientific research that is conducted in whole or in part by non-professional scientists, has gained popularity lately, e.g., for the purpose of crowdsourced data collection. Smartphones with their abundance and ubiquity are perfectly suited and have been widely used for crowdsourced data collection in real life settings. The ongoing, EC-funded research programme named BigO exploits the citizen-science paradigm to collect behavioral (eating, sleeping and physical activity) and affective (mood) data from children populations by means of a novel smartphone application with the intention of developing a decision support system to assist public health authorities in effective policy making against childhood obesity. This paper presents the development – in the context of BigO – of the myBigO app, one of the first citizen-scientist smartphone applications addressed to children for behavioral and affective data collection. This includes the design, implementation, and deployment of myBigO app in a number of data collection studies as well as its preliminary evaluation with respect to technical robustness and user experience in the context of these studies.

Keywords: mHealth · Citizen-science · Crowdsourced data collection · Behavioral informatics · Children behavior

© ICST Institute for Computer Sciences, Social Informatics and Telecommunications Engineering 2020
Published by Springer Nature Switzerland AG 2020. All Rights Reserved
G. M. P. O'Hare et al. (Eds.): MobiHealth 2019, LNICST 320, pp. 294–302, 2020.
https://doi.org/10.1007/978-3-030-49289-2_23

1   Introduction

Citizen-science, a relatively new scientific paradigm where the general public is actively engaged in scientific research [1], has gained popularity during the last decade. A popular application of citizen-science is the *crowdsourced collection of data* (for example in hydrology [2]) for a variety of research purposes, in cases where conventional data collection methods are impractical or even impossible. Nowadays, smartphones demonstrate an unprecedented abundance and, owing to their continuous presence in everyday life, are perfectly suited for *ecological momentary data collection* tasks [3]. For this reason, smartphones are commonly exploited by citizen-science initiatives when crowdsourced data collection is needed. However, designing smartphone applications (or apps) for citizen-science projects is a challenging task, since the user engagement and effectiveness need to be taken into account [4].

Focusing on crowdsourcing, there are several citizen-science studies that have employed smartphone apps for the collection of *behavioral data*. For example, the SMART study [5] has used the Ethica[1] smartphone app to collect (1) self-reported physical activity and sedentary behavior data, and (2) sensor-acquired data such as location, inertial measurement unit (IMU) recordings, image/audio files, etc. from 317 adult citizen-scientists. The objective of the SMART study has been to analyze the collected data so as to translate the gained knowledge about active living into policy interventions. The Ethica app itself has been employed in the past by citizen-science initiatives in epidemiology [6]. When it comes to children, there exist past studies where they have been engaged as data collecting citizen-scientists (e.g., [7]). However, to the best of our knowledge there are few – if any – citizen-science efforts that developed smartphone apps specifically designed for children.

Using a similar rationale to [5], the ongoing research programme named BigO[2] relies on the citizen-science paradigm to collect data concerning the *eating, sleeping and physical activity behavior* of children populations by means of a novel smartphone app. BigO undertakes extensive crowdsourced data collection in 6 European cities. The behavioral patterns of the local children populations that will be extracted from the collected data will then be associated with a number of local extrinsic conditions as well as the local prevalence of childhood obesity. These associations will be employed by the decision support system of BigO so as to inform public health authorities about promising policies against childhood obesity.

This paper presents the development of one of the first citizen-scientist smartphone apps that are addressed to children, namely the *myBigO app*. The myBigO app has been developed to support the crowdsourced data collection activities of the BigO programme. The behavioral and affective data that are collected by the app are intended for further analysis in the scope of the BigO programme. The current paper covers (1) the design and implementation of the app; (2) the deployment of the app in a series of data collection studies; and (3) the preliminary evaluation of the app through the aforementioned studies with respect to technical robustness and user experience.

---

[1] https://www.ethicadata.com/about.

[2] https://bigoprogram.eu/.

2 Methods

The design of the myBigO app has been guided by (1) its *intended usage*, i.e., the collection of behavioral and affective data that are associated with obesity, (2) its *intended user group*, i.e., school-aged children, and (3) its *intended research paradigm*, i.e., citizen-science. These three guides have majorly impacted the eventual functionalities (see Sect. 2.2) and user interfaces (see Sect. 2.3) of the app. For instance, the modern design of the screens and the included features of the app were considered to be appropriate for the age group of its users, while two extra tabs (Maps and Stats tab) were inserted in the Main Screen of the app for the purpose of providing feedback to the users. The data to be collected were carefully selected (see Sect. 2.1) on the basis of unobtrusiveness (e.g., keeping popping questions to a minimum and promoting data collection in the background). All aforementioned design decisions were made with the objective of maintaining the engagement of the users so as to eventually maximize their effectiveness in data collection [4].

2.1 Collected Data

The myBigO app is able to collect data concerning a variety of behaviors of its users (namely, sleeping, eating and physical activity behavior) as well as their emotional state (or mood). Table 1 provides the specification of the behavioral and affective data that are collected. Regarding the data collection process, a hybrid approach was adopted, which includes:

- **Passive data collection.** Collection of objective data from smartphone sensors in the background (e.g., accelerometry measurements).
- **Active data collection.** Collection of objective and subjective data that requires active input from the user; this is further classified as: (1) the user-initiated collection of sensory data such as meal and food advertisement photographs, and (2) the self-reporting of subjective data through ecological momentary assessment (e.g., user mood).

2.2 Functionality

The functionalities that are offered by the myBigO app can be organized into 3 categories based on the context of use and these are outlined in the following subsections.

Registration
This refers to initial, one time use of the app to register the user into the BigO platform. The users go through a typical registration procedure (e.g., reviewing and agreeing to the terms and conditions, entering their registration code and selecting their nickname). The registration functionality entails a certain amount of data collection as well through a series of self-assessment questions. For instance, the sleep and wake-up times for weekdays and weekends (see Table 1) are reported by the user as part of the present functionality.

Table 1. Specification of the behavioral and affective data collected by the myBigO app.

Target data	Collected data description	Collection mode	Collection frequency
Sleep duration	Sleep & wake-up times in weekdays, sleep & wake-up times in weekends	Active; self-reported	Once (at registration)
Mood	User rating in a revised 5-point Wong-Baker scale [8]	Active; self-reported	Once daily
Location	Latitude, longitude, altitude, accuracy, bearing, speed	Passive; sensory	Every minute
IMU data	Measurements from accelerometer & gyroscope	Passive; sensory	5–25 Hz
Annotated meal photos	Meal photo with meal type, temperature, preparation & main ingredients	Active; sensory & self-reported	User defined
Annotated food ad photos	Food ad photo with location, size and context	Active; sensory & self-reported	User defined

Main Usage

This functionality becomes available through the *Main Screen* of the myBigO app, as soon as the registration is completed. The Main Screen consists of 4 tabs:

1. the *Action Tab* (default) initiates the process of meal and food advertisement photo acquisition and annotation (see Table 1)
2. the *Maps Tab* displays the locations where food advertisement photos have been captured
3. the *Stats Tab* presents statistics about the contribution of the user and her peers in photo collection, and
4. the *Settings Tab* allows the users to change their preferences and access app-related info.

Background Data Collection

This is a separate, non-interactive functionality of the myBigO app which transparently acquires measurements from the smartphone IMU and GPS receiver (see Table 1). This functionality covers the entirety of passive data collection by the myBigO app.

2.3 User Interfaces

The user interfaces (UI) of the myBigO app, i.e., the set of screens that implement the human-computer interaction within the app, have been carefully designed with the help of a professional usability expert. The screens that have been designed for the Main Usage functionality of the myBigO app are presented in the figures that follow with the help of screen captures from a running instance of the app. More specifically, Fig. 1 lists the tabs of the Main Screen, while Fig. 2 presents the screens that are associated with the active data collection in the myBigO app.

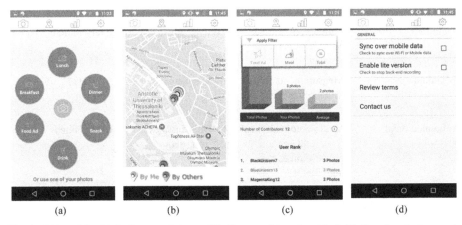

(a)   (b)   (c)   (d)

Fig. 1. Tabs of the Main Screen of the myBigO app – (a) action tab, initiating the photo acquisition and annotation functionality; (b) maps tab, displaying the location of the contributed food advertisements; (c) stats tab, presenting statistics about photos contributions; (d) settings tab.

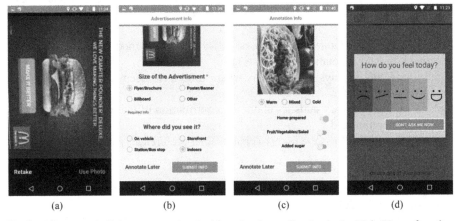

(a)   (b)   (c)   (d)

Fig. 2. UI screens & dialogues associated with active data collection in the Main Usage functionality of the myBigO app – (a) photo preview screen; (b) food advertisement annotation screen; (c) meal annotation screen; (d) mood dialogue.

2.4 Implementation Details

The myBigO app has been developed for Android smartphones running on Android 5.0 to 9.0. Before being released, the app was thoroughly tested in a number of iterative test cycles simulating actual use and putting emphasis on app stability. During the testing phase, SonarQube[3] and Firebase[4] were leveraged for static code analysis and bug tracking, respectively.

3 Results

This section provides information about the deployment of the myBigO app so far for data collection in the context of the BigO programme, along with the preliminary evaluation of the app with respect to the technical robustness and user experience.

3.1 Deployment Studies

Up to this point, the data collection activities of the BigO programme revolved around 3 private schools, namely the *Internationella Engelska Gymnasiet* (IEGS) in Stockholm (Sweden), *Ellinogermaniki Agogi* (EA) in Athens (Greece), and *Ekpaideutiria Mpakogianni* (EKP) in Larissa (Greece). Each school organized and conducted a number of different data collection actions (8 in total) with the myBigO app being the main data collection instrument. Informed consent was acquired from all the participating students in the high school, while in the case of the primary school (EA) informed ascent and consent was acquired from the participating students and their parents, respectively. For the most part, an organized participation strategy relying on school projects (e.g., short-term projects as part of the Physical Activity class) was employed for student recruitment. The overview of the 3 participating schools and the corresponding data collection actions is provided in Table 2.

Table 2. Overview of the 3 participating schools and the corresponding data collection actions.

School	Level	Location	Dates	Nr. participants
IEGS	High school	Stockholm (SE)	11.2017–05.2018	84
EA	Primary school	Athens (GR)	03.2018–06.2018	83
EKP	High school	Larissa (GR)	03.2018–06.2018	38

---

[3] https://www.sonarqube.org/.
[4] https://firebase.google.com/.

3.2 Technical Robustness

From a technical standpoint, the myBigO app performed considerably well in the previously described deployment studies. No major issues (e.g., problems rendering the app unusable) were reported, while minor issues, such as occasional crashes, were constantly monitored with the help of Firebase and/or reported by the school personnel via Redmine[5]. The recorded issues were investigated, prioritized and then resolved through regular updates of the app. The performance of the myBigO app in its primary task is indicated by the volume of behavioral and affective data that were eventually collected during the deployment studies. Table 3 summarizes the volume of data collected from each school using an abstract categorization of the main types of collected data. In the particular case of the primary school (EA), the food advertisements and the accelerometry data were not part of the data collection actions that were organized by the school – thus the corresponding N/A entries in Table 3.

Table 3. Volume of the main categories of behavior data that were collected per school during the deployment studies.

	Students (#)	Ad photos (#)	Meals photos (#)	Accelerometry (days)
IEGS	84	1886	122	93.2
EA	83	N/A	411	N/A
EKP	38	9	472	196.1
Total	**205**	**1895**	**1005**	**289.3**

3.3 User Experience

User experience is a concept from the field of Human-Computer Interaction which refers to the attitude and emotions of a user towards a product or system. The User Experience Questionnaire (UEQ) is a validated instrument for evaluating user experience [9] and it consists of 26 questions which are rated on a 7-point Likert scale [10]. The questions are grouped in 6 scales associated with distinct aspects/dimensions of user experience. Concerning the standard interpretation of a scale, scores between -0.8 and 0.8 represent a neural evaluation, while scores >0.8 (< -0.8) represent a positive (negative) evaluation [11]. The high-school students participating in the previously described deployment studies were asked to fill in the UEQ after they have stopped using the myBigO app. In total, 30 students completed the questionnaire. The aggregated results along each scale of the UEQ are visualized in Fig. 3. One can observe that the myBigO app received a positive reaction for half of the scales and a neutral reaction for the other half. In brief, the app was considered to be adequately efficient in what it does, easy to use and attractive; however, it did not provide enough stimuli or novel features to the users. Surprisingly,

---
[5] https://www.redmine.org/.

given the small amount of logged and reported technical problems, the users were not convinced about the dependability of the app.

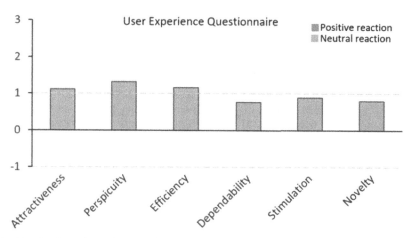

Fig. 3. Results from the evaluation of the user experience of the myBigO app along with 6 scales of the UEQ.

4   Conclusions

This paper has presented one of the first citizen-scientist smartphone apps that have been designed for children, namely the myBigO app. The app has been developed in the context of the BigO research programme with its primary goal being the collection of behavioral (eating, sleeping, and physical activity) as well as affective data from children populations. The myBigO app has already been successfully deployed in a series of data collection studies (in 3 European cities), providing the opportunity for the preliminary evaluation of the app with respect to technical robustness and user experience.

Additional evaluation covering other aspects of the myBigO app is still needed. This evaluation will be conducted in conjunction with the upcoming data collection actions of BigO, which will scale up the volume of collected behavioral and affective data. The successful utilization of the scale-up data for associating the behavioral patterns of the studied populations with local extrinsic conditions and local childhood obesity prevalence – to the aid of public health policy makers – will automatically validate the myBigO app. On top of that, our future plans include the enhancement of the app with features to support user engagement and more detailed logging of the collected data volume. Regarding user engagement, the need to improve user experience, especially with respect to stimulation and novelty, has been made evident from the conducted preliminary evaluation. To this direction, a gaming feature revolving around a data collection competition among citizen-scientists will be integrated in the myBigO app. The aforementioned detailed logging of the collected data will be also used for score calculations within the game.

Acknowledgements. The work leading to these results has received funding from the European Community's Health, demographic change and well-being Programme under Grant Agreement No. 727688, 01/12/2016–30/11/2020.

References

1. Socientize Consortium: Green paper on citizen science. Citizen Science for Europe. Towards a better society of empowered citizens and enhanced research, Brussels (2013)
2. Lowry, C.S., Fienen, M.N.: CrowdHydrology: crowdsourcing hydrologic data and engaging citizen scientists. Groundwater **51**, 151–156 (2013). https://doi.org/10.1111/j.1745-6584. 2012.00956.x
3. Burke, L.E., et al.: Ecological momentary assessment in behavioral research: addressing technological and human participant challenges. J. Med. Internet Res. **19** (2017). https://doi. org/10.2196/jmir.7138
4. Wald, D.M., Longo, J., Dobell, A.R.: Design principles for engaging and retaining virtual citizen scientists. Conserv. Biol. **30**, 562–570 (2016). https://doi.org/10.1111/cobi.12627
5. Katapally, T.R., et al: The SMART study, a mobile health and citizen science methodological platform for active living surveillance, integrated knowledge translation, and policy interventions: longitudinal study. JMIR Public Health Surveill. **4**, (2018). https://doi.org/10.2196/ publichealth.8953
6. Hashemian, M., Stanley, K., Osgood, N.: Leveraging H1N1 infection transmission modeling with proximity sensor microdata. BMC Med. Inform. Decis. Mak. **12**, 35 (2012). https://doi. org/10.1186/1472-6947-12-35
7. Eastman, L., Hidalgo-Ruz, V., Macaya-Caquilpán, V., Nuñez, P., Thiel, M.: The potential for young citizen scientist projects: a case study of Chilean schoolchildren collecting data on marine litter. Rev. Gestão Costeira Integrada - J. Integr. Coast. Zone Manag. **14**, 569–579 (2014)
8. Wong, D.L., Baker, C.M.: Smiling face as anchor for pain intensity scales. Pain **89**, 295 (2001). https://doi.org/10.1016/S0304-3959(00)00375-4
9. Laugwitz, B., Held, T., Schrepp, M.: Construction and evaluation of a user experience questionnaire. In: Holzinger, A. (ed.) USAB 2008. LNCS, vol. 5298, pp. 63–76. Springer, Heidelberg (2008). https://doi.org/10.1007/978-3-540-89350-9_6
10. Likert, R.: A technique for the measurement of attitudes. Arch. Psychol. **22**(140), 55 (1932)
11. Schrepp, M., Hinderks, A., Thomaschewski, J.: Applying the User Experience Questionnaire (UEQ) in different evaluation scenarios. In: Marcus, A. (ed.) DUXU 2014. LNCS, vol. 8517, pp. 383–392. Springer, Cham (2014). https://doi.org/10.1007/978-3-319-07668-3_37

Data Management within mHealth Environments

Intelligent Combination of Food Composition Databases and Food Product Databases for Use in Health Applications

Alexander Muenzberg[1,2(✉)], Janina Sauer[1,2], Andreas Hein[2], and Norbert Roesch[1]

[1] University of Applied Science Kaiserslautern, Amerikastr. 1, 66482 Zweibrücken, Germany
{alexander.muenzberg,janina.sauer,norbert.roesch}@hs-kl.de
[2] Carl von Ossietzky University Oldenburg, Ammerländer Heerstr. 114-118,
26129 Oldenburg, Germany
{alexander.muenzberg,janina.sauer,andreas.hein}@uni-oldenburg.de

Abstract. The necessity of using food data in mobile health applications is often linked with difficulties. In Europe no standardized and quality-controlled food product databases are accessible. Data from third party sources are often incomplete and have to be checked carefully before use for errors and inconsistencies. The purpose of this approach is to improve data quality and to increase information density by developing a dedicated food data warehouse. By using the extract, transform and load processes known from data warehouse technologies, multiple data sources will be combined, inserted and evaluated. The data is cleaned up by using data profiling techniques. Data mining methods are used to merge the datasets from food composition databases and food product databases to increase information density. The aim is to analyze, if and how Big Data technologies can increase performance of data processing significantly.

Keywords: Food data · Data analysis · Data mining · Big Data

1 Introduction

The use of mobile health applications (health apps) is constantly increasing in the app stores of mobile platforms and many of them are focused on nutrition. However, no standardized sources of food product data are available in Europe with complete information of available food products on the market. Most app developers are dependent on their own data or on data collections of third parties. Such datasets are often incomplete or have not been sufficiently checked to guarantee a data quality which is sufficient for medical use. Missing or incomplete datasets can have negative effects on the data quality and therefore on the quality of the app. This circumstance reduces the user's trust in the app to a high degree. Provider of quality-controlled and verified food datasets are limited to a few and usually offer their data at a very high fee [1, 2].

Within the project "Digital Services in Nutritional Counselling" (DiDiER) [3], funded by the German Federal Ministry of Education and Research (BMBF), a food data

G. M. P. O'Hare et al. (Eds.): MobiHealth 2019, LNICST 320, pp. 305–319, 2020.
https://doi.org/10.1007/978-3-030-49289-2_24

warehouse system was developed, which combines the food data of different, mostly free or public data sources and stores them in a uniform data format and data structure. Using data profiling tools, errors and duplicates were detected and eliminated [1]. By combining food composition databases with food product databases and creating ontologies between their data elements, inconsistencies among the data are detected and the datasets are completed. In order to obtain hidden information of useful value from the data and ontologies, data mining methods are used.

2   State of the Art

2.1   Food Data Warehouse

The Food Data Warehouse (FDWH) contains a collection of information about natural foods, packaged foods and branded products. The data was obtained from the sources of various platform operators and food manufacturers. The data was extracted from the external data sources, transformed into a uniform data structure as well as data format and then loaded into a central relational database by the Extract, Transform and Load process (ETL process) known from data warehousing. The FDWH currently contains data with information about approximately 40,000 foods from the following extern data sources [1].

– Food Composition Databases

- German Federal Food Key (Bundeslebensmittelschlüssel [4]
- Swiss nutrition database (Schweizer Nährwertedatenbank) [5].

– Food Product Databases

- WikiFood.eu [6]
- das-ist-drin.de [7]
- OpenFoodFacts.org [8]
- FoodRepo.org [9]
- Danone and its subsidiary Nutritcia [10, 11].

Data profiling methods were used to detect and correct defective characters, incorrect data formats and duplicates of data records. Data profiling includes the following tasks in detail.

– Checking patterns and data types
– Outlier detection
– Characterization of missing and preset values
– Data rule analysis (e.g. recognition of values corresponding to certain regular expressions)
– Analysis of column properties (validity check of all values in a table column)
– Analysis of value dependencies across columns
– Recognition of functional dependencies or foreign key dependencies in databases.

Using special metrics, which enable data quality to be measured, quantifiable quality values in terms of completeness and consistency were determined in order to obtain an initial assessment of the data quality improvement using the above-mentioned data profiling methods [1].

2.2 Food Information for Health Applications

For the analysis of food intolerances and allergies, correct and complete lists of ingredients are required e.g. for the detection of related elicitors. Although it is required in the EU that information on 14 major allergens must be labelled by manufacturers on food packages, also other ingredients and additives have the potential to provoke allergic reactions [1]. In the field of Frailty Syndrome, the focus is on energy intake. Information about nutrition facts, in particular of energy, fat, protein and carbohydrates is needed. Information about Nutrition Facts is important for a wide range of health fields, such as healthy nutrition and fitness as well as the prevention of diseases such as obesity, cancer, diabetes, heart attack or stroke [12].

2.3 Differences Between Food Composition and Food Product Databases

Food Composition Databases (FCDB) provide the name of foods in conjunction with their nutritional information. Unlike Food Product Databases (FPDB), FCDBs do not provide branded products but natural food without branding. The following nutritional information is provided using FCDB data [5].

- Energy value in kilo joules (kJ) and kilo calories (kcal)

  - calculated from the sum of the kJ values of

    - carbohydrates 17 kJ/g
    - protein 17 kJ/g
    - fat 37 kJ/g
    - alcohol 29 kJ/g
    - food fibers 8 kJ/g.

- values of macronutrients

  - carbohydrates, food fibers, fat, cholesterol, protein, alcohol, water.

- values of vitamins

  - vitamins a, b1, b2, b6, b12, c, d, e, etc.

- values of the minerals among other things

  - sodium, salt, potassium, chloride, calcium, magnesium, iron, iodine, zinc, etc.

In contrast to the FCDB, the FPDB data also provides the information in the following.

- brand
- origin
- Global Trade Item Number (GTIN)
- information about packaging and special features
- content quantity (for packaged products)
- ingredient lists
- allergens requiring labelling.

2.4 Food Information Service

The Food Information Service (FIS) is a webservice that provides FDWH data via an Application Programming Interface (API) [13]. The FIS receives a request from the application with username and salted password hash [14] (for secure authorization) as well as a search string. Within the FIS, the identifiers (IDs) of suitable foods with reference to the search string are selected and returned to the requesting application. A reference of the food to the search string exists if the search string completely or partially corresponds to the food name, the manufacturer name or the category as well as the soundex values (code generated by the sound of a name) [15] of the search string and the food name correspond. Based on the selected IDs, the application can now request more detailed information about the associated food. Both the requests and the answers provided by the FIS are in the human- and machine-readable JavaScript Object Notation Format (JSON format) [1, 16].

2.5 Ontologies Between Food Data

In the context of information theory, ontologies are special data models that formally define data objects of a subject area [17]. When evaluating the data of the FDWH such data models are generated in order to extract specific knowledge about individual data elements, with the help of which it can be recognized whether it concerns a consistent value. Furthermore, in many cases missing values in the databases can be derived with the help of such models.

In the following, the ingredient lists, which are available in text form, are preprocessed using Text Data Mining (Text Mining) [18] so that further ontologies can be formed between the FCDB and FPDB datasets and their attributes in order to extract missing information in data as far as possible from other similar or identical datasets.

3 Methods

3.1 Preprocessing of Ingredient Lists by Text Mining

Before information about the ingredients can be generated by the food data records, the ingredient lists, which are available in text form, must be processed using text mining methods. The supplied ingredient lists of the external data sources were also stored in the FDWH as comma separated text strings, for presentation in health apps. In the further course, the individual ingredients are extracted from these strings.

By tokenization [18], the ingredient lists are split into individual ingredient character strings at the points where a predefined character (in this case a comma) occurs. The ingredient strings are stored separately related to the food ID to which the ingredient belongs. All strings are stored in lower case. These strings, or parts of them, that correspond to numeric values, special characters, and specific words from a stopword list are then removed. Stopwords are filler words, adjectives and articles (e.g. with, a, the, big, etc.) as well as words that describe a processing form of an ingredient (e.g. cooked; for the entry "cooked egg"). Ingredient lists often contain additional explanations on quantity relationships using numerical or percentage values. After removal of stop words, double ingredients may appear in the tokenized table and will be deleted afterwards (Fig. 1).

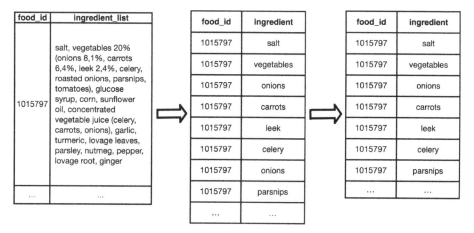

Fig. 1. Tokenization of the content list including stopword removal and removal of duplicates

Stemming generate the word stem of a certain word [18]. In order to be able to compare ingredients and FCDB Food names, the word stems of the ingredients are generated by using the snowball stemmer method [19]. Differently named ingredient words of the same meaning are linked language-spreading to a representative english term. For example, the North German word "Apfelsine" means "Orange" in Southern Germany. These two words are combined with the corresponding English translation "orange". Thereby the library Thesarus [20] helps, which contains synonyms of many words. In addition, the Google Translate Library [21] is used to translate and a specially created library with synonymous food names. By linking the words of the same meaning and the stemmed words a new linking table is created (Fig. 2). Using this linking table, all individual ingredients can now be converted into a standardized main term. This will later help to identify the same ingredients in different ingredient lists.

main_term	synonym
orange	orange
orange	apfelsine
orange	orang
orange	apfelsin
...	...

Fig. 2. Linking of ingredients with synonyms and word stems

3.2   Method for Similarity Analysis Between Datasets

In order to achieve a higher information density of the food data, a scheme was developed that combines the information from the FCDB and the FPDB. To explain it, the following scenario is considered.

Scenario. A user of a health app, which provides information on food ingredients and nutritional values, uses the app's search function to search for the drink named "Cola" and enters this name in a search mask of the app. In the background, the app receives various results from the FDWH via the FIS, including the food named "Coladrink" from the FCDB and the two (fictitious) branded products named "Cola X" and "YZcoke". By selecting one of the displayed foods, the user can display its information on ingredients

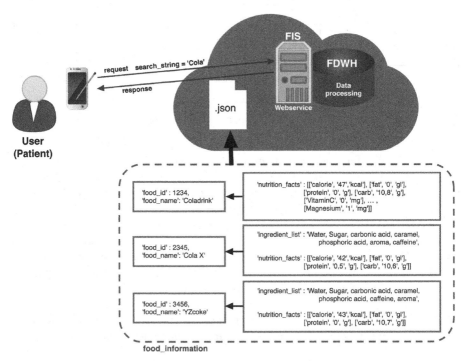

Fig. 3. FIS response (from food information from the FDWH) in JSON format, which matches to the search term "Cola"

and nutritional values. However, the food Coladrink from the FCDB does not provide any ingredients and the two foods from the FPDB, Cola X and YZcoke do not provide all Nutrition Facts that Coladrink provides (Fig. 3). It would be useful if the different information of similar foods would be combined and contained in each food dataset. For example, the information of the ingredient lists would then also be contained in the food data set of Coladrink and the information about vitamin C and magnesium (among others) would also be contained in the food data sets of Cola X and YZCoke (see Fig. 6). However, for this must be developed a method that recognizes similar foods on the basis of the given information.

In order to develop a scheme that links the information of such similar foods with each other, the attribute ranges presented in the following list are analyzed to identify similarly composed foods.

– Food names:

  • Parts of the food names are identical

– Ingredient lists:

  • products with the same or to a large extent the same ingredients

– Nutrition values:

  • The nutrition values are in the same range.

For the foods in the above scenario, the analysis of the food names shows that in the textstrings "Coladrink" and·"Cola X" the same substring "Cola" is contained. The ingredient lists of Cola X and YZcoke are only different in the order of the last two ingredients (see Fig. 3). Furthermore, the distance between the nutritional values of energy, fat, proteins and carbohydrates among the foods is small, so that all three foods are similar in this attribute range (see Fig. 3).

With the help of the data mining method of decision tree generation [22], decision trees were developed on the basis of 1000 food test data (Fig. 4 and Fig. 5), with the help of which it is determined to what extent the individual ingredients and nutritional values may differ, so that the foods can be regarded as similar in these attribute ranges.

The two ingredient lists of a food pair, food X and food Y, are transmitted to the decision tree in Fig. 4. First, it will be checked if both ingredient lists contain more than two ingredients (the length of the lists must be greater than two). The first three ingredients of both lists must be identical. If the lists are greater than three elements and do not differ in the number of elements by more than three elements, all other elements (from the fourth to the last ingredient) are compared with each other. Finally, the food pair is classified as similar in the attribute range of the ingredient lists, if the number of elements of the ingredient in the larger of the two ingredient lists is less than 15 and the ingredients are contained in both ingredients lists except for a maximum of one element (the order does not matter). If the number of elements in the smaller of the two ingredient lists is greater than 15 elements, the ingredients must be contained in both ingredients lists up to a maximum of two elements.

The decision tree in Fig. 5 receives as input the nutritional values carbohydrates, fat, proteins (each in gram per 100 g) and energy (in kcal per 100 g) of food X and food Y. These values of the both foods are compared with each other. The foods are similar in the attribute range of the nutritional values if none of the compared nutritional value pairs differ by more than the value 10. The nutritional values for carbohydrates, fat, proteins and energy are the most widely contained nutrition facts in the food data sets.

For the similarity analysis of the food names, the individual words of the food names of two foods are tokenized and filtered with the help of stopword lists (as already described in Sect. 3.1). The words of both food names are then compared with each

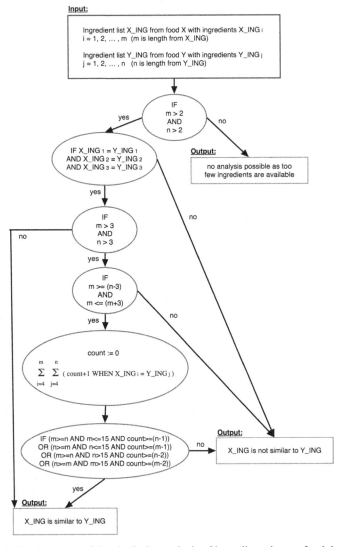

Fig. 4. Decision tree of the similarity analysis of ingredients in two food datasets

other. If at least two words in the two food names are identical, the food is classified as similar in the name attribute range.

If two foods are similar in at least two of the attribute ranges, their data sets are considered to be similar overall. This fact is true by the pairs Coladrink and X Cola as well as with X Cola and YZcoke (see Fig. 3). The similarity of X Cola to the other two foods results in a transitive dependency, so that the foods Coladrink and YZcoke are considered similar to each other. Finally, the following scheme is summarized with the help of which all food pairs of the FDWH can be analyzed for their similarity.

1. Similarity analysis of food names between all foods of the FPDB among themselves
2. Similarity analysis of the ingredients between all food products of the FPDB using the decision tree in Fig. 4
3. Similarity analysis of the nutritional values between all foods of the FPDB using the decision tree in Fig. 5
4. Similarity analysis of the food names between all foods of the FCDB among each other
5. Similarity analysis of the nutritional values between all foods of the FCDBs among themselves whose similarity of the food names is already confirmed by the analysis in 4. using the decision tree in Fig. 5
6. Similarity analysis of food names between FPDB and FCDB foods
7. Similarity analysis of nutritional values between all foods of FPDB and FCDB whose similarity of food names is confirmed by the analysis in 6. Already confirmed using the decision tree in Fig. 5
8. Determination of foods that were classified as similar in two of the similarity analyses in different attribute ranges
9. Determination of transitive dependencies between similar food pairs.

If no similarity is confirmed after the analysis according to 4. or 6., an analysis according to 5. or 7. is no longer necessary because at least two similarities must occur in different attribute ranges and the foods of the FCDB have no lists of ingredients and can therefore only be analyzed in two attribute ranges.

The IDs of the foods whose data sets were classified as similar overall are stored in a special database table linked with each other. The FIS is modified so that it obtains missing information of a food data set from a linked food data set and delivers it to the requesting app (Fig. 6).

In the above scenario, this means that when the user selects the entry Coladrink, the ingredients of the other two linked foods are also displayed. If he selects one of the other two foods, additional nutritional values of the FCDB data set Coladrink will be displayed which are not contained in the selected data set.

If a specific nutritional value of the linked data sets Y and Z (e.g. carbohydrate value of Y and carbohydrate value of Z) is to be displayed for a data set X, the mean value of the supplied information (mean value of carbohydrate value of Y and Z) is calculated. Ingredients are only obtained from linked data sets if the ingredient list of the selected food dataset is missing, so that no existing entry is falsified. For FCDB foods where ingredient information is missing, all ingredients from linked data sets are included. Now it can happen that this information does not correspond exactly to the food the user is looking for in the health app, but the user still has the important information which ingredients might be present in the food (this circumstance must be specially marked by the FIS or the displaying app). Now, for example, a nutritionist who looks at this information, in the case of a food allergy, can take a closer look at such a food data set if an occurrence of the allergen is apparent from the ingredient list (even if the occurrence was only vaguely determined) and the user of the app who suffers from the allergy can avoid eating the food for its own safety.

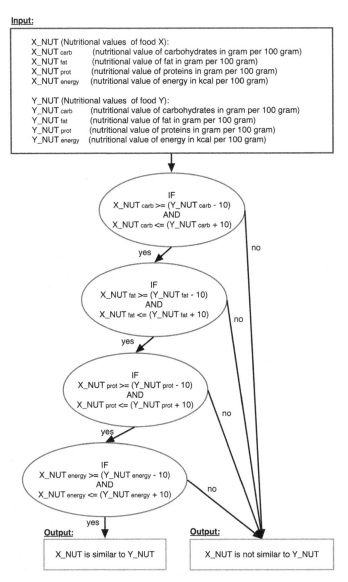

Fig. 5. Decision tree of the similarity analysis of nutrition values in two food datasets

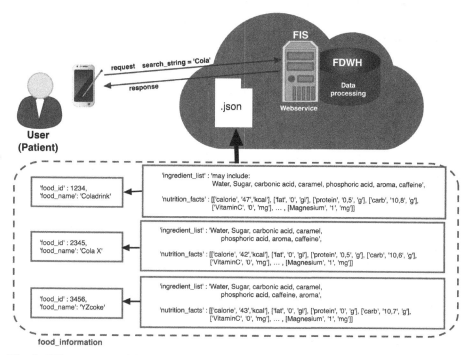

Fig. 6. FIS response which matches the search term "cola", with foods whose information has been completed with the help of similarity analysis

3.3 Using Big Data Technologies to Increase Performance

By comparing and mapping all data sets with each other using decision trees, conventional data analysis frameworks and tools quickly reach their performance limits. For example, the similarity analysis of the food names of 1000 food data sets already took more than 15 min. With an increased number of food data sets, the time taken by nested iterations during data processing increases exponentially. By using the Big Data Framework Spark of the Apache Foundation [23] it is possible to process the data sets very quickly with the help of special techniques (map, reduce, filter, text mining methods, etc.) and so-called lambda functions (anonymous functions without names that directly provide the return value) [24]. With Spark the data can be processed on different computing clusters directly in the main memory with the help of resilient distributed datasets (RDD) [23]. For example, RDDs can be represented and edited as data frames, which are known to developers of the programming language Python [25], which is often used in the data science field. Spark can be integrated into Python using the library PySpark. By operating on the data frames with the help of the PySpark library, the execution time is minimized many times over. Figure 7 shows a code snippet, as example for the similarity analysis of food names, in the programming language Python, using the PySpark library and using lambda functions. The food names were selected from a comma separated values file (csv file) and stored as RDDs. Further, the names were tokenized (splitted in single terms by space character) and stopwords were eliminated in each tokenized term.

The terms were compared to each other to determine similar name parts. The results, which name pairs are similar to each other, are written into a new csv file.

```
rdd = sc.textFile(
        ,data.csv').map(lambda line :line.split(,,`))
data_frame = rdd.toDF(['x_food_id', 'y_food_id',
                      'x_food_name', 'y_food_name'])
tokenizer = Tokenizer(inputCol=,x_food_name`,
                      outputCol=,x_vector')
data_frame = tokenizer.transform(data_frame)
tokenizer = Tokenizer(inputCol="y_food_name",
                      outputCol="y_vector")
data_frame = tokenizer.transform(data_frame)
remover = StopWordsRemover()
remover.loadDefaultStopWords('german')
remover.setInputCol("x_vector")
remover.setOutputCol("x_vector_without_stopw")
data_frame = remover.transform(data_frame)
remover.setInputCol("y_vector")
remover.setOutputCol("y_vector_without_stopw")
data_frame = remover.transform(data_frame)
differencer = udf(lambda x, y: list(set(x) - set(y)), Ar-
rayType(StringType()))
data_frame = data_frame.withColumn(
        'difference', differencer('x_vector_without_stopw',
        'y_vector_without_stopw'))
comparer = udf(lambda x, y, z: not len((set(x) - set(z)))
              == 0 and not len((set(y) - set(z))) == 0)
data_frame = data_frame.withColumn(
            'comparing', comparer('x_vector_without_stopw',
            'y_vector_without_stopw', 'difference'))
result_data_frame = data_frame.filter(
                    data_frame["comparing"] == True)
result_data_frame.toPandas().to_csv('new_data.csv')
```

Fig. 7. Code snippet as example for the similarity analysis of food names

4 Evaluation

To evaluate the similarity analysis, 1000 food test data, of which 200 dataset pairs had to be classified as similar, were evaluated by computer-based similarity analysis. The result shows that the analysis of the ingredients of 1000 foods has classified 249 dataset pairs as similar in this attribute range. The analysis of the nutritional values identified 207 similar dataset pairs and those of the Food Names 502 pairs. A total of 196 food data set pairs were classified as similar, including transitive dependencies. Only four data sets were not classified. This results in a recognition rate of 98% for the overall similarity analysis (Fig. 8). An incorrect similarity classification of dissimilar data sets did not take place.

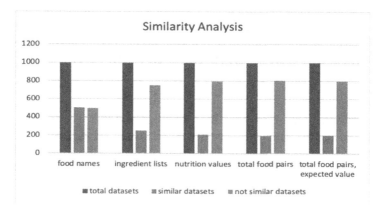

Fig. 8. Results of similarity analysis using test data

By using the Big Data Framework Spark and the additional Lambda functions used, the execution time of the similarity analyses was reduced by a factor of 90[1] (Fig. 9).

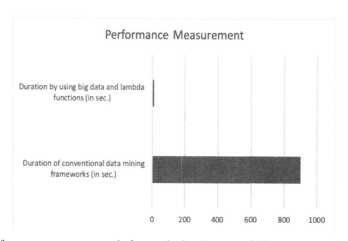

Fig. 9. Performance measurement before and after the use of big data technologies for the similarity analysis of food names

---

[1] On a single cluster system with 4×2.5 gigahertz (GHz) processor and 16 gigabyte (GB) main memory.

5 Conclusion and Outlook

In order to deliver food data sets of sufficiently good data quality to e-health apps, the data sets of several data sources from both FCDBs and FPDBs were standardized and stored in a standardized data format in the FDWH. The FIS is used to deliver the data in the FDWH to the respective apps. Using data profiling methods, erroneous and duplicate data sets were detected and corrected or eliminated [1]. Data mining methods were used to link information from similar data sets in order to achieve a significant increase in information density. The evaluation with test data showed that the methods used achieved a high degree of recognition of the similarity analyses. By linking data sets through the similarity analysis, it can happen that ingredients and nutritional data are not determined 100% accurately. Nevertheless, these data can serve the experts in medical settings (nutritionists, physicians) as clues for a diagnosis [26]. The processing of food data records has shown that the time taken to process data increases exponentially with conventional data mining methods, as the amount of data records increases and thus the performance of the data processing system decreases, even if the 40,000 data records already stored are not yet classified as "Big Data". The number of food data records is constantly increasing as the amount of data in the data sources increases and new data sources are added. For these reasons, the use of Big Data technologies is unavoidable. This use has already resulted in a considerable increase in data processing performance.

In the further course of the DiDiER project, the quality improvement of the data sets is to be further promoted with the help of machine learning and the detection of inconsistencies. The aim is to achieve the greatest possible coverage of high-quality food information. In a study of the project, the methods used will be evaluated progressively.

References

1. Muenzberg, A., Sauer, J., Hein, A., Roesch, N.: The use of ETL and data profiling to integrate data and improve quality in food databases. In: 2018 14th International Conference on Wireless and Mobile Computing, Networking and Communications (WI Mob), pp. 231–238 (2018). https://doi.org/10.1109/wimob.2018.8589081
2. Arens-Volland, A., Roesch, N., Feidert, F., Herbst, R., Moesges, R.: Change frequency of ingredient descriptions and free-of labels of food items concern food allergy sufferers. Allergy: Eur. J. Allergy Clin. Immunol. **65**, 394 (2010). https://doi.org/10.1111/j.1398-9995.2010. 02393.x
3. Elfert, P., Eichelberg, M., Tröger, J., Britz, J., Alexandersson, J., et al.: DiDiER digitized services in dietry counselling for people with increased health risk related to malnutrition and food allergies. In: IEEE Symposium on Computers and Communications (ISCC), pp. 100–104. IEEE (2017)
4. Max Rubner Institue (MRI) Karlsruhe: Bundeslebensmittelschlüssel. https://www.mri.bund. de/de/service/datenbanken/bundeslebensmittelschluessel/. Accessed 10 May 2019
5. Schweizer Nährwertedatenbank. https://www.naehrwertdaten.ch/. Accessed 10 May 2019
6. WikiFood: Knowing what's inside, the Wiki for foodstuffs. http://www.wikifood.eu/wikifood/ en/struts/welcome.do. Accessed 10 Mar 2019
7. snoopmedia GmbH, das ist drin: gemeinsam besser leben. http://das-ist-drin.de/. Accessed 12 May 2019
8. OpenFoodFacts – World. https://world.openfoodfacts.org. Accessed 12 May 2019
9. The Open Food Repo. https://www.foodrepo.org/. Accessed 12 May 2019

10. Danone GmbH. http://www.danone.de/. Accessed 12 May 2019
11. Nutricia GmbH. http://www.nutricia.de/. Accessed 12 May 2019
12. Biesalski, H.K., Pirlich, M., Bischoff, S., Weimann, A.: Ernährungsmedizin: Nach dem Curriculum Ernährungsmedizin der Bundesärztekammer, 5th edn. Thieme, Stuttgart (2017)
13. Upwork. https://www.upwork.com/hiring/development/intro-to-apis-what-is-an-api/. Accessed 12 May 2019
14. Eckert, C.: IT-Sicherheit: Konzepte – Verfahren – Protokolle, 7th edn. Oldenbourg Verlag, München (2012)
15. Ourcodeworld. https://ourcodeworld.com/articles/read/249/implementation-of-the-soundex-algorithm-function-in-different-programming-languages. Accessed 12 May 2019
16. Friesen, J.: Java XML and JSON, 1st edn. Apress, New York (2016)
17. Hochschule Augsburg: Glossar. https://glossar.hs-augsburg.de/Ontologie. Accessed 12 May 2019
18. Hotho, A., Nuernberger, A., Paaß, G.: A brief survey of text mining. LDV Forum - GLDV J. Comput. Linguist. Lang. Technol. **20**, 19–62 (2005)
19. Korenius, T., Laurikkala, J., Järvelin, K., Juhola, M.: Stemming and lemmatization in the clustering of finnish text documents. In: Proceedings of the Thirteenth ACM International Conference on Information and knowledge management (CIKM 2004), pp. 625–633. ACM, New York (2004). http://dx.doi.org/10.1145/1031171.1031285
20. Thesarus. https://www.thesaurus.com/. last accessed 2019/05/12
21. Google Cloud. https://cloud.google.com/translate/docs/. Accessed 12 May 2019
22. Cleve, J., Lämmel, U.: Data Mining, 1st edn. De Gruyter Verlag, Berlin (2014)
23. Apache Spark. https://spark.apache.org/. Accessed 12 May 2019
24. Python-Kurs. https://www.python-kurs.eu/lambda.php. Accessed 12 May 2019
25. Python. https://www.python.org/. Accessed 12 May 2019
26. Roesch, N.: Der Einsatz von Informations - und Kommunikationstechnologie bei Nahrungsmittelallergie. Shaker Verlag, Aachen (2010)

Labeling of Activity Recognition Datasets: Detection of Misbehaving Users

Alessio Vecchio$^{(\boxtimes)}$, Giada Anastasi, Davide Coccomini, Stefano Guazzelli,
Sara Lotano, and Giuliano Zara

Dip. di Ingegneria dell'Informazione, University of Pisa, Pisa, Italy
alessio.vecchio@unipi.it

Abstract. Automatic recognition of user's activities by means of wearable devices is a key element of many e-health applications, ranging from rehabilitation to monitoring of elderly citizens. Activity recognition methods generally rely on the availability of annotated training sets, where the traces collected using sensors are labelled with the real activity carried out by the user. We propose a method useful to automatically identify misbehaving users, i.e. the users that introduce inaccuracies during the labeling phase. The method is semi-supervised and detects misbehaving users as anomalies with respect to accurate ones. Experimental results show that misbehaving users can be detected with more than 99% accuracy.

Keywords: Activity recognition · Wearable device · Machine learning

1 Introduction

In the last years, we assisted to the proliferation of a large variety of wearable devices such as smart-wristbands, smart-watches, and smart-shoes. All these devices are equipped with sensors and are thus able to provide a rich amount of information about their users. In this context, a significant effort has been devoted to the design and development of methods useful to automatically recognize the activities carried out by people [14,17]. By recognizing the activities of daily living (ADLs), higher-level goals can be achieved. Examples include customization of the environment depending on users' actions (e.g., in a smart-home or in a smart-factory), monitoring of patients' conditions (e.g. to detect an increased sedentary style or falls of elderly citizens) [1,6,7,25], or automated logging of training sessions [4,26]. Many methods rely on machine learning techniques, which must be properly trained to operate successfully. In general, a dataset is collected in a controlled or semi-controlled environment and used to train a system. Then, the trained system is used to recognize the users' activities during the operational phase. Rather obviously, the availability of training datasets characterized by high quality is a necessary condition for obtaining accurate recognition results [27].

© ICST Institute for Computer Sciences, Social Informatics and Telecommunications Engineering 2020
Published by Springer Nature Switzerland AG 2020. All Rights Reserved
G. M. P. O'Hare et al. (Eds.): MobiHealth 2019, LNICST 320, pp. 320–331, 2020.
https://doi.org/10.1007/978-3-030-49289-2_25

Training datasets are generally produced by collecting movement data from a set of users, and then by manually annotating the resulting traces. This process is time consuming and characterized by inaccuracies. The presence of errors in the ground truth negatively impacts the learning phase, and in turn the accuracy of the whole method. Some tools have been proposed to ease the annotation process, e.g. by suggesting the most probable labels to the operator who, most of the time, must simply confirm one of the options [9]. The operator may also be assisted by tools which, during the labeling phase, show a video recorded at the time of the data collection, as an easy way to detect possible errors. Studies demonstrated that assisted labeling is less error-prone and less time-consuming in comparison to a completely manual procedure.

In other cases, the dataset is generated according to a crowdsourcing-based approach, with normal users responsible for both collecting movement data, by means of miniaturized Inertial Measurement Units (IMUs), and labeling the traces. On one hand, crowdsourcing makes possible the creation of large datasets characterized by the presence of a significant number of individuals. On the other hand, the chances of introducing inaccuracies in the dataset get increased by the inclusion of non-professional operators in the process.

In this paper, we propose a method for automatically recognizing the presence of inaccuracies in the labeling phase. In particular, we suppose that users may introduce errors during the labeling phase of their own data. Such inaccuracies can be deliberately introduced by a malicious user who wants to corrupt the dataset, or simply as a consequence of the lack of care during the annotation process. The proposed method relies on one-class classification techniques to understand if one of the users labels his/her data in a way that is significantly different from the other users. Results show that such anomalous users can be identified with more than 99% of accuracy.

2   Related Work

As mentioned, some tools have been proposed in the last years for reducing the effort during the annotation process.

In [16], a data collection tool that allows semi-automated labeling is presented. The tool includes the possibility to manually check and correct labels, and focuses on activity data collected by means of inertial measurements units, pressure insoles, and cameras. The smart annotation tool relies on edge detection, concerning the signal produced by pressure sensors, to achieve a reduction of annotation costs. The tool also helps the operator to synchronize videos and IMU-generated data with the traces produced by pressure sensors. According to the study, the labeling time can be reduced by 83% when using the tool.

The consistency of annotations related to data collected by sensors on a smartphone was studied in [10]. The main goal was to relate the daily behavior of students with their academic performance, using information about their locations and movements. The analyzed data consist of a label, which represents the user's annotation, and the physical location saved by the GPS. First, clusters are obtained by grouping physically close locations. Then, for each user, the consistency of obtained clusters is calculated. Consistency is based on entropy, which considers the number of different labels within a cluster and the number of their occurrences. Considering that the annotations are made by inexperienced users, the results obtained have a reasonable level of consistency (69%). However, by means of semantic analyses, it is possible to obtain a slightly higher level of consistency, equal to 74%. The study mostly focuses on correct labeling of locations.

A method for filtering inaccuracies in a training dataset is described in [2]. In the considered scenario, a trained wearable device – the source device – is used to train a new device – the target device The motivation is that people change wearable devices rather frequently and the knowledge of past devices could be transferred on new ones to reduce the effort required from the user. Initially, source and target device work together while the user carries out his/her activities of daily living. During this period, the predicted label of the source device is transferred to the target device. Then, self-paced learning is used to reduce the impact of inaccuracies [13].

Other tools useful to ease annotation of videos are described in [15,18]. An evaluation of different annotation methods is presented in [23].

In the end, the vast majority of the above mentioned studies, try to reduce the amount of errors introduced during the labeling phase, by assisting the user in different forms. Little attention has been devoted to automatic detection of inaccuracies in datasets, which are used in an always increasing number of studies in the e-health domain.

3   Method

The idea behind the proposed method is to recognize misbehaving, untruthful users as anomalies with respect to a set of truthful ones. In particular, a model of truthful users (TUs) is defined using one-class classification (OCC) methods. Then, the model can be used to recognize untruthful users (UUs) as instances that do not belong to the truthful class.

3.1   One-Class Classification

In machine learning, OCC methods are able to define a model of a single class – the positive class. Training of OCC methods is semi-supervised and requires only samples of the positive class. The absence of non-positive instances during the training phase makes the problem harder with respect to traditional classifiers, as defining the boundaries of the positive class cannot rely on counter-examples [11,12].

OCC methods are particularly useful whenever obtaining non-positive instances is difficult. For example, the normal operational status of an aircraft can be easily observed, while instances of faulty ones are typically unavailable or not common. Another situation where OCC methods are particularly useful is when the negative class is not well-defined: while a news website can be

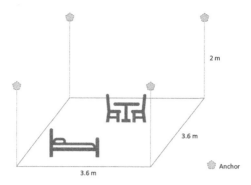

Fig. 1. Room setup.

reasonably identified, all non-news website belong to a such large and diverse set of possible categories that they cannot be easily modeled using traditional classification methods.

The proposed approach relies on OCC mostly because UUs may behave in many different ways, and this makes UUs not easily classifiable. For instance, some malicious users could tag all running activities as walking ones, i.e. they could be systematical in introducing errors during the labeling phase. Sloppy users, on the other hand, could label a given activity as another one, randomly picked, just because of their lack of care.

3.2   Data Collection

We collected a dataset where ten users performed some activities of daily living. Users' movements were captured using both IMUs and Ultra-WideBand (UWB) transceivers. IMUs have been extensively used for this purpose during the last years, as accelerometers and gyroscopes are effective and characterized by reduced costs. UWB transceivers have also been used as they recently became increasingly popular in similar healthcare-related contexts [19,20,22]. In particular, each UWB transceiver is able to determine the distance between itself and another UWB transceiver. If wearable devices are equipped with UWB tranceivers, distance data can be used to obtain information about users' movements.

To collect users' movements we used both Shimmer devices [3], equipped with accelerometers and gyroscopes, and an MDEK Decawave kit [8], whose devices are equipped with transceivers compatible with the IEEE 802.15.4-2011 UWB standard.

In a lab, a room with size 3.6 m × 3.6 m was set up (Fig. 1). Four MDEK sensors were placed at the corners of the room, 2 m above the ground. Such devices operated as "anchors", i.e. nodes whose position is known, and which can be used to compute the position of mobile wearable nodes, called "tags". Each user wore five MDEK devices, and two Shimmer sensors. Devices were attached

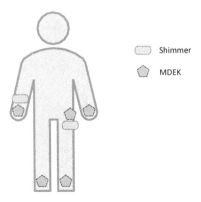

Fig. 2. Position of devices on users' body.

to the users' body according to the scheme illustrated in Fig. 2. MDEK devices were configured to estimate their position with a frequency of 10 Hz, whereas Shimmer devices where set up to collect acceleration and angular velocity at 102.4 Hz. The position of tags in the 3D space of the room was not directly used to understand which was the activity that was currently carried out by the user. 3D positions of tags were used, instead, to compute the distance between couples of wearable devices, e.g. between ankle and wrist or between ankle and pocket. Then, the distances between devices were used to observe user's movements. The rationale for this choice originates from the need to characterize users' movements independently from the position of users in the room. A similar approach was followed in [7], where the reader can find more details.

In the end, for each user, a trace containing the following data was collected: the tri-axial acceleration at the wrist and at the waist, the tri-axial angular velocity at the wrist and at the waist, the ten distances between all the possible couples of UWB-enabled devices (left wrist - left ankle, left wrist - pocket, left wrist - right wrist, etc).

Each user performed six different activities of daily living. Each activity was carried out for one minute. The sequence of activities was: i) walking in circle, ii) standing in the middle of the room, iii) picking up an object repeatedly from the ground, iv) sitting, v) simulated eating, and vi) lying supine.

The main characteristics of the ten users involved in the experiments are shown in Table 1.

3.3　Feature Extraction and Selection

Each user's trace is six minutes long, and contains, as mentioned, 22 signals. Traces have been segmented using fixed size windows, with a duration of 2 s. Then, for each window, a set of functions was computed for all the 22 signals. The adopted functions are: mean, min-max, standard deviation, mean cross ratio, average absolute variation [5], and mean absolute deviation. These functions are

Table 1. Main characteristics of the users involved in the experiments.

User	Height (cm)	Weight (kg)	Age	Gender
1	182	62	29	M
2	158	50	24	F
3	156	65	24	F
4	180	85	23	M
5	182	63	24	M
6	186	78	24	M
7	173	60	28	M
8	176	65	28	M
9	185	62	27	F
10	168	80	24	M

frequently used for signal processing or in the context of activity recognition. Thus for each window, a vector containing 132 features was produced (the feature vector). The number of features was then reduced to 30 using the *relieff* method [21]. This step is generally followed, in activity recognition methods, to avoid overfitting problems and to obtain more efficient systems.

3.4   Identifying Untruthful Users

The resulting dataset contains the feature vectors of all the users. Each feature vector is correctly labelled according to the activity that the user was performing during that time window. The dataset is divided in two parts: one used for training and one used for evaluating the performance of the trained OCC method. In particular, the data of eight users out of ten are used to train an OCC method using only the samples belonging to the positive class, i.e. TUs. The trained OCC method is then evaluated on previously unseen data using the traces of the two remaining users. The OCC method must be evaluated in terms of correct identification of TUs and UUs as truthful and untruthful respectively. To this purpose the data of one of the two remaining users is given as input to the OCC method as it is, and the OCC must identify the user as a truthful one. The data of the last user is transformed to obtain an untruthful one by assigning a wrong, random label to all his/her feature vectors. The transformed data is finally given as input to the trained OCC, which must recognize the user as an untruthful one. This procedure is repeated using all the possible sets of eight users for training, and using all the possible permutations of the remaining two users for the evaluation.

In this context, a true positive means that a TU is classified as a TU, whereas a true negative means that a UU is classified as an UU. Similarly, a false positive means that a UU is classified as a TU, whereas a false negative means that a TU is classified as a UU (Fig. 3).

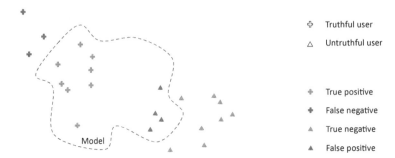

Fig. 3. The model is built using the data of eight users. The remaining data is used to evaluate the trained system.

4   Results

We evaluated the performance of the proposed method when changing some parameters of operation and OCC techniques.

4.1   Impact of the Fraction of Rejected Positive Instances During Training

OCC methods are trained using only positive instances, in our case truthful users. One of the main parameters of OCC methods is the fraction of rejected positive instances during training (*fracrej*). When this parameter is equal to zero, the training phase produces a boundary that includes all positive instances. Such boundary correctly includes all the positive instances provided during the training phase, but it may be prone to generate a number of false positives during the operational phase (some of the positive instances may be particularly far from the "core" of the model). When *fracrej* is greater than zero, a fraction of positive instances are rejected during the training phase. This increases the chances to obtain false negatives during the operational phase, but at the same time reduces the number of false positives (as the boundary is tighter).

We evaluated the performance of the proposed method when *fracrej* is varied in the [0, 0.1] range, when using a Gaussian one-class classifier. Figure 4 shows the obtained false negative rate (FNR) and false positive rate (FPR) of the method. As expected, FPR decreases when *fracrej* increases, whereas FNR increases for larger *fracrej* values. When *fracrej* is equal to zero, the FPR and FNR values are relatively balanced, thus a *fracrej* value equal to zero is used to compute the results presented in Sect. 4.2.

4.2   Combining Results Obtained from Different Windows

The FPR and FNR, obtained by a Gaussian one-class classifier with *fracrej* equal to zero, are 0.20 and 0.14 respectively. Such values suggest that a UU can be reasonably identified, but with some chances to classify a TU as a UU and

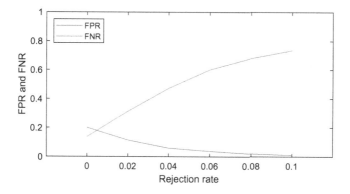

Fig. 4. FPR and FNR when varying the rejection rate.

vice-versa. To improve the performance of the proposed method, we adopted a technique based on majority voting: the results of a set of windows are considered, and the global result is equal to the result obtained in the majority of the windows. Let us define n the number of windows (odd) and k the number of results that indicate the user as an untruthful one. The global result is UU only if $k \geq \lceil \frac{n}{2} \rceil$.

The probability of obtaining k correct results out of n windows can be modelled as a binomial random variable, with probability mass function

$$P(k) = \binom{n}{k} p^k q^{n-k} \tag{1}$$

where p and q are the success and fail probabilities (with $q = 1 - p$). For UUs, q is 0.20 (the FPR on a single window) whereas for TU q is 0.14 (the FNR on a single window). The probability of obtaining the correct result when using n windows is equal to

$$\sum_{k=\lceil n/2 \rceil}^{n} P(k) \tag{2}$$

i.e when the majority of results in the single windows is correct.

Figure 5 shows the results for different values of n, in the [1, 15] interval (obviously, a value of n equal to one corresponds to the case described in Sect. 4.1). When using 15 windows, corresponding to 30 s of user's movements, UUs and TUs can be reliably identified, with a FPR and FNR equal to 0.0042 and 0.0003 respectively.

4.3 Different OCC Techniques

The analysis described in Sect. 4.1 was repeated considering a set of different OCC techniques, besides the Gaussian one. The set of additional methods is: Principal Component Analysis (PCA), Autoencoder, k-means, and Minimum

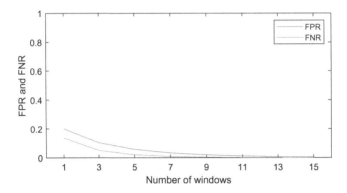

Fig. 5. Incorrect identification (FPR and FNR) of UU and TU with majority voting.

Table 2. Results obtained when using a set of OCC techniques.

OCC method	FPR	FNR	*fracrej*
Gaussian	0.20	0.14	0.0
PCA	0.16	0.15	0.02
Autoencoder	0.19	0.18	0.02
k-means	0.24	0.19	0.08
Minimum Spanning Tree	0.31	0.27	0.08

Spanning Tree [24]. Table 2 shows the obtained results, in terms of FPR and FNR. For each OCC technique, also the *fracrej* value that provided the best result is indicated. The overall best result is achieved by the OCC version of PCA, with FPR and FNR values equal to 0.16 and 0.15 respectively. When the majority voting technique is applied to the OCC PCA classifier, the final values of FPR and FNR are equal/below $1 \cdot 10^{-3}$ (when using 15 windows). This confirms that correct identification of TUs and UUs is possible with high accuracy when using just 30 s of data.

5   Conclusion

Automatic recognition of user's activities by means of wearable devices is a key element of many e-health applications, ranging from rehabilitation to monitoring of elderly citizens. Human activity recognition generally relies on supervised machine learning, where an annotated dataset is used to train the system. An annotated dataset requires the users or the operators to manually specify a label associated to the activity performed during a specific time interval of the training traces.

The proposed method is able to reliably identify untruthful users (or opera-tors), i.e. the ones who associate wrong labels to trace segments. Given a set of positive examples, the method is able to detect untruthful users as anomalies, thus without the need of counter-examples. As far as we know, this problem received very little attention despite the importance of training datasets, used as ground truth, in the context of human activity recognition.

Presented results have been obtained under the assumption that a set of truthful users is initially available to train the OCC method. Future work will study the impact caused by the presence of a fraction of untruthful users also in the initial set. Finally, to better assess the performance of the proposed method, further studies will include a larger dataset, both in terms of users and duration of performed activities.

Acknowledgment. This work was partially funded by the Italian Ministry of Education and Research (MIUR) in the framework of the CrossLab project (Departments of Excellence).

References

1. Abbate, S., Avvenuti, M., Bonatesta, F., Cola, G., Corsini, P., Vecchio, A.: A smartphone-based fall detection system. Perv. Mobile Comput. **8**(6), 883–899 (2012). https://doi.org/10.1016/j.pmcj.2012.08.003, http://www.sciencedirect.co m/science/article/pii/S1574119212000983, special Issue on Pervasive Healthcare
2. Bao, Y., Chen, W.: Automatic model construction for activity recognition using wearable devices. In: 2018 IEEE International Conference on Pervasive Computing and Communications Workshops (PerCom Workshops), pp. 806–811, March 2018. https://doi.org/10.1109/PERCOMW.2018.8480411
3. Burns, A., et al.: Shimmer^{TM} - a wireless sensor platform for noninvasive biomedical research. IEEE Sens. J. **10**(9), 1527–1534 (2010). https://doi.org/10.1109/ JSEN.2010.2045498
4. Chambers, R., Gabbett, T.J., Cole, M.H., Beard, A.: The use of wearable microsensors to quantify sport-specific movements. Sports Med. **45**(7), 1065–1081 (2015). https://doi.org/10.1007/s40279-015-0332-9
5. Cola, G., Avvenuti, M., Vecchio, A., Yang, G., Lo, B.: An unsupervised approach for gait-based authentication. In: 2015 IEEE 12th International Conference on Wearable and Implantable Body Sensor Networks (BSN), pp. 1–6, June 2015. https://doi.org/10.1109/BSN.2015.7299423
6. Cola, G., Vecchio, A., Avvenuti, M.: Improving the performance of fall detection systems through walk recognition. J. Ambient Intell. Humanized Comput. **5**(6), 843–855 (2014). https://doi.org/10.1007/s12652-014-0235-x
7. Aliperti, A., et al.: Using an indoor localization system for activity recognition. In: Sugimoto, C., Farhadi, H., Hämäläinen, M. (eds.) BODYNETS 2018. EICC, pp. 233–243. Springer, Cham (2020). https://doi.org/10.1007/978-3-030-29897-5_19
8. Decawave: www.decawave.com. Accessed 15 July 2019
9. Diete, A., Sztyler, T., Stuckenschmidt, H.: A smart data annotation tool for multi-sensor activity recognition. In: 2017 IEEE International Conference on Pervasive Computing and Communications Workshops (PerCom Workshops), pp. 111–116, March 2017. https://doi.org/10.1109/PERCOMW.2017.7917542

10. Giunchiglia, F., Zeni, M., Bignotti, E., Zhang, W.: Assessing annotation consistency in the wild. In: 2018 IEEE International Conference on Pervasive Computing and Communications Workshops (PerCom Workshops), pp. 561–566, March 2018. https://doi.org/10.1109/PERCOMW.2018.8480236
11. Khan, S.S., Madden, M.G.: One-class classification: taxonomy of study and review of techniques. Knowl. Eng. Rev. **29**(3), 345–374 (2014)
12. Koppel, M., Schler, J.: Authorship verification as a one-class classification problem. In: Proceedings of The Twenty-First International Conference on Machine Learning, p. 62. ACM (2004)
13. Kumar, M.P., Packer, B., Koller, D.: Self-paced learning for latent variable models. In: Lafferty, J.D., Williams, C.K.I., Shawe-Taylor, J., Zemel, R.S., Culotta, A. (eds.) Advances in Neural Information Processing Systems, vol. 23, pp. 1189–1197. Curran Associates, Inc. (2010). http://papers.nips.cc/paper/3923-self-paced-learning-for-latent-variable-models.pdf
14. Lara, O.D., Labrador, M.A.: A survey on human activity recognition using wearable sensors. IEEE Commun. Surv. Tutorials **15**(3), 1192–1209 (2013). https://doi.org/10.1109/SURV.2012.110112.00192
15. Liu, C., Freeman, W.T., Adelson, E.H., Weiss, Y.: Human-assisted motion annotation. In: 2008 IEEE Conference on Computer Vision and Pattern Recognition, pp. 1–8, June 2008. https://doi.org/10.1109/CVPR.2008.4587845
16. Martindale, C.F., Roth, N., Hannink, J., Sprager, S., Eskofier, B.M.: Smart annotation tool for multi-sensor gait-based daily activity data. In: 2018 IEEE International Conference on Pervasive Computing and Communications Workshops (PerCom Workshops), pp. 549–554, March 2018. https://doi.org/10.1109/PERCOMW.2018.8480193
17. Mukhopadhyay, S.C.: Wearable sensors for human activity monitoring: a review. IEEE Sens. J. **15**(3), 1321–1330 (2015). https://doi.org/10.1109/JSEN.2014.2370945
18. Palotai, Z., et al.: LabelMovie: semi-supervised machine annotation tool with quality assurance and crowd-sourcing options for videos. In: 2014 12th International Workshop on Content-Based Multimedia Indexing (CBMI), pp. 1–4, June 2014. https://doi.org/10.1109/CBMI.2014.6849850
19. Qi, Y., Soh, C.B., Gunawan, E., Low, K.S., Maskooki, A.: A novel approach to joint flexion/extension angles measurement based on wearable UWB radios. IEEE J. Biomed. Health Inform. **18**(1), 300–308 (2013)
20. Qi, Y., Soh, C.B., Gunawan, E., Low, K.S., Maskooki, A.: Using wearable UWB radios to measure foot clearance during walking. In: 2013 35th Annual International Conference of the IEEE Engineering in Medicine and Biology Society (EMBC), pp. 5199–5202. IEEE (2013)
21. Robnik-Šikonja, M., Kononenko, I.: Theoretical and empirical analysis of ReliefF and RReliefF. Mach. Learn. **53**(1), 23–69 (2003). https://doi.org/10.1023/A:1025667309714
22. Shaban, H.A., El-Nasr, M.A., Buehrer, R.M.: Toward a highly accurate ambulatory system for clinical gait analysis via UWB radios. IEEE Trans. Inf. Technol. Biomed. **14**(2), 284–291 (2010). https://doi.org/10.1109/TITB.2009.2037619
23. Szewcyzk, S., Dwan, K., Minor, B., Swedlove, B., Cook, D.: Annotating smart environment sensor data for activity learning. Technol. Health Care **17**(3), 161–169 (2009)
24. Tax, D.: Ddtools, the data description toolbox for Matlab, January 2018. Version 2.1.3

25. Vecchio, A., Cola, G.: Fall detection using ultra-wideband positioning. In: 2016 IEEE SENSORS, pp. 1–3, October 2016. https://doi.org/10.1109/ICSENS.2016. 7808527
26. Vecchio, A., Mulas, F., Cola, G.: Posture recognition using the interdistances between wearable devices. IEEE Sens. Lett. **1**(4), 1–4 (2017). https://doi.org/10. 1109/LSENS.2017.2726759
27. Yordanova, K., Krüger, F., Kirste, T.: Providing semantic annotation for the CMU grand challenge dataset. In: 2018 IEEE International Conference on Pervasive Computing and Communications Workshops (PerCom Workshops), pp. 579–584, March 2018. https://doi.org/10.1109/PERCOMW.2018.8480380

Mobile App for Optimizing Home Care Nursing

Virginia Sandulescu[1(✉)], Sorin Puscoci[1], Monica Petre[1], Sorin Soviany[1],
Mirabela Chirvasa[2], and Alexandru Girlea[2]

[1] National Communications Studies and Research Institute-INSCC, Bucharest, Romania
virginia.sandulescu@inscc.ro
[2] QuickWeb Info, Bucharest, Romania

Abstract. The paper presents a mobile app designed to be used by health care providers, mainly by the nurses that pay visits to the homes of the clients/patients of the health care providers. The app should optimize the nurses activity and also the communication between the nurses and the coordinators and between the nurses and the patients. The described mobile app is part of a larger software platform as will be described in the article.

Keywords: Home care · Home nursing · Health care · Mobile app · Point of care documentation

1 Introduction

As life expectancy grows we are faced with an aging population all across Europe and beyond. The effects of an aging population are expected to become more and more visible over time, as the number of the elderly divided by the working age population grows. It is expected that in 2050, the ratio of elderly to the active population in Europe will reach 2:1 [1].

The elderly need assistance in the daily living, in performing their routine activities and most of them also need health care services, be it for a chronic illness, for a specific incident for a short while or for preventive care.

The care services may be offered a) in an institution: in a nursing home for long term care; b) in the hospital for short term or ambulatory care; c) at home. There are multiple benefits in delivering health care or different care services to the elders at home and avoiding having them long/short term institutionalized. These benefits are related to the quality of life of the elders that get to live in their own homes, in the same environment that they are accustomed with.

There are studies suggesting that living at home with support, compared to getting care at a different location improved health and functional status, mortality rates and, at least, delayed hospitalization and institutionalization in nursing homes [2, 3].

A review of the research regarding the best point of care for elders [3] shows that the results are heterogeneous, depending on the degree of dependency of the subjects. The growth of the user segment of home care services and the diminishing workforce that provides them leads to a need to optimize the delivery of such services.

G. M. P. O'Hare et al. (Eds.): MobiHealth 2019, LNICST 320, pp. 332–339, 2020.
https://doi.org/10.1007/978-3-030-49289-2_26

The work described in the current paper is part of an ongoing research project implemented in Romania that aims to address this problem: optimizing the activity of home care services providers (HCPs) through an integrated software and hardware platform.

The platform is called CDMS [2] and it presents a multilayered architecture. Components at the top level are designed to be implemented by an agent that offers services to multiple HCPs, so that an HCP may enter the market with minimum investments and start offering services in an organized and optimized manner. At the top level is the center for dispatching and management for multiple home care providers, consisting of servers running dedicated software: web applications dedicated to the home care providers.

The next level is the HCP level and, because of the multiple functionalities implemented at the top level, it consists only of Internet enabled terminals. These terminals do not require high computing power or large storage capacity, as these functionalities are implemented at the CDMS level.

Every assistant that performs home visits is required to use a mobile device during the visits. The device (a smartphone or a tablet) runs a mobile app that communicates with the servers at the CDMS level in order to offer information to the assistant and to record information about the visit. There is also another level consisting of remote monitoring devices designed to be located at the homes of the clients/patients.

A general and functional description of the CDMS platform is available in [4].

The current work presents the mobile app for the nursing staff: a mobile app, called Homeassis, designed for Android and iOS devices, that targets the employees of home health care providers. The app should ease the activity of the nurses that pay home visits to the clients/patients, by providing them with the information and assistance that they need during the visits.

2 State of the Art

As stated in the introductory paragraphs, there is a need for solutions that deal with taking care of the elders. The need is reflected in an abundance of research projects motivated by the problems involved by dealing with an aging society.

Most of the research is split in two major directions: a) independent living at home (aided by home care systems) or b) solutions for nursing homes for the elders. The current work focuses on c) living at home while receiving care from specialized nursing staff. The following paragraphs will study solutions from all three groups, with focus on the latter category: living at home while receiving home care services. Of course, this category does not exclude getting help from solutions from category a) or b) like ambient assisted living or short term institutionalizations in different situations. Also, the main focus will be on the mobile solutions.

The research in category a) is mostly centered on smart home and ambient assisted living solutions. This area has been a research subject for a long time, although the health care aspect is not studied in all the research available, many of them focusing more on user comfort and optimizing energy usage. Research suggests that this type of implementation of technology may have positive impacts on health status and quality of life of the assisted subjects [5–7] although the level of technology readiness for smart homes and home health monitoring technologies is found to still be low [5]. The CDMS platform also proposes the use of health monitoring solutions implemented in the homes of the clients, but this part of the research is not the subject of the current paper.

Much of the current research considers offering care services in institutions like nursing homes. Again, most of the research is related to ambient assisted living and smart environments. In this paragraph, only solutions related to mobile apps available for care services will be presented. More precisely, to what is called point of care documentation. The work presented in [8] describes an app developed to aid the staff of a nursing home in Portugal and describes all the steps involved in developing the app: starting from analyzing the ICT used by the nursing home before, analyzing the needs of the staff, the activities performed and so on. The app offers access to the electronic health records of the patients at the point of care, replacing the need for handwritten charts and medical records. The technologies used for the development of the mobile app are based on React Native – a Javascript framework developed by Facebook, MySQL for the database and a PHP Rest API to allow the communication between the client – the mobile app and the server side – where the database is stored. There are some commercially available solutions for point-of-care documentation like Medsys2 [9]. Medsys2 is a solution for managing the process of offering health care in any location (hospital or outside of the hospital) tailored for the legislation and workflow of the medical domain in the United States. It allows recording information about the visits performed and, afterwards, reporting it in predefined or customized format pdf documents. By allowing the creation of customized documents, it might allow also reporting of the materials used in each activity.

The proposed app described in this paper is using native technologies for each of the two targeted platforms: Android and iOS. The communication with the server is based on a PHP Rest API. Along with access to the patients' electronic charts, the proposed app offers aid in performing the required procedures and in registering information on the necessary supplies.

The proposed solution offers more than point of care documentation by offering support to the assistant in: contacting the patient, navigating to the patient's home, keeping track of the used supplies, allowing integration of medical documents generated by other health care providers. Also, the integration of the proposed app in a more complex ecosystem of hardware and software components offers other advantages not just to the nursing staff but also to the administrative personnel of an HCP.

3   General and Functional Description

The proposed mobile app is designed to run on Android and iOS devices: smartphones or tablets that the home assistant wears during the home visits.

The app is designed to act as a client in the architecture of the whole CDMS platform, Fig. 1. It will be used by the assistants during home visits and it will synchronize the acquired data with servers located at the CDMS level.

For the moment, as the research project that funds the development of the CDMS platform and of the presented mobile app is a Romanian research project, the app's interface is designed in Romanian language, but during the programming stages, internationalization tools have been used to allow for easy translation of the strings presented on the screens of the app.

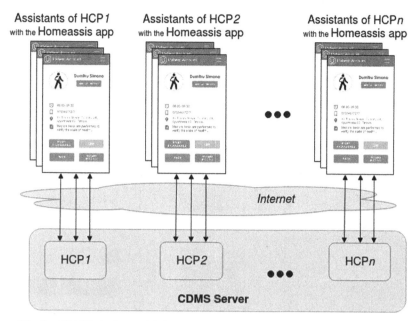

Fig. 1. CDMS platform with the Homeassis app for the assistants of each HCP

The database used for the app is SQLite, encrypted using AES128. Data are only temporarily stored on the device and deleted after each successful upload to the server. For security reasons, communication between the CDMS server and the device (the client) is performed only on mobile data, not on Wi-Fi. The server is offering an HTTPS connection.

The app allows access to information about the clients/patients, information about the visits or help regarding certain procedures. In the first stages of the project, multiple research visits were conducted in the field in order to interview and gather data from HCPs and home assistants, so that the functionalities reflect the needs of the intended users. All along the development of the whole CDMS platform, feedback from HCPs has been received: in the design, development and testing phases, to ensure the fact that the platform meets the needs of the intended users.

The app offers the following functionalities:

- View of the program of the visits for the current day;
- Navigation using the GPS to the homes of the clients/patients;
- Management of the applied procedures:

  - Log details about the applied procedures;
  - Edit the elements about the supplies used for the procedures.

- Record physiological measurements;
- Add medical documents to the electronic charts of the patients.

Figure 2 presents different screens of the mobile app. The usage scenarios may be synthesized as in the following paragraphs.

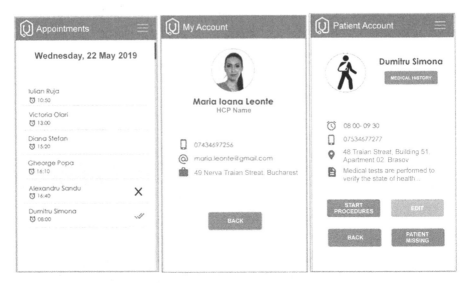

Fig. 2. Different screens of the mobile app: a) list of the scheduled appointments; b) profile screen of the logged in caregiver; c) patient information screen (Color figure online)

3.1 First Time Usage of the App: Authorization of the Device on the CDMS Platform and User Login

In order to use the app, the mobile device must be authorized by an HCP. The authorization of a device is based on a two factor authentication. At the first usage of the app, the user is requested to input the URL of an HCP (in a screen of the app only available if the device is not paired with any HCP). An administrator of the HCP must then use the web app available through the CDMS platform to generate a validation code that must be input in the mobile app.

After the authorization of the device, the user – a caregiver must authenticate by using a username and a password. After a successful login, the user data stored on the server are synchronized on the device. The data consist of the following appointments along with the information regarding them: the required procedures, the necessary materials, information about the patients (contact information like address and phone number, medical history of the patient).

After this first data synchronization, next synchronizations take place after each successful login, after each visit, daily at midnight or at a user request for synchronization.

3.2 Manage the List of Scheduled Appointments for the Current Day

An authorized caregiver consults his list of scheduled appointments. This is the first screen available to the user after a successful login.

An example of this screen is depicted in Fig. 2a). Already performed visits are marked with a tick and visits that could not be performed (for different reasons: client refused certain procedures, client was not at home/not available) are marked with a red cross. Once a visit has been performed, it is moved to the end of the list. There is the case that there is no appointment scheduled for the day, in this case a message is shown to the user, along with a button that allows for a resynchronization with data on the server.

Starting from this screen, by pressing on a client's name, a caregiver may view information about the visit and about the client that is to be visited, as seen in Fig. 2c).

3.3 Perform a Visit at a Client

Presuming a caregiver is logged in and has synchronized the data on the device with the CDMS server, he may start performing the scheduled visits.

Starting from the screen presented in Fig. 2c) the user may get all the information needed to perform a visit. The screen presents information about the patient and about the visit: scheduled time of the visit and client's address.

Also, the screen allows the caregiver to directly make a phone call to the client, start the navigation app to see the recommended route to get to the client's home, see the medical chart of the patient; mark the patient as unavailable for the visit or start applying the requested procedures.

In order to record the performed procedures, the assistant selects the "Record procedures" button shown in Fig. 2c) and a list of the procedures requested by the client/recommended by the medic is shown. For each procedure the assistant may view a description, record it as applied or refused, input comments/observations about it and record the supplies used for the procedure. New procedures may be added to the list of already requested procedures, following a request from the patient or as considered necessary by the caregiver.

The app allows the assistant to input the vital parameters measured during the visit, parameters like: arterial tension, glucose level, pulse, temperature and others. The app allows the input of several predetermined vital parameters. The list of vital parameters that may be recorded was defined by medical personnel consulted during the design phases of the whole CDMS platform (and, implicitly, of the mobile app). The list of available procedures to be performed is also predetermined and developed during the design phase of the platform after consulting with medical personnel and home nurses. Using the web components of the CDMS platform (not directly through the described mobile app) new procedures and new physiological parameter types may be added to the corresponding lists.

For each of the medical procedures the necessary materials along with typical quantities are predefined. The assistant may change these values according to each situation.

While performing a visit, the assistant may add documents specifically to the current visit or to the electronic file of the patient, by adding a file: a picture or a different type of file considered relevant to the visit, or to the medical history of the client.

4   Results

An experimental model of the whole platform has been deployed as an experimental model at a possible CDMS center in Alba County, Romania. For the moment, the platform is tested by the personnel of the CDMS and the mobile app by the personnel of an HCP. Neither is being used with real clients' data.

The potential users have expressed requests for alterations either directly for the app or alterations for the platform that are reflected in the app. These functionalities are currently being implemented and testing activities are performed in close relation to the development activities.

The prototype of the whole platform, containing also the model app is scheduled to be released in March 2020. Different screens of the app are available in Fig. 2. As observed during use of the experimental model, the designed features improve both the activity of the home nurses and of the adminsitrative personnel of HCPs.

One of the most important advantages that arise from using the proposed mobile app is a clear and standardized workflow that all nursing staff must adhere to, which also leads to fewer errors in performing and reporting the activities and in filling information in the patients' medical charts. It also improves communication between different nurses attending to the same patients and between patients and the nursing staff. It also aids reporting and monitoring the activity of the nursing staff and optimizing and monitoring the use of needed supplies for the home care procedures.

5   Conclusions and Future Work

In conclusion, the paper presents a mobile app for Android and iOS devices, designed to be used by health care providers, mainly by the nurses that pay visits to the homes of the clients/patients of the health care providers. The app should optimize the activity of the nurses by allowing them to: remotely access clients'/patients' data; manage the applied/requested procedures for each patient; record the supplies used for every procedure.

Also, the app facilitates the interaction between workers and coordinators and between workers and patients. The usage of the app optimizes and eases the activity of the home nurses and also the activity of the administrative personnel of the HCP, by allowing for a better and close to real time knowledge of the visits and procedures applied by their nurses and of the supplies used during visits.

As mentioned before, the app is currently in testing, as it is deployed as part of the experimental model to a CDMS and HCP in Alba County, Romania.

Although multiple targeted users were consulted during the design phase of the platform and of the app, during the first months after deploying the experimental model, multiple requests have been made by the users regarding different functionalities of the app and these requests are currently being implemented.

The testing and polishing of the experimental model continues until March 2020 when a pilot for the whole platform is programmed to be released at the same CDMS and HCP in Alba County. A training period is scheduled for the pilot through multiple workshops planned for the employees of each HCP.

The pilot is set to run until September 2020, when the implementation of the research project is over.

After that, there are plans for translating the software into more languages, as internationalization was taken into account during the development phase of all the components of the CDMS platform, including the presented mobile app. Further developments include creating a mobile app dedicated for the patients and several improvements to the web components of the CDMS platform, which may reflect in changes in the presented mobile app.

Acknowledgements. This work has been supported by Project Dispatching and Management Center for Optimizing Home Care Integrated Services, from Operational Competitiveness Program 2014-2020 Axis 1 – Romanian Research Ministry.

References

1. Eurostat: People in the EU -population projections – Statistics Explained (2019)
2. Boland, L., et al.: Impact of home care versus alternative locations of care on elder health outcomes: an overview of systematic reviews. BMC Geriatr. **17**, 20 (2017)
3. Markle-Reid, M., Browne, G., Weir, G., Gafni, A., Roberts, J., Henderson, S.: The effectiveness and efficiency of home-based nursing health promotion for older people: a review of the literature. Med. Care Res. Rev. **63**, 531–569 (2006)
4. Sandulescu, V., Puscoci, S., Petre, M., Soviany, S., Chirvasa, M., Girlea, A.: Dispatching and management center for optimizing home care integrated services. In: Proceedings of the 5th International Conference on Information and Communication Technologies for Ageing Well and e-Health ICT4AWE, vol. 1, pp. 255–261. Scitepress, Heraklion (2019)
5. Liu, L., Stroulia, E., Nikolaidis, I., Miguel-Cruz, A., Rincon, A.: Smart homes and home health monitoring technologies for older adults: a systematic review. Int. J. Med. Inf. **91**, 44–59 (2016)
6. Memon, M., Wagner, S., Pedersen, C., Beevi, F., Hansen, F.: Ambient assisted living healthcare frameworks, platforms, standards, and quality attributes. Sensors **14**, 4312–4341 (2014)
7. Queiros, A., Dias, A., Silva, A., Rocha, N.P.: Ambient assisted living and health-related outcomes—a systematic literature review. In Informatics, MDPI (2017)
8. Esteves, M., Esteves, M., Abelha, A., Machado, J.: A mobile health application to assist health professionals: a case study in a Portuguese nursing home. In: Proceedings of the 5th International Conference on Information and Communication Technologies for Ageing Well and e-Health ICT4AWE, vol. 1, pp. 338–345. Scitepress, Heraklion (2019)
9. Medsys2: Work flow process. http://medsys2.com/?page_id=1960. Accessed 01 Sept 2019

Author Index

Alfi, Gaspare   153
Almeida, Nuno   140
Altamirano, Sara   18
Anastasi, Giada   320
Andersen, Björn   127
Arakawa, Yutaka   60
Arcarisi, Lucia   249
Aschan, Tuulevi   281

Baake, Merle   127
Blankenhagel, Kim Janine   229
Boumpa, Eleni   171
Boyle, Daniel   97
Brás, Susana   140
Burriel, Verónica   18

Carbonaro, Nicola   153, 249
Casalino, Gabriella   43
Castellano, Giovanna   43
Cesari, Valentina   86
Charmandari, Evangelia   294
Chen, Jingbo   36, 163
Chen, Mingsheng   36, 163
Chirvasa, Mirabela   332
Coccomini, Davide   320

Delopoulos, Anastasios   294
Diou, Christos   294

Echevarria Mateu, Humberto   75

Ferreira, David   112, 140
Gallach-Solano, Elisa   75

Gemignani, Angelo   86, 153
Girlea, Alexandru   332
Guazzelli, Stefano   320

Hayashi, Masayuki   256
Hein, Andreas   3, 305
Hembroff, Guy C.   97
Higashino, Teruo   256

Ingenerf, Josef   127
Ioakimidis, Ioannis   294

Kakarountas, Athanasios   171
Karhula, Maarit   281
Kassari, Penio   294
Kilintzis, Vassilis   294

Laurino, Marco   86, 153, 249
Lekka, Eirini   294
Li, Gen   36
Linker, Miriam   229
Lotano, Sara   320

Magal-Royo, Teresa   75
Maglaveras, Nikolaos   294
Männikkö, Minna   281
Maramis, Christos   294
Marinai, Carlotta   249
Marinari, Elena   86
Martínez-Alzamora, Nieves   75
McHugh, Daniel   201
Melo, Daniela   112
Menicucci, Danilo   86, 153
Muenzberg, Alexander   3, 305

Nagar, Atulya Kumar   201
Nawaz, Anum   267
Nguyen Gia, Tuan   267

Otsubo, Atsushi   60

Papapanagiotou, Vasileios   294
Partala, Timo   281
Pasquadibisceglie, Vincenzo   43
Peña Querata, Jorge   267
Petre, Monica   332
Prefasi-Gomar, Salvador   75
Puscoci, Sorin   332

Qin, Mingxin   36, 163

Reid, David 201
Roesch, Norbert 3, 305

Saar, Laura 281
Sandulescu, Virginia 332
Santo, Andreia 112
Sauer, Janina 3, 305
Secco, Emanuele Lindo 186, 201, 212
Sierra San Miguel, Pilar 75
Siewert, Laura 3
Silva, Pedro 112
Silva, Samuel 112, 140
Soares, Sandra C. 112, 140
Soviany, Sorin 332
Stefanopoulos, Leandros 294
Suwa, Hirohiko 60

Tadesse, Andualem Maereg 186, 212
Teixeira, António 140
Tenhunen, Hannu 267
Teppati Losè, Massimo 249

Thorsteinsdottir, Gudrun 18
Tognetti, Alessandro 153, 249

Uchiyama, Akira 256

Vecchio, Alessio 320

Wagner, Timothy Van 97
Westerlund, Tomi 267

Xu, Jia 163

Yang, Jun 36
Yasumoto, Keiichi 60
Yoshikawa, Hiroki 256

Zara, Giuliano 320
Zarnekow, Rüdiger 229
Zaza, Gianluca 43
Zhang, Haisheng 163

Printed in the United States
By Bookmasters